# Foundations of Rope Bondage

## A Fun and Friendly Introduction to Rope Fundamentals

**TheDuchy**

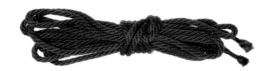

# Foundations of Rope Bondage

## A Fun and Friendly Introduction to Rope Fundamentals

### TheDuchy

Green Candy Press

*Foundations of Rope Bondage*
*A Fun and Friendly Introduction to Rope Fundamentals*
Published by Leabhar Inc
Toronto, Canada
greencandypress.com

Copyright © 2023 Lazarus Redmayne
ISBN: 978-1-937866-43-3
eBook ISBN: 978-1-937866-44-0

Photography © Lazarus Redmayne

Editorial: Virginia Haze and Breda Lezha
Production Editor: Thomas Whitcomb
Design and illustration: Ian Phillips

Printed in China by 1010 Printing

Massively Distributed by P.G.W.

Before we begin, I want to give a huge shout out and my effusive thanks to the BDSM and rope communities around the world. "The Scene" is full of amazing, deeply knowledgeable people. They are passionate about the art and science of rope. They love to experiment, find innovative and interesting ways to apply rope, and share what they discover. What you find in this book is my way of explaining the collected experience and wisdom of thousands of people across the globe sharing what they know.

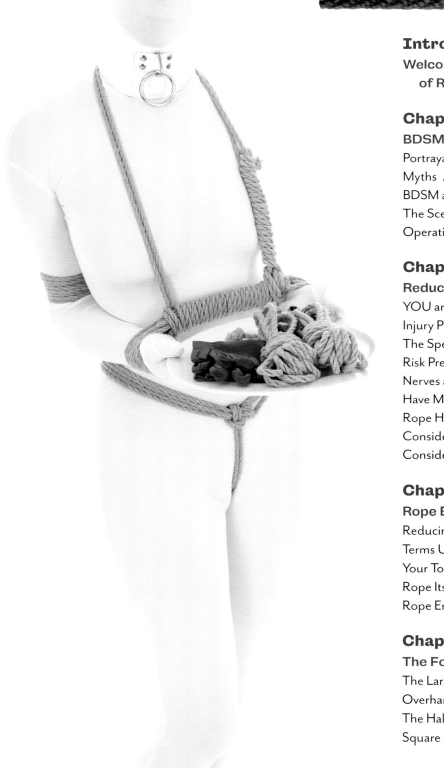

# Contents

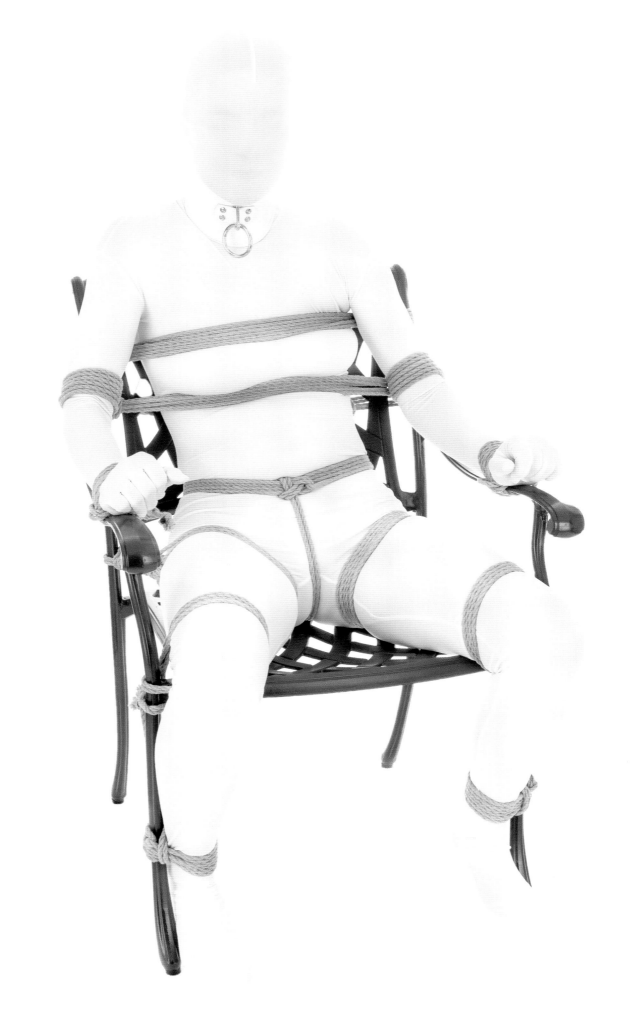

# Welcome to the Wonderous World of Rope Bondage!

People are drawn to rope bondage for a wide variety of reasons. Perhaps you love the artistic appeal of rope around a human form; perhaps you see bondage as erotic (true for many practitioners, but not for all); perhaps you are attracted to the idea of building a skill that requires discipline and practice to master. Regardless of what brought you here, know that your interest is shared by all kinds of people from around the world.

## About this Book

Bondage is everywhere — movies, TV, books, your neighbor's bedroom. And while most people just watch and wonder "What if...?", *you* have done more than that. You had the courage to pick up this book and to take a first step toward learning more.

If you want to be the person *doing* the tying, this book is for you! It's not difficult to get started with rope bondage, but there are important things you need to know in order to do so without causing injury.

If you want to be the person *being tied*, this book is also for you! Receiving rope bondage is an active skill, and understanding the basics of rigging is critically important for your safety and your ability to advocate for yourself. Many rope bottoms are fantastic riggers in their own right.

In this book you will find a series of ties that are fun, easy to learn, and — when done properly — low risk. They can be combined and layered to create thousands of different kinds of scenes; see Chapter 11 (p. 383) for a few fun ideas!

Much of the material in this book is also available on TheDuchy.com, where you can find video tutorials as well as a huge library of ties.

## What Attracts a Person to Bondage?

There are as many reasons as there are people. You might do it for the fun, excitement, thrill, danger, identity exploration, or to find acceptance by connecting with others that have the same interests. You may have simply stumbled on pictures of someone tied up and found yourself intrigued. You may have been introduced to the idea by an intimate partner, a lover, or a friend.

There are also many people that indulge in rope bondage for non-sexual and non-kink reasons. They just love the artistic aspects of it, they find the detail-oriented nature to be meditative, or the deep communication, care, and focus required to be therapeutic.

Whatever *your* reason is for picking up this book, welcome! We're glad you're here.

## How to Use This Book

This book is designed to be accessible to anyone who is completely new to rope bondage. It assumes zero knowledge and builds from the foundation up. But it can also be useful to people that already have some experience. It can be helpful to see how someone else does things, the things they emphasize and do that may be different from the way that you currently do it. Take from these tutorials what is valuable to you.

If you are new, start at the beginning and go through everything sequentially. The concepts in this book build on themselves, so skipping to the end may lead to a bunch of jumping back and forth.

### Start With Risk Management/Safety

You don't need to know *everything* in this book before you start, but *before* you put rope on anyone with a pulse — including yourself — you *do* need to understand the risks involved and how to manage them.

I know you're excited to get your hands on rope and begin tying, but DO NOT SKIP THE *REDUCING RISK* CHAPTER (p. 49). It contains information that it is crucial for you to understand.

### This Book is Helpful for Both Tops and bottoms

Rope bottoming is not a passive activity. It is a skill that is honed with practice and education. The information in this book is just as important for the person who is being tied as it is for the person doing the tying. It is especially important for a rope bottom to know safety procedures and knots so they can advocate for themselves during negotiations and in a scene itself. Also, a knowledgeable rope bottom is incredibly valuable in helping new Rope Tops learn and grow.

Top or bottom, if you want to be capable of giving informed consent, **you need to read the risk and safety section**. Education is a key component to consent. You cannot give informed consent from a place of ignorance. You need to understand the information in the safety section because without that understanding, *informed* consent is not possible.

### Pace Yourself

When you understand the risks and safety guidance, continue through the book — in order. Master each technique. **Practice** each one over and over until you are doing it correctly and no longer need to refer to the book for the next step. Then keep doing the techniques over and over to build muscle memory and confidence through experience and practice. With repetition, the techniques will begin to feel natural and more intuitive. Start off tying slowly so you can master the movements to be able to tie faster and cleaner later on.

Enjoy the journey.

There are many people who love rope bondage and are completely satisfied using only the techniques found in this book. You can create thousands of different scenes using nothing more than what you will learn here. That said, if you reach the end of this book and you want to know more, head to TheDuchy.com.

If you have questions about any of the techniques in this book, you can also check out the tutorials found at TheDuchy.com/foundations. URLs are provided for each tie to make it easy to get more information.

### Find and Meet With Other People That Love Rope. Learn From Them

We strongly recommend that you join your local rope community (p. 10) if you can. Find a local mentor. Getting live feedback from an experienced Rope Top or bottom is incredibly valuable!

*Better than a thousand days of diligent study is one day with a great teacher.*

Books cannot point out that you have the rope too loose or too tight. They cannot point out that you are doing the opposite of what is being shown in the picture, and are reaching through from the wrong side of the knot. There are so many things, large and little, that an experienced person might notice and help you understand.

If you do not have a local rope community, consider joining online forums where people share information about rope (p. 10).

At whatever level you are comfortable, reach out and find others. You will make better progress if you do.

### Disclaimer

The information in this book comes from the collected experience generated by thousands of rope enthusiasts from all around the world, working together to find and share fun and amazing techniques while managing risk to an acceptable level. But new methods may supplant those in this book.

Let this book be the *beginning* for you. Don't rely on this book to be your only source of information. There is so much out there that is absolutely amazing. Even if you don't want to go further than these foundational techniques, you can still get better at them. Find ways to continue to learn.

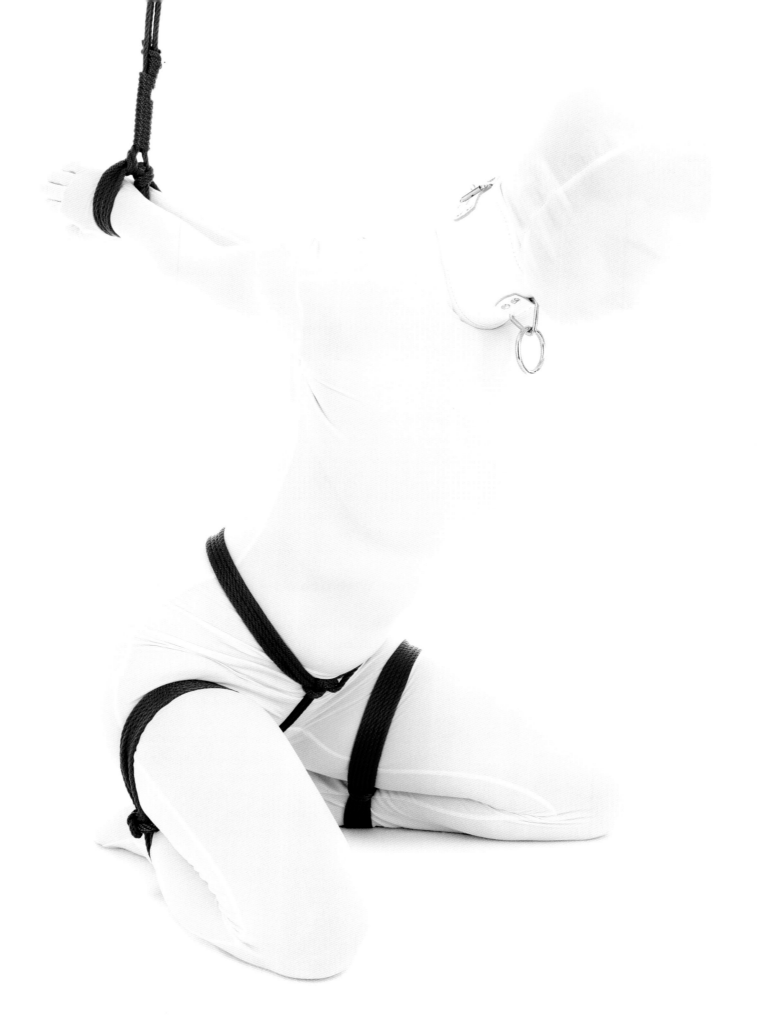

# 1

# BDSM and Rope

For most people, rope bondage is an activity to be shared with another person, maybe more than one. The rest of this book covers rope bondage information and techniques, but this chapter is focused on people: How to find other people that are interested in rope, how to interact with them socially and, if you should progress to wanting to tie with them, how to talk with them about *that* and negotiate a scene.

But first, let's talk about rope bondage as a whole, and some basics and myths. Starting at the beginning, what is rope bondage?

Rope bondage is often thought of as an aspect of the bondage part of "BDSM" — an acronym that combines B&D (Bondage and Discipline), D/s (Dominance and submission), and S&M (Sadism and Masochism) into a single umbrella term. For many, BDSM is often assumed to involve overt sex, but this is not always true. While sexuality and eroticism often are incorporated into BDSM, they are not an *inherent* part of it. The same is true for rope bondage.

People may be interested in rope for many reasons:
- The desire to restrain someone or be restrained for the sake of sexual gratification.
- The desire to restrain someone or be restrained with some other kinky activity in mind.
- An attraction to its artistic or visual appeal.
- The desire to have a fun and useful skill.
- Etc.

There is nothing wrong with BDSM or rope bondage done with sexual overtones/activities in mind. However, it is important to understand that just because you might want to do rope bondage or some other BDSM activity with someone, that does not imply that you want to have any type of sexual activity with them, nor they with you. Consent to do rope is *not* consent to participate in sexual activity.

If you are interested in trying rope with someone, talk to them, find out what they want and need out of it, and come to an agreement about what you each are willing to do. If you want to do *more* to/with them while they are in rope, talk about that specifically and agree to all those details beforehand. More on this when we talk about negotiation (p. 32).

# Portrayal in Media

Rope bondage is hilariously popular in Western media. From restraining the protagonist in action films to tying up a distressed damsel in children's cartoons, rope bondage is everywhere. However, it is quite rare to find rope bondage executed correctly in non-kinky media, and even within the kink world the skill in execution varies wildly.

When we say "correctly," we mean rope bondage that would actually be effective — would be difficult, if not impossible, for the bottom to get out of — *and* that is unlikely to cause injury. In most cases on-screen, rope that is used for the sake of restraint would be laughably easy to get out of, or it is applied in such a dangerous way that it could seriously injure someone. This is often even true in erotic media, where you would think they would want to get it right!

For that reason, while media portrayals can be fun to look at and can give you general inspiration for things you might want to try, don't rely on them for procedure or instructions. Do your research first. Learn how to do the things that piqued your interest, but in ways that control and limit risk. Safety — understanding risk and what you can do to manage that risk — is a major part of doing rope properly. It is part of RACK, or Risk Aware Consensual Kink.

As you explore this world, it is important to educate yourself on the differences between the fantasies that you have seen or read, and what works in a practical sense in the real world.

# Myths

There are lots of myths about rope and rope bondage.

| | |
|---|---|
| Using rope is easy and safe. "I see rope used in movies and TV all the time, so it must be easy." | For most people, learning to use rope in a way that reduces risk is not difficult, but you *do* still need to learn about it. There are many risks you need to understand and you need to learn the proper techniques you can use to lower those risks. Much more on this may be found in Chapter 2 (p. 49) and throughout the rest of this book. |
| Rope is so dangerous that you should never engage with it. | It is true that many kink practitioners consider rope bondage to be "edge play" — more extreme or risky BDSM activities — because rope bondage carries a significant risk of physical injury, especially in more advanced practices like suspension. Being aware of those risks and adjusting how you use rope in order to minimize some of them is only possible through education. However, those risks can be minimized. Millions of people around the world play with rope and have a wonderful time. |

**Rope is a "sex" thing.**

One of the most important things to keep in mind when dealing with anything related to BDSM is that sex is NEVER implicit. Really, honestly, truly. Never.

First of all, "sex" is a highly subjective concept. What constitutes sexual touch and sexual activity varies highly; every person has their own definition. In order for rope to be a "sex" thing, we would all have to agree on what constitutes sex.

An interest in tying someone does not imply a sexual interest in them, and neither does an interest in being tied by someone. All it means is that you want to tie or be tied. That is all. If you want it to be a "sex" thing, make that abundantly clear to the person you want to tie with.

**Talk about everything you would like to do *clearly and explicitly*. Everything. In detail.** "I would love to lick your nipple while you are in bondage; would you like that?" That is the level you want to get to. No implications, no inuendos. Clear statements of interest for the other person to clearly accept or decline. More on this when we talk about negotiation (p. 32).

**Rope bondage is slow.**

Okay, sure, rope *can* be slow. It is objectively true that it takes longer to tie someone in a **Double Column** than it does to lock them in a pair of handcuffs, although with practice and experience, ties can be surprisingly fast! There are some that can be put on in less than 30 seconds.

That said, the fact that it takes time can be a *good* thing. You are providing extra attention — taking that time to communicate via touch and rope tension alone — and that can be very erotic. If sex is a planned part of the scene, the act of tying itself can be a very powerful form of foreplay.

**There is only one right way to do rope, or to engage in BDSM.**

Laughably, no. You will often hear the phrase "There is no 'One True Way.'"

Every relationship/dynamic is a custom job. If you and your partner(s) are being responsible, communicating clearly, behaving ethically, and educating yourselves on the things you want to explore so you know the risks and how to manage them, you can build whatever works for you.

**I have to find a partner before I can begin learning rope.**

You don't need a partner to practice rope. You can tie on yourself (e.g., cross your ankle on your knee and practice **Single Columns** on it), a pillow, stuffed animals, a mannequin, etc. If your rope is pure art, all you need to know is procedure.

If you want to apply rope to a human, however, you're going to need some feedback. Pillows can't tell you if the wraps are too loose or too tight, or if they're experiencing nerve compression or rope burn. The number of nerves in a human being is well over 7 trillion; the number of nerves in a pillow is zero. That's a big difference.

# Psychology, Motivation, and Profiles

| | |
|---|---|
| You're a sick fuck if you want to tie people up. | No. All kinds of no. There are *many* reasons that a person may want to tie or be tied. It is a demonstration of trust. For the bottom, it can be a release of responsibility, allowing them the freedom to simply feel and react without their anxieties or concerns getting in the way. For the Top, it can be an expression of skill and control, both over the rope and over their very willing partner. It can be primal. It can be artistic. It can be a playful vacation from the norm. It can be cathartic. It can be a way to connect with your partner more powerfully. |
| If you want to tie someone up and have them restrained and helpless in any way, that means that you don't care about them. | One cornerstone of ethical/responsible rigging is being very aware of, and responsive to, the needs of your bottom. One of the most important things we do before, during and after a scene is communicate. A responsible partner cares. They listen and they design an experience intended to fulfill the needs of everyone involved. Not just their own. |
| If you want to have someone restrained and helpless, you must want to do something to them that they don't want you to do. | Again, no. Done right, bondage is something that everyone involved wants. Rope bottoms love being tied and the feeling of being restrained. And yes, they may want other sensations while being restrained, too! But those are things that both Top and bottom need to discuss beforehand, so everyone involved is getting what they want and need from the scene and nothing is happening that was not previously agreed upon. No surprises, no hidden agendas. |
| Only a certain kind of person would want to be tied/tie someone up. | This myth extends to gender, sexual orientation, D/s dynamics, and more. The validity of who you are and how you identify is in no way lessened by an interest in bottoming or Topping for rope bondage.

  Within the context of BDSM, some may have it in their head that a "real Dom" would never want to bottom for a rope scene. This is ridiculous. Read the definition of both "Top" and "bottom" in the vocabulary section (p. 8). Being a bottom only refers to being on the receiving end of sensation during a given activity. Being a Top means that you are the one giving sensation to another person. Neither one of these roles has anything to do with who is in control or directing what goes on. Therefore, they are separate ideas/roles from D/s. As someone once said, "It is possible to suck dick in a very dominant way."

  If you want to experience the feeling of being restrained, that does NOT mean that you aren't really a Top/Dom.

  Rope can be applied to any person no matter what they look like or who they are. Rope is for everybody and every body that is interested. Any person of any ethnicity, gender, biological sex, sexual orientation, D/s role, and physical ability can experience rope. The flexibility and customizable nature of any rope experience is part of its beauty. |

# Rope Itself

There is only one kind of rope that should be used for rope bondage.

No. Different ropes bring different qualities and are good for different things. There is much more on this in Chapter 3 (p. 85).

I should invest in a good set of ropes and, once I have them, I will never need to buy rope again.

Nope. Rope is a consumable.

Over time, friction and wear will reduce the strength of your rope, no matter how good it is. This will happen more quickly if you are doing any load-bearing ties where the friction is higher. Sometimes individual fibers get caught on something, or rope becomes contaminated in a way that can't be remedied (paint, dye, bodily fluids, wax), or the bight gets worn over time.

If you are using your rope, it will wear out and you will eventually need to replace it.

Rope can be sanitized.

Rope can be cleaned, but sanitization is tricky. If rope comes into contact with bodily fluids, there is no guarantee that you will be able to remove all traces of those fluids. This is especially important when tying multiple partners.

Use barrier methods or make a piece of rope dedicated to a particular partner if it's going to come into contact with bodily fluids other than sweat.

Cleaning rope is still a good practice even if you have rope dedicated to a particular partner or use barrier methods. See *Rope Hygiene* (p. 78) for more.

Rope is only for people of a certain body type or below a certain weight.

No. Rope is for everybody and every body that is interested in it. It is amazingly customizable and can be adapted to an almost limitless degree.

A person's build or size has no bearing on whether or not they are a good candidate for a rope bottom. Different bodies may require different things in order for you to tie them comfortably and safely. See *Body Type Considerations* (p. 324).

This book does not cover suspension as that is an advanced skill, but we are going to use it as an example to make this point more intuitive.

When doing a suspension, a person's weight must be distributed on a series of straps that you create using rope and then connect to an overhead hard point.

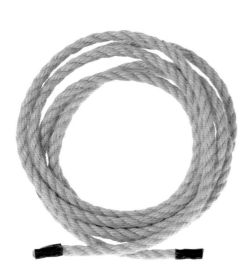

- If you are suspending a short gymnast, they have low overall mass and require only a few straps to distribute that mass comfortably.
- If you are suspending a huge wrestler, they have much more mass. There will be much more pressure on the straps suspending them. In order to make that comfortable, the straps need to be wider and it can be helpful to create more of them. It is simple physics: When you distribute force over a larger area, there is less pressure. So wider straps and more straps make it more comfortable and less risky, allowing you more flexibility in whom you can suspend. *But this is a skill that is up to you, as the Top, to learn.*

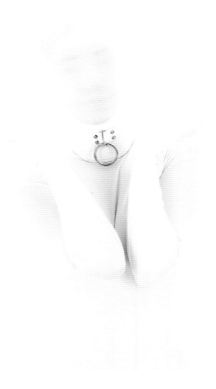

The point is that the ability to suspend someone is dependent on the skill of the rigger, not the physical build of the bottom. If you do not feel you have the skill to safely suspend someone, then do not do it.

But that is a reflection of your skill and experience as a rigger; don't make it their problem by telling them that they are too big. Tell them instead that you are still building your skill and are not confident that you would be able to do it safely. Make it clear that it is you, not them. Then, if you still want to do something with them, do something with less risk that will help you learn more about each other. Start with floor work (non-suspension), then move to partial suspension (one foot stays on the ground to support them) and build from there.

A word on body type and this book: Most of the pictures in this book are of one of your authors, Kajira Blue, a person with one specific body type. Do not take this to mean that we are implying that rope is only for that body type. Far from it. Almost every technique in this book can work equally well on almost any body. For ties that may require some modification, there are a few simple techniques that allow you to do so. See *Body Type Considerations* (p. 324).

## Another Myth

Once I finish this book, I will know all I need to know.

This book is a great *start*. It contains a fusion of the collected wisdom and experience of thousands of people in the rope community all over the world.

When you are done with this book, you will have the building blocks needed to create *thousands* of different scenes.

But this is just us sharing the best information that we know *at this moment*. Information is subject to change, and the community may have found better techniques and information by the time you read this.

Continue your rope education by connecting with your local community and by going to TheDuchy.com for updated information.

# BDSM and the Law

What happens between consenting adults is no one else's business.

Understand that *there are places where bondage and other BDSM activities are not legal.* In many places activities involving restraint and/or impact are classified as *assault* and, while *authentic consent* to such activity is what they call an "affirmative defense" against a charge of assault in many jurisdictions, this is not true everywhere. Research your local, state, and federal laws.

There are places where law enforcement can independently charge you with assault if they see you restraining or striking another person, even if both of you state clearly that all parties consented. This is why some locations do not have public dungeons and all parties are private and require that you be vetted.

If your jurisdiction does not recognize consent as an affirmative defense, it is up to you to decide if you are going to take part in these activities despite that. Doing so carries legal risk in those locations.

It should go without saying; however, touching someone sexually in any way *without* their authentic consent, especially in a context where restraint is involved, *is assault — or worse —* in most jurisdictions.

# *The Scene & The Community*

If you are here just to learn to tie on yourself, or to tie on a mannequin or other inanimate object, you can skip to the next chapter. The rest of this chapter is dedicated to those of you who would like to tie or be tied by other people, or would like to meet other shibari enthusiasts.

If you are interested in shibari purely for artistic/aesthetic purposes, be aware that some rope lovers are coming into this from a BDSM background. If you are coming at this from a BDSM background, be mindful that some rope lovers are in it purely as an artistic endeavor. Keep this in mind when interacting with others. If you are unclear about a person's specific motivations, interests, or desires, ask.

The rope community can be found in every part of the world and many places online. Like all kink, it used to be hidden deep underground, but the internet has made people aware that they are not alone, and the community continues to grow and become more open. Rope people love to share what they have learned, but the community does have expectations and etiquette standards that are important to know.

# Common Vocabulary Terms

Here are a few selected terms used commonly in the scene. There are many others, but this should get you started.

## BDSM

BDSM is a compound initialism combining B&D (Bondage and Discipline), D/s (Dominance and submission), and S&M (Sadism and Masochism). While its exact origin is unclear, the common use of the term dates back to 1969. The terms "BDSM" and "kink" are often used interchangeably.

Regardless of its origin, BDSM is used as a catch-all phrase to include a wide range of activities, forms of interpersonal relationships, and distinct subcultures. Historical and artistic records show such activities dating back to approximately 3000 BC and they are assumed to date back to the start of humankind as a species.

BDSM is a variety of erotic practices involving power exchange, bondage, role-playing, and other interpersonal dynamics. Given the wide range of practices, some of which may be engaged in by people who do not consider themselves as practicing BDSM, inclusion in the BDSM community and/or subculture is usually dependent on self-identification and shared experience.

Interest in BDSM can range from one-time experimentation to an ongoing lifestyle and is considered by some to be a distinct sexual identity/orientation.

## Bondage

Bondage is consensually tying, binding, or restraining a partner (usually physically) for erotic, aesthetic, and/or somatosensory stimulation. Rope, cuffs, chain, tape, or many other types of restraints may be used for this purpose.

Bondage may be used as an end unto itself. The active partner can derive visual pleasure from seeing their partner tied up, and the restrained partner can derive tactile pleasure from the feeling of helplessness and immobility. A common reason for the active partner to tie up their partner is so both may gain pleasure from the restrained partner's submission and the feeling of the temporary transfer of control and power.

It may also be used as a part of sex or in conjunction with other BDSM activities. It is common to have sexual activities as part of a bondage scene, but they do not have to be involved.

For sadomasochistic people, bondage is often used as a means to sadomasochistic ends, where the restrained partner is more accessible to other sadomasochistic activities.

## Rope Bondage

An umbrella term for all styles of applying rope to human participants. It can be done for erotic appeal, visual enjoyment, physical restraint, or as a part of other plans.

## Shibari

Also called "Japanese rope bondage," *shibari* — the Japanese word for "to tie" — is a style of rope bondage generally characterized by being visually appealing. While not technically the same thing, the term "shibari" is often used interchangeably with the general term "rope bondage." Shibari is more about the attractive appearance of the rope itself or position of the person in rope, or both. It may or may not include elements of physical restraint.

## A Scene

A scene is a mutually agreed upon encounter during which two or more people engage in kink/BDSM-related activities. The activities that will take place during a scene are pre-negotiated. They may or may not involve sexual activity. A scene is not over until any aftercare (p. 45) has ended.

   Activity that takes place during a scene may be referred to as "play." A scene may also be referred to as a "session" to set a more professional tone, especially if it is conducted as part of a professional transaction, by a "Pro Dom" or "Pro Domme" (usually pronounced the same).

## The Scene

*The* scene is distinctly different from "a scene." It refers to the community of people who engage in kink/BDSM-related activities. It can refer to the community in a given geographical area, the events in that area or, more generally, to the larger population of kink-minded people as a whole.

   Ex: "The rope scene around here tends to focus on Eastern style bondage. I only know two riggers who regularly use Western ties," or, "I stepped away from the kink scene for a few years due to some things outside of my control. I'm excited to reconnect with my community!"

## Types of Bondage

- Decorating a partner for sensual and/or artistic reasons.
- Binding body parts, such as arms and/or legs, together.
- Spreading out body parts, such as arms and/or legs, so they are unable to touch each other.
- Binding the restrained partner to an outside object, such as a bed, chair, or table.
- Suspending the restrained partner from an overhead hard point.
- Hindering and/or slowing down the movement of the restrained partner, such as with a hobble skirt or a corset.
- Wrapping the entire body of the restrained partner up, mummification.
- Binding the body in such a fashion as to cause pain for the purposes of S&M.

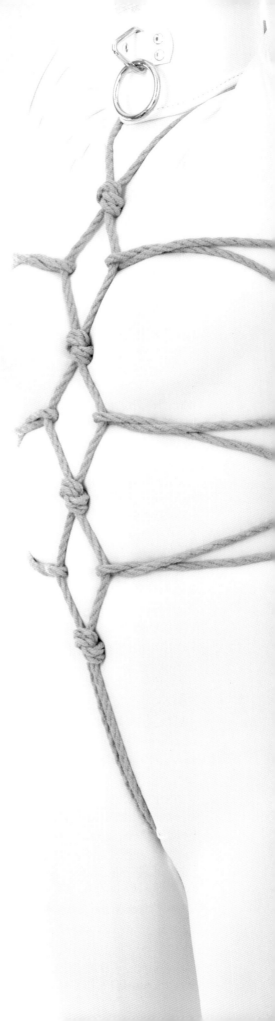

# Finding Your Local Scene or Community

At the time this book was written, a popular resource for finding local contacts, and for socializing and learning about anything kink-related from real life practitioners was FetLife.com.

FetLife is a social networking site focused specifically on connecting kinksters. It is designed to help build a community, so it purposefully does not include the features of a dating site; you cannot search for people based on their profile or demographics. It allows people to create profiles, yes, but it then focuses on *groups* and *events*. This is an important and powerful difference that has made it popular with kinksters all over the world, so it can be a useful tool for connecting with your local rope/kink community. It is free and, if you use a separate email, anonymous to create an account.

Once you create an account, first look for a "munch" by searching FetLife using this term:

"(Name of your closest larger city) Munch"

(For example, "St. Louis Munch", "Cincinnati Munch", "Leeds UK Munch", "Rome Munch", "Singapore Munch").

A "munch" is the term for a meeting that takes place in a public place so that people can meet and get to know one another and talk about kink without doing something risky like going to an unknown person's house. Munches are often a combination of a community outreach and early/ continuing education venue. Most larger cities tend to have multiple munches put on by different groups with different interests. Every group is different and you may find yourself connecting more naturally with the people in one over another, so try several before you settle on one to attend more regularly. For example, if you are under 35 years old, you may find that you connect better with a "TNG munch" than you do with the "rope munch" because members of the TNG group are all under 35, too. (TNG stands for "the next generation".) Or you may find that you like the local rope group better because it has people with more experience that are willing to teach. Or you may find you prefer the wider range of topics offered in a general munch or group vs. one focused on a particular activity.

If you are wary of using an online tool, consider heading to your local sex/kink shop and asking for resources. Sex/kink/rope-friendly retail establishments tend to be few and far between, so they can serve as important centers of information about the local scene. The same goes for some alternative nightclubs. It may be worth talking to the employees of such places on your quest for information. Be specific with the questions you ask. If you are looking for rope groups/ practitioners, say so. Take note of the recommendations you get and look for trends and patterns. Eventually you will find your crowd. It just might take a little digging.

## Use Common Sense

It is important to understand that the kink scene (online and in-person) is a collection of individuals. The vast majority are good people, constructive,

**Some Other Helpful Search Terms and Links:**

**"City Name Rope Munch"**
A munch for people particularly interested in rope.

**"City Name Rope"**
A more general search for rope groups even if they don't do munches.

**fetlife.com/events/near**
A list of events in or near your area.

well-meaning, and willing to help. But, as with any other community, it also has members who are not trustworthy. You *will* come across ignorant people who think that kinksters are all "easy" and that they can get easy sex if they just pretend to be an uber-Dom or sex kitten. Do your research. Vet any individual before meeting them (p. 22); make sure they are known in the community and have a good reputation. If a person says that they don't like to do things with the local community, many consider that to be a red flag, no matter what reasonable-sounding excuse they might offer. Protect yourself. Use good internet and real-life safety skills.

# Find a Local Teacher or Mentor

One other reason to connect to your local scene: For most people, an important step in growing new skills is having an experienced person watch what you are doing and give you feedback, which is a valuable part of the process that a book alone cannot give you. Regardless of how detailed and precise we try to be in this book, there will be things that you may miss or may not understand until someone shows you in person. Also, maybe another rigger's style of tying or the way they phrase the instructions clicks better for you and that's great! Again, there is no "one true way" and if you find a way that works better for you, run with it!

### How Do You Find a Local Teacher or Mentor?

First find your local rope community. Start going to rope munches, rope practice labs, or parties put on by a rope group. At those events, ask people who they respect that might be willing to teach you, or to watch you and provide feedback. Ask for *honest* feedback and accept any comments you get gratefully, like the gifts they are. Learn from them. Over time, you may find yourself connecting with someone, and that may lead to more.

Your local rope group or adult store may also put on formal classes or be able to recommend classes taught by other groups in the area. These can also be tremendously helpful.

### Not Necessarily Local, but Still Worth it!

There are also various conferences and conventions focused on kink in general or on rope specifically. These can be great opportunities for learning and socializing — and realizing just how *big* the scene really is!

Just Google "BDSM rope convention" or "rope bondage convention" to find options near you or within reasonable traveling distance.

# Understanding Types of Participants

## Top

A "Top" is the person primarily performing the actions or giving the sensations, as contrasted with the "bottom," the person receiving the action of sensation in a BDSM scene.

The term "Top" is not the same as "Dom" or "Master/Mistress"; the person providing the sensation may not be the one in control of what is happening in the scene.

A Dom of whatever gender might enjoy the sensation of being penetrated with a strap-on dildo and tell a sub to wear one to give them pleasure. In this case, the Top is the *submissive* (following the direction of the Dom who controls the scene) and the bottom is the *Dom* (receiving the sensations given by the sub).

## Rope Top/Rigger

Within the context of rope bondage (aka rigging), the person applying rope is the Rope Top. Another term for this role/person is rigger.

## Service Top

A Service Top might be a D-type (Dominant, Dom, Domme), M-type (Master, Mistress), or s-type (submissive, sub, slave) that performs topping skills on a willing bottom primarily for the benefit of the bottom (as a service to them). A Pro-Dom or Pro-Domme is a Service Top.

## Bottom

A bottom is a person receiving the action or sensation provided to them by the "Top" in a BDSM scene. The term "bottom" is not the same as submissive or slave, as they are not necessarily relinquishing control.

For example, during flogging, the person swinging the flogger implement would be the Top, while the person being struck with the flogger would be the bottom.

## Rope Bottom/Bunny

Within the context of rope bondage, a person who is having rope applied to them is called a rope bottom. Another common term for this is rope bunny.

## Dominant/Dom/Domme

A Dominant, or Dom, is the person in control, the one with the power or authority in a power exchange situation or relationship. They practice some form of domination, whether it be physical, mental, emotional, spiritual, or a combination.

"Dom" is the most commonly used form and does not imply anything about gender, orientation, etc. Some people use the form "Domme" to specifically identify a Dominant that identifies as female.

"Domme" is pronounced "dom" by some and "dom-may" by others. Occasionally the word "Domina" or "Dominatrix" is also used to describe a female/feminine Dominant or Mistress.

### Submissive/Sub

A submissive, or sub, is a person that gives up some degree of authority and/or control to a Dominant for the duration of a specific scene or all the time. It is not to be confused with the term "bottom."

The term "sub" is synonymous with submissive and does not imply anything about gender, orientation, etc.

### Switch

A person who participates in relationships, scenes, and activities as a Top/Dominant or bottom/submissive depending on their mood, partner or the situation. Some Switches enjoy changing their power dynamic during a scene.

A Switch is a person who enjoys both sides of the coin, so to speak. Some Switches choose a specific role with particular partners or activities, others decide based on their mood.

Within the context of rope, someone who enjoys both Topping and bottoming may refer to themselves as a Rope Switch.

## A Few Guidelines

Your first kink or rope event will probably be a "munch"— a meeting of kinky people in a public place like a restaurant so that people can feel safe meeting other new people.

All social groups have their unique norms and expectations. It is always best to be observant at first and learn the rules of a new group before barreling in, but here are a few expectations and general guidelines that will be helpful as you begin.

### Privacy is Vitally Important

Depending on where you live, the prevailing culture there, and your particular lifestyle, you may feel free to be open about the fact that you like rope or kink. Or you may be very serious about keeping that side of yourself private.

Regardless of your personal views, never make assumptions about the relative privacy of others. This is their secret to keep.

**No "Outing." What Happens at Any Kink Event,**
*Stays at that Kink Event*

If you meet a person at a kink event and then later run into them at a work event or anywhere else, *you do not know them* until they introduce themselves. Such an encounter can be *very* jarring; worlds colliding. The best thing to do is to act as you normally would. If it would be awkward to avoid them, then don't. Introduce yourself in a neutral way and do not make any assumptions about whether or not they want to acknowledge that you have met before: "Hi, my name's _____ . Good to meet you. I'm trying to remember, have we met before?" Let them decide how to proceed.

That said, sometimes it can be helpful to *out yourself.*

If you are engaged in kink, particularly if you become really into it, there may be times when other people need to know about it.

It can be helpful to be open about this interest to your doctor, therapist, chiropractor, etc. If you come out to them *before* you have an issue, they are less likely to be concerned if you later come to them for help with an injury or if they see something that might otherwise be concerning. If you have already told your doctor that you are into spanking, for example, they will better understand if they later see you with a bruised ass from a heavy session. They will probably still ask you about it. It is their job to make sure you feel safe and to offer help if you do not. But if you reply clearly and without embarrassment that this was the result of a consensual and very fun scene, that will hopefully be the end of it.

If you are concerned about having such a conversation with your doctor (perhaps they are the same doctor that sees your grandma, and you just can't), you might find a different one using the Kink-Aware Professionals list (KAP), published and maintained by the National Coalition for Sexual Freedom:

Kink-Aware Professionals list (KAP): kapprofessionals.org

## Don't Make Assumptions About Anything

You enter the room. You see a tiny, cute girl, dressed in pink chiffon, smiling brightly as she perches on the knee of some huge, fuck-off boxer type dressed in heavy black leather, his hand resting possessively on the small of her back, gazing imperiously at the world around him. Do *not* assume she is the sub and he the Dom. Do *not* even assume that "she" identifies as a "she" or "he" a "him." It could easily be that the person in pink is giving the orders and uses he/him or they/them pronouns.

One of the most ruthless Doms I have ever met was an 80 pound, 22-year-old woman who liked to dress like a baby doll.

She looked like she wouldn't hurt a fly, but she just *loved* to bring people to floods of tears. Her thing was to lean into stereotypes and then shatter expectations.

The BDSM world respects the fact that physical characteristics, gender identity, gender expression, sexual identity, sexual expression, and sexual preferences are all *different* things.

Don't assume a person's role, ability, intentions, pronouns, gender identity; just ask! If you want a straight answer, ask a straight question. Innuendos and metaphors are breeding grounds for confusion. Asking for clarification or posing a "stupid question" is rarely offensive when done in a *conscientious* and *respectful* way. Remember that you are talking to a human being, just like you.

Example of how you might talk to the couple in pink and black: "Hi, I'm _____. Great to meet both of you. Love the outfits! What would you like me to call you? What are your pronouns?"

Don't bat an eye if the person in pink answers with "Oh, I am Gozer the Destructor. [tinkling laugh] I own this lovely hunk of deliciousness here. You can just call them 'Gatekeeper' [nod of genial acknowledgment] Pleasure to meet you. First time here?"

Just roll with it, call them Gozer and Gatekeeper as asked. All names and all words were made up at one time, so don't let it bother you that these ones sound a little different to your ear. You will get used to it surprisingly quickly.

You can be charming and witty, ask them where the Keymaster is, but don't cross the line to being creepy, don't immediately ask them if you can be the Keymaster.

[If these names didn't make you smile, go treat yourself: Watch the 1984 film *Ghostbusters*]

## Be Honest

Generally and always: Be honest about what you choose to share. You don't have to share anything you don't want to share, but if you choose to speak, let your words be true. Let people learn they can trust you. This is just a general statement that can apply to almost anything, but in the world of rope it is critically important. If you are asking someone to allow you to tie them, you are *literally* asking them to trust you with their life. Be worthy of that trust.

Beyond the general statement of "be worthy of trust," there are some specific things to call out:

### Be Honest About Your Level of Experience

If you are not experienced in something, don't try to hide that fact or embellish your skill level. If you cannot admit that you have things to learn, how will you learn? Being honest about your experience level is critical to consent, safety, and being an ethical player.

Yes, experience *is* an attractive trait, but a lack of experience does not make you unattractive. Some people try to come off as some sort of shibari master or the ultimate bottom even when they are just beginning. Yes, it can be hard to admit you don't know something. It can be hard to ask for help, but you will gain the respect of those around you by doing so. Even if the question feels repetitive or basic, ask it. A good teacher will never make you feel inferior for trying to learn.

There is no shame in being a beginner. Every expert was once a beginner, including the authors of this book. Be honest about your experience level and, if you are interested in changing that, make that happen. Do more research, tie yourself, practice on inanimate objects, ask your best friend to help, find your local rope community and attend their events, ask to observe a rope scene done by a rigger you admire, ask them to watch you tie and provide their input, go to a convention or other event. Every experience will add to your knowledge in some way.

A note for bottoms: Be skeptical of a person who makes boastful claims to be an expert. People with big egos sometimes think they have nothing left to learn. The best riggers are continually learning, refining and honing their skill. They understand that it is always possible to get better. Humility is a sign of wisdom and integrity. Keep that in mind when vetting potential Rope Tops.

**Be Honest About What You Want**

Even if you are not yet comfortable talking about your deepest desires, be honest with *yourself* about them. Over time, as you build trust in the people you are meeting and begin to really understand the huge spectrum of people out there, you can begin sharing more and more of yourself. You can become comfortable enough to share the really important things and find others who are also into what you are into. *That* is the path to amazing things.

Yes, it can be intimidating to admit things about yourself, even privately, especially if they fall outside traditional roles. To give a classic example: Perhaps you are a manly man, ex-Marine from a family who have *all* been Marines since the Corps was created in 1775. But you long to feel what it would be like to be made to dress in a corset, thigh-high stockings, and stiletto heels. Perhaps you want to tie or be tied while in that outfit. Don't let the messages from society stop you from exploring! There are many people out there that would be just as into that as you are. You just need to find them. And to find them, you need to be honest about what you want and become part of that community.

**Don't Come Off as Desperate**

Desperation is not a good look ... unless it is part of a pre-negotiated scene (a look of desperation in the eyes of their bound partner can be a huge turn-on for some riggers).

If you are just beginning your rope/kink journey, it may feel like your options and opportunities are few and far between. You may feel like you will never find what you crave. This *will* change with time. Accept that things take time and enjoy the journey as you go. Rushing to find a rope partner can make for cringe-worthy messages or interactions.

Confidence is sexy, desperation is not.

Take your time. Meet in public places, at munches, at events, learn the community, let them learn about you. Eventually you will find someone that you connect with, and you can build from there.

## Build Confidence Through Experience

One thing you can do to build confidence is to build an interesting technical skill. That is something this book can help you with. Build your skills by practicing on yourself or some inanimate object. Build your confidence so that when you find an opportunity to try rope on a person, you are not fumbling with the technique itself, but rather simply trying a technique you have already practiced. The two experiences will feel quite different to the person you are tying.

Seek out experienced rope bottoms. They are incredibly valuable to new riggers. Experienced bottoms know how rope should feel and can give you excellent feedback.

It is generally not a good idea for two inexperienced players to be learning exclusively together. If you are a new Rope Top, it would be good for you to find an experienced rope bottom to work with. If you are a new rope bottom, it would be good to find an experienced Rope Top. If you are both new, you are more likely to run into problems that could have been avoided if either one of you had a better idea of what to look out for.

An example of how you might approach someone respectfully:

*At a party, having watched two people do rope together, speaking first to the Top:*
"Hi! I loved your rope scene! I am new to rope and find it fascinating. I have been learning from online sources and am trying to master the Somerville Bowline. Would you be willing to watch me do it and give me feedback?" Or, after some conversation, "...I have been trying to master the Shinju. Would you be willing to allow me to tie one on your partner, if they are okay with it, and let me know if I am doing it correctly?" If they agree, thank them and then ask for help from the volunteer bottom as well: "I have not tied it on another person before, so I would love feedback from you, too, if you are willing."

Online:
"I am new to the world of rope and am interested in finding a partner to practice with. I have been practicing on myself and I would love to try what I have been learning on someone else so I can get their feedback. If you are interested in having a conversation to see if we click, let me know. If not, no worries. I hope you have a nice day."

### Treat Everyone with Respect

No one owes you anything. They don't owe you their time or knowledge. If they choose to gift you either, respect that. Value it as the gift it is. Thank them.

#### The Folly of Playing a Numbers Game

Copying and pasting the same message into 20 different message boxes may seem like it will increase your chances of connecting with someone, but it won't.

Treat people like they are real people that you may someday have a relationship with and care about. Be respectful of their time and put some effort into how you reach out. Read profiles, reach out to people you find genuinely interesting and with whom you *actually* have real points of connection. Show that interest in your messages. They are not fantasy dispensers. Catch their interest with those real points of connection. Give them a reason to want to respond.

Go to events and meet people in real life. Moving the relationship from virtual space to real life space is the only way you will be able to actually do rope together, and you have a much better chance of doing that if you genuinely connect with the other person.

And never send unsolicited pictures of your genitals. Seriously. That is an instant turn-off.

### There is no "One True Way" Despite What Some May Try to Say

There are a few generally accepted rules and expectations, but there are many variations amongst people, protocols, and practices. Don't be afraid to think a little outside the box.

Practices, expectations, and cultures often vary by location. Every place has its own kink scene culture that is a product of the people who make up that scene. If you don't mesh with people in one group or location, try another.

We feel we have to say this because "the community" is made up of individuals. As with every community, there will be some individuals who have very strong opinions and will want to tell you that what you are doing is wrong (according to them). Listen to what they have to say. Be respectful of their time. If what they say makes sense to you, great! Take it onboard. But just because some random person says that "This is how it is" doesn't necessarily make it true, or true for you. Don't be intimidated. Talk to other people, too. Do further research. Learn how others in your local community see things and make up your own mind about what works for you.

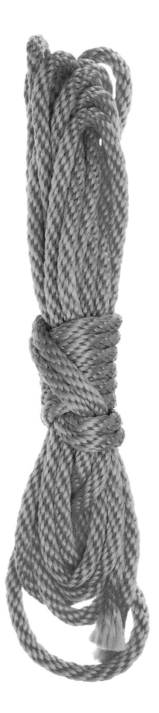

## Ask Permission Before Touching Another Person or Their Belongings. Always.

Explicit consent is the cornerstone of trust in our community. Keep your hands to yourself until you ask for and receive explicit permission. A few examples of doing this well:

- "Oh! That rope looks sooo silky! What kind is it? May I touch it?" *"Help yourself!"*
- "I've never seen carabiners like that before, how do they work?" *"Here, let me show you."* (Demonstrates) *"You want to try it?"*
- "OMG, that paddle is amazing? Did you make it?" *"I did, yes! Fun Project. Feel free to pick it up and feel its heft if you want to."*
- (After negotiation) "Okay, we planned to do a Shinju and turn that into a **Box Tie**. This is going to be just practicing the technique and seeing how it feels to both of us. We are not going to be doing this as a 'scene,' agreed?" *"Yes."*
  "Great! Are you ready? May I put rope on you?" *"Absolutely!"* Enthusiastic, authentic consent.

More on this in *Consent* (p. 24).

## Your Safety is Your Responsibility

You make the decision to trust people with your safety. People only know what you tell them. If you have a hard limit or some condition that may become a problem during a scene and you do not tell your partner about it, the responsibility for that does not fall only on them if it becomes an issue. You are responsible for your physical and mental well-being and providing the information needed to care for you.

No one truly has "no limits" and saying you have no limits is not an attractive quality. It isn't fair, reasonable, or responsible to place your well-being in the hands of another person without giving them some sense of how to take care of you.

Communicate your needs and limits before and during a scene. For example, nerve compression can happen in seconds and the only one who will know when it's happening is the person experiencing it. It is your responsibility to do sensory and motor tests (p. 73), and to tell your rigger there is an issue. Because if you don't, that's on you.

# Operating Within the Scene/Community

## A General Framework for BDSM (and other) Encounters

In the BDSM world, we like to talk about several elements that are important to having a successful encounter. Many people find this framework useful for other relationships as well.

We like to help people see every encounter as having the same general framework:

1. Find someone you'd like to play with.
2. Vet your potential play partner to confirm if you do, in fact, want to scene with them.
3. Negotiate together to find common interests and agree on what will happen in that scene.
   - Plan what you will do — what is permitted — and how.
   - Plan what you will *both* do if things go according to plan.
   - Plan what you will *both* do if things go awry.
   - Be clear about what is *not* permitted.
4. Do the scene.
   - React to positive and negative things, address issues.
5. Provide aftercare to everyone involved.
   - Tops and bottoms all have needs.
   - Make sure everyone is okay and back to themselves.
6. Process your emotional and other reactions after the scene has ended.
   - You may experience heightened or lowered emotions, ebullience or drop, or both.
   - Note lessons learned, both positive and negative. Learn from your encounter.
7. Decide if you want to do more with that person or not.
   - If things went well, this may have been a step toward establishing an ongoing relationship.

## Find Someone You'd Like to Play With

Perhaps you are reading this book to learn new skills with your intended play partner. If so, great! This part is done already!

But perhaps you are looking for a partner, or if you have one, you both are interested in "opening" your relationship and exploring with others, too.

The good news is that this world does exist in real life! If you have only ever seen this world through movies or TV, it is not what you think it will be. It is filled with curious, passionate people that love to explore and have that indefinable something that gives them the courage to do so. We like to say that it is filled with sex nerds and adventurers!

There are many online tools that can be very helpful to begin your search.

General dating apps and sites *might* work, but it can be difficult figuring out if someone you are interested in might be into kink. More and more, people are just being up front with it, but that can be risky, so many include code phrases in their profiles. These will change over time, but some that are common as of the writing of this book include: *50 Shades* or *The Secretary*, Ethical Non-Monogamy (ENM), compersion, macrame, rope, shibari, etc.

As discussed in *Finding Your Local Scene or Community* (p. 10), FetLife.com can be a useful resource for meeting potential partners. It is *not* set up as a dating tool, although some do try to use it that way. It's intended purpose is better. We believe that if you are looking to form a real relationship, it is best to move things from virtual space to real-life space as quickly as you can. Staying online will only get you so far. Here is where FetLife can be helpful. Its primary goal is to connect people with the real-life community, helping you find local groups of real people that share your interests. Sign up for free and go to the Events Page. If you love rope and want to find other people who love rope, go where those people are!

## Be Realistic. We are Still Part of the Real World, for Better and for Worse

There are people who hear about our world and try to join it because they think they can get easy sex or they are predators hoping for easy prey.

For both Tops and bottoms: Check references and don't accept a person's word without the corroboration of someone you trust, preferably more than one person.

- Bottoms: There are dangerous Tops, people who play outside their ability, who don't respect boundaries, are careless, or may even be predators.
- Tops: There are also dangerous bottoms, people who are not honest about their abilities or what they want and can thus contribute to getting one or both of you physically and emotionally hurt. This can violate your consent. It could also hurt your reputation.

Use all the "keep me safe" skills you have learned as part of a wired world:

- Ask for and check references. Vet the person through well-known people in the local scene, look up local groups on FetLife and talk to the leaders there, and/or get the opinion of another bottom who has played with them, if possible.
- Meet in public or at events put on by local BDSM groups first.
- Play at parties or events first, establishing trust before ever meeting alone.
- Set up a safe call (p. 39) when you are meeting someone alone.

# Vetting

Rope bondage often entails some form of restraint. Therefore, it is important to vet anyone you plan on doing it with. Vetting is different from negotiation in that it is mostly about getting a feel for the person you may be tying with, common interests, etc. Vetting is about answering the question, "Do I want to scene with this person at all?" Negotiation focuses mainly on the details of the scene itself.

Vetting can take many forms:

- Asking them questions.
  - This helps you determine compatibility for engaging in play.
  - You can also probe into their experience and other information important for informed consent. See questions below.
- Asking them for references.
  - This is iffy, they may only tell you about people they have had a positive experience with, but it does show that there *are* people they have had positive experiences with.
- Asking leaders of groups in their local area if the person is known to them.
  - This can be helpful if the person is known in the community, but not everyone is known.
  - You can often do this through FetLife.com.
- What if the person isn't part of their local community?
  - "Oh, I prefer to stay away from the community because [reason or excuse]."
  - This is a little controversial, because there can be good, legitimate reasons for not engaging with the local community, but many people see it as a red flag if a person does not engage with the local community at all.
  - Perhaps they say it is "too cliquey" or there's "too much drama." Perhaps this is true, or perhaps they are known in the local community and have a bad reputation, so they claim otherwise.

Listen to your gut. If something seems off, even if you can't quantify it or articulate why you feel that way, pay attention to that sense. You have years of experience in reading others; use it. If a person is unknown, you should insist on attending multiple public scene events (munches, parties, etc.) first. Get to know them in a monitored environment, play with them in such a place first, before you play with them in private.

## Questions to Ask When Vetting a Potential Rope Top:

- Have you ever Topped for rope before?
- What, specifically, would you like to try? What is your experience with that/those thing(s)?
- Are you involved in the local community or scene? What kinds of community events do you go to?
- What do you check for to ensure the safety of your bottom?
- How do you clean your rope?

- Tell me about a time when a scene went wrong. How did you handle it?
- Do you have past play partners I can talk to?
- What kinds of educational resources do you use to continue learning about rope?
  - Remember, informed consent is not possible if one is not informed. It is necessary for both Tops and bottoms to learn about the potential risks that come along with rope bondage.
- What are your hard/soft limits?
- I'm interested in being tied by you; would you be interested in doing a scene with me?

## Questions to Ask When Vetting a Potential Rope Bottom:
- Have you ever bottomed for rope before? If yes, what was that experience like?
- Are you involved in the local community or scene? What kinds of community events do you go to?
- Do you have references or other partners I can talk to who have tied you?
- What, specifically, would you like to try? What is your experience with that/those thing(s)?
- What kinds of educational resources do you use to continue learning about rope?
  - Remember, informed consent is not possible if one is not informed. It is necessary for both Tops and bottoms to learn about the potential risks that come along with rope bondage.
- What are your hard/soft limits?
- I'm interested in tying you; would you be interested in doing a scene with me?

## Moving from Vetting to Negotiation
Once you have decided that you are interested in more, you move to a negotiation, which is about the scene itself. This may happen at a different time or as part of or following the above conversation.

Here are some beginning questions that are more related to negotiation than vetting. These questions apply to both Top and bottom. This is just a beginning; see *Negotiation* (p. 32) for more.
- What are you looking to get out of doing a rope scene with me?
  - The answer to this question will help inform what kind of scene you might do as well as if you think you may be compatible with this person.
  - Potential answers: Education, trying a new thing, increasing experience, taking pretty pictures, bottoming before learning how to rig for themselves, tying for sex, etc.
- Are you aware of any triggers so I can avoid them?
- Is sexual touch something that you want to be included in this scene?
- What kind of aftercare do you need?
- ...and more, see *Negotiation* (p. 32).

# Consent

## Consent is the Cornerstone of Everything We Do

Touching someone without their authentic consent, especially in a context like this where restraint is involved, is legally *assault* in many jurisdictions.

Depending on where you live, consent may not be a viable defense against assault charges in a court of law. See *BDSM and the Law* (p. 7) for more on this.

Get used to asking for consent. With practice, it becomes second nature.

*Agreement* is **not** the same thing as *consent*.

Consent is a type of agreement, held to a much higher standard.

## Consent Must be Authentic, Informed, and Explicit

There are many definitions and models of consent out there, but this is the one we prefer:

Affirmative Consent: "An informed, authentic and explicit agreement, freely given between two legal adults in a non-altered state of mind to allow a specific set of activities to happen during a specific time frame."

Every word in that definition is important:

- Informed – You must know what you are agreeing to and the possible risks and implications you are exposing yourself to. Education and understanding are critical to consent. If you don't understand the potential risks and implications of an activity, how can you authentically state that you accept those risks? Top or bottom, you need to understand everything in the *Reducing Risk* chapter (p. 49), because without that understanding, informed consent is not possible. *Without knowledge, you are not informed.*

- Authentic – Actively interested and willing to participate in the activities proposed. To be authentic, agreement must be informed and freely given. Some people like to use the phrase "enthusiastic consent" because when someone is truly into something, that often comes across as enthusiasm, but we like the term "authentic" better because not everyone displays enthusiasm, even under conditions of great excitement. And it is pretty common for a sub to be anything but enthusiastic if they are on their way to a punishment they know they have earned.

- Explicit – All people involved, having clear understanding of all the activities being proposed — everything on or off the table — all clearly state that they agree to take part in those activities. No assumptions. No implications. No innuendos.

- Freely given – Consent is only valid if it is freely given, with no coercion; be it physical, emotional, social, psychological, or chemical (drugs or alcohol).

- Legal adult – Any person who is not a legal adult in the jurisdiction in which an activity is taking place cannot legally consent to any sexual activity or activity related to sex.
- Non-altered state of mind – A person under the influence of any mind-altering influence or substance cannot consent to anything, *even if they agree to it*. A person who is asleep cannot consent.
- *Specific* set of activities – If someone consents to a chest harness scene, that is not consenting to a waist harness and certainly not to being groped or penetrated in any way. Consent to one type of sexual contact doesn't mean consent has been given for any other type of sexual contact. Don't include any activity that you did not specifically and clearly include in the negotiation before the scene.
- During a *specific time frame* – Just because someone consented to something yesterday does not mean you get to do that same thing again today, or ever.

If you have never seen the "Tea and Consent" video, treat yourself! ConsentIsEverything.com

The National Coalition for Sexual Freedom has much more on this. This link will take you there: TheDuchy.com/ncsf-consent-counts/

## Silence Does Not Mean Consent!

There is a phrase sometimes used in the corporate world: "*Qui tacet consentire videtur.*" It is part of a larger phrase that translates as "He who is silent, when he ought to have spoken and was able to, is taken to agree." Project managers feel clever in throwing that quote around as a way to try to drive conversation and agreement. Sort of like "speak now or forever hold your peace."

To be very clear: That does *NOT* apply to *any* activity related to sex or physical restraint in *any* way.

Silence, or simply the lack of a "yes," should ALWAYS be taken as a "no."

## Implicit/Implied Consent

This is a situation where a person's *actions* are taken to indicate their consent. This is risky and more likely to result in consent violations than explicit consent, though it does have its place.

For example, if you choose to walk into a cupcake shop, you are implying that you consent to seeing cupcakes on display. You are also implying that you consent to seeing cupcakes being made, sold, and even eaten by other customers in the shop. If you were to see someone messily eating a cupcake in a way that made you feel uncomfortable, you would be well within your rights to leave the cupcake shop to avoid seeing such things. However, your consent was not violated because you implied that you were okay with seeing cupcakes, and the activities that are associated with them, by choosing to walk into the cupcake shop. If you were to walk into the cupcake shop and see two people engaging in a sexual act in the back corner, your implied consent *would* be violated. Walking into a cupcake shop does not imply that you are interested in watching someone pierce a cupcake with their penis, because that kind of activity is not usually expected in a bakery.

When going to a kink event or party it is expected that the event will have published rules about what is and is not permitted at that event or venue, AND for all attendees to have read and to abide by those rules. Therefore, by choosing to attend that event, you are implicitly consenting to possibly seeing any activity permitted by the rules.

This does NOT mean that by attending an event in such a space you are implicitly consenting to *engage* in any of those activities *yourself*. When it comes to any person's bodily autonomy, rely on *explicit* consent, not implicit. No person at that event should attempt to do anything with or to you without your *explicit*, authentic consent. Nor can you do anything with or to another person at that event without first getting *their* explicit consent. Just *ask*.

## Common Consent Models

There are several models out there. In the kink world, the two most popular are SSC and RACK.

### SSC - Safe, Sane, Consensual

This was used for years, but it has a few issues: Who defines safe? Who defines sane?

### RACK - Risk Aware Consensual Kink

This one recognizes that many things we do involve risk and that a critic could easily label them as "unsafe" or "not sane."

This model places more responsibility on the individuals involved. You are entering into a situation in which you are aware of the potential risks and accept that what you are choosing to do may not necessarily be "safe" to some people.

This consent model is built upon the awareness and knowledge of all parties involved. Under RACK, one cannot ethically consent without knowing and understanding the risks involved in what they are doing. This is especially important in the context of rope, as rope bottoming can be quite dangerous, especially if a bottom does not know the signs and symptoms that could indicate a problem that could lead to injury.

## Yes, No, Maybe — Translated

"Yes" means yes, "no" means no, "maybe" means no!

- "Yes" means yes.
  - Even better is: "Hell, yes!" We love authentic, enthusiastic, eager consent!
  - Do not say "yes" if you are not sure. Tell them you aren't sure, then invite them to keep talking if you are open to considering a proposed activity.
- "No" means **no**!
  - ONE exception: If people have explicitly agreed to change that word for purposes of a specific scene. For example, someone

wants to have a more primal scene and they negotiate to be able to scream "No! Stop it, you monster!" In a case like that, they explicitly agree to replace "no" with a safe word (p. 36) instead, so they can use "no," "stop," etc., freely in the scene.

But the meaning of the word "no" is only altered during the specific time frame that is outlined in negotiations. **During a negotiation, "no" always means no.**

- Accept a "no" gracefully. Don't badger them or make them defend their answer. That is a slippery slope to coercion.
  - "Totally fine. Is there something you *would* be interested in trying?"
  - "I appreciate you considering it. I hope you have a great evening (or party)!"
- "Maybe" also means *no*!
  - With a "maybe," they may be leaving the door open to be asked again some other time, but they might just be trying to not be rude by shutting you down entirely. We try to help people gain the confidence to just say what they really mean, but not everyone is comfortable with that.
  - If you get a "maybe" try saying this: "I am going to take that as a 'no' for tonight. I am still interested though, so feel free to reach out if you change your mind. Would you mind if I asked you again some other time, or would you prefer I not?"
  - This gives them the comfort of seeing you take their answer gracefully, which may make them feel better about the whole idea. But it also gives them a graceful way to change that "maybe" to a "no" smoothly in a way that is safer, emotionally speaking. If they ask you to not ask them later, they really meant "no" all along. Thank them for their honesty and move along.
- Verify *everything*.
  - My definition for a word may not be the same as yours.
- Get used to asking for clarification. Make sure you understand.
  - "What does that mean to you?"
  - "Can you say more about that?"
  - "Can you give me an example?"

**Empower Your Bottom to Say "No" During a Scene**

In a power exchange context (D/s, M/s) it can be hard for a sub or slave to say "no" when they want to please their Top/Dom/Master/Mistress. Be aware of this potential hurdle if you are in a power exchange dynamic and talk about it with your partner beforehand. Command them to tell you if they sense an issue that could result in injury, physical or otherwise. Reassure them that telling you is the right thing and is required. Make it clear that you care more about them than you do about one little scene.

If a person has difficulty saying "no," it can be helpful to set up words or signals that feel easier or safer to say. More on this in *Safe Words/ Gestures/Actions* (p. 36).

### Revoking Consent

- Consent may be withdrawn at *any* time *before* or *during* an activity.

  If consent is withdrawn, all activity must stop *immediately*.

**Consent may *not* be withdrawn *after* the activity has ended.** If you are not comfortable with something and you make that clear, a responsible, ethical player will respond immediately. But you cannot revoke consent *after* something has already happened that you had given consent to.

### Consent Violation:

- Something is done to you that you did not explicitly and authentically agree to doing.
- You said to stop doing something that you had previously consented to and your statement was ignored.
- An activity that you previously consented to is done at a time when you did not consent to it.
- Someone does something with you that you had consented to doing with a person other than them.

### Not a Consent Violation:

- If you *explicitly* and *authentically* consent to a specific thing, that thing is done to/with you and you feel badly afterwards, your consent was *not* violated. It may be that you regret your decision. You learned something new about yourself and it is your responsibility to move forward with that knowledge.
- There are also some things that cannot be controlled, even by the most conscientious Tops. If, for example, a rope bottom requests that no rope marks be left behind after a rope scene, a Rope Top may not be able to prevent that from happening entirely. This is why RACK is a useful consent model to follow. Clarifying that risks *can* be mitigated, but not completely prevented when engaging in these activities, is a critical part of the negotiation process. In this case, if the bottom were to consent to a rope scene knowing that rope marks were a risk, their consent would not be violated if they walked away with a few marks despite the Top's best efforts.

## Consent Violations

It is important to understand that consent covers actions that are taken, not the outcomes. A person can control their actions, they cannot always control the outcome. Sometimes negative things happen despite everyone's best intentions and efforts.

An example:

During your negotiations for your first spanking scene, you tell your Top that you don't want to get bruised. Your Top states that they understand and will take it step by step so you can feel each level and give them feedback. They start light and you love it. You ask

them to go a little heavier and they do. You love that. They ask if you want to feel a slightly heavier impact, and you do. Your Top tells you that they could go much harder, but that they are going to stop here because this is your first time and they want to keep things relatively light until you both learn how your body reacts. You have a warm, satisfied feeling. The next morning you look at yourself in the mirror and see a few light bruises. You are surprised; you didn't think that you had been hit hard enough to bruise. You said you did not want to be bruised, but you were. Unless there are other circumstances involved, this would not normally be considered a consent violation. Everyone was doing their best, communication was good, but there was an unfortunate *outcome*. Both you and the Top can learn from it that your skin is more sensitive to bruising than average — at least for now — and you can take that knowledge with you into future planning.

**But make no mistake, actual consent violations can and do happen.** There are several different levels and how they are handled is usually determined by which level they fall into.

### Categories of Consent Violations:

*Levels in red are malicious.*

1. Innocent – One/both/all involved didn't know that the infraction would be an issue. This is closely related to accidental, but the person that took the action had no way of knowing and would not have been expected to know that the action was unwelcome.

2. Accidental – A simple mistake. People are not perfect and sometimes important details slip our minds or tools don't behave as expected: Perhaps they slip or break. Unfortunately, this can result in a violation of someone's consent.

3. Misunderstanding – Perhaps certain terms were not clearly defined during negotiation. Example: "When I said I did not want to be touched below the waist, that included my stomach. That may not have been clear to you since I didn't explicitly say that, but that is what 'below the waist' means to me." This is a consent violation, but some responsibility falls on both parties here. The person being violated could have more clearly defined what they meant, and the violator could have asked them to specify what they meant.

4. Neglect – As a Top, NEVER leave a person alone while in bondage. They are unable to help themselves if something happens. Neglecting them is irresponsible. It is a safety violation at the very least and, depending on the circumstances, might be judged to be malicious.

5. Ignoring – If the bottom reports an issue and the Top ignores it, that can quickly lead to injury. Especially with rope bondage where nerve compression can happen in a matter of seconds.

   Even worse is if the bottom says to stop an activity — revokes

consent – and the Top does not respond appropriately. What was an activity happening between consenting adults then becomes a case of legal assault* or false imprisonment*.
*Never* ignore your bottom.

6. Sexual Assault* – Any sexual contact of any type without affirmative consent*.

7. Rape* – Any unwanted sexual penetration of any area, no matter how slight, by means of force or coercion. If someone is tied up and you have sex with them without their affirmative consent*, you are guilty of rape. Period.

* The actual legal definition of these terms varies from jurisdiction to jurisdiction, but the spirit is generally the same.

**How to Respond to a Violation of Your Consent**
Check in with yourself. Try to understand what kind of an effect the consent violation may have had on you. Consent violations do not always affect the person who was violated in a negative way. Sometimes they can present an opportunity for growth and self-reflection. Other times they can wreak havoc on an individual's well-being. Whatever they happen to be, your feelings are valid. You have the right to express them and be heard.

As general guidelines:

**#1-3.** Stop everything and talk. Be specific about what happened, how you felt, what you had consented to, and what you had not. Depending on how you feel, you can either address the violator directly or you may want to speak to somebody more removed from the situation like a friend or, if you met in a group setting, the moderator of the group. It may also be helpful to write down your immediate thoughts and feelings after the fact.

Sometimes all this requires is a conversation, but sometimes more. Perhaps some education on the topic in question is warranted, perhaps some closer monitoring by the monitors of the venue or event for a while until it is clear that this is a one-time issue and unlikely to recur.

**#4.** This is more serious and indicates a lack of education or due care. A violation of this nature certainly warrants education and closer monitoring for a time. Perhaps more in specific cases or if there are repeated violations.

**#5.** This is very serious and, depending on the details, may become criminal activity. If the Ignoring was a safety issue only, education and monitoring is certainly warranted. Some groups might consider expelling a person who does this, especially if they receive more than one report about a particular person. If it crossed the line into criminal activity, see #6-7 below.

**#6-7.** These are serious crimes and should be treated as such. You have the full set of options to report this to law enforcement and, if you met the person through a local group, to report it to the moderators of that group. Do not worry about outing the person who criminally violated your consent. If you would like to take legal action against them, you are well within your rights to do so. If you would prefer not to pursue legal action, that is also okay. The highest priority in this situation should be your safety and well-being.

## If Someone Approaches You Saying You Violated Their Consent

If this happens, how you respond will demonstrate your character. People will be watching and they will make their decisions about you based on your actions and reactions.

### Listen

Regardless of how you feel, take the time to listen to what the person being violated has to say. Do not interrupt or attempt to correct them. This is a chance to learn about the person who is talking to you. They are demonstrating a lot of courage, agency, and self-advocacy by choosing to bring this up with you. Respect that by giving them the floor and listening intently to what they have to say.

### Seek to Understand Before Responding

Demonstrate your respect and concern for them by listening carefully and attempt to understand where they are coming from. If you need some time to think before responding, ask for it. The way in which you respond to this situation will demonstrate the content of your character.

### Own it

If you did, in fact, violate this person's consent, own it. Accept that you made a mistake. Understand that you may feel bad about the situation for a while and make peace with that. Sometimes we have to feel those negative feelings in order to grow into better versions of ourselves.

### Seek to Repair the Relationship, if Possible

Ask about what you need to do to help address the situation. Tell them what you *will* do to make sure the issue does not recur. Tell them that you will be doing this regardless of whether they choose to play with you again or not and ask if there is something you can do to help them feel better.

### Seek Education

If the person would still like to interact with you, seek to learn from their experience. What was it that went wrong, and how might you have prevented the situation you are in now? Were there questions you could have asked? Assumptions you could have refrained from making? Take some time to reflect on your past experiences and look for patterns. Has this kind of violation happened before?

Remember, consent is a highly nuanced and ongoing conversation. Do your best to communicate honestly and authentically, respect your boundaries and those of the people around you, ask questions when you aren't sure, and treat yourself with the same kindness and grace that you extend to others.

## Negotiation and Planning

This is the foundation of authentic, informed consent.

After going through the vetting process, you have decided that you would like to do a rope scene with someone. The next step is NOT to just pick up a rope and put it on them or allow them to put it on you. There are many things you both need to know in order to do so ethically and safely. You both need to:

- Agree on what activities will be permitted.
- Understand the risks of those activities.
- Figure out how you will know if something is going wrong.
- Plan for what you both will do if something does go wrong.
- Understand what you need to do for each other after the session ("aftercare"). Discuss and prepare for what you need.

### You Need a Plan

Yes, spontaneity can be fun and sexy, but it is not responsible to be looking for spontaneity with a brand-new partner, especially when there are as many risks to manage as there are with rope. Spontaneity is something that can come with time, experience, and trust with a specific partner. But when you begin playing with someone new, or with an unfamiliar activity, you need to revert to detailed negotiation until you both learn enough about each other to *agree* to introduce spontaneity.

### Be Honest and Complete About the Things You Choose to Share

The root of ethical and effective negotiation is honesty.

BE HONEST. Be complete. Don't hide important things, including your level of experience.

This is critical. Without real understanding of (1) the people involved and their needs and limits, and (2) the planned activities and their associated risks, it is impossible to give informed consent. This begins with being honest with yourself. What do you want out of bondage? Tell your partner(s) what you really want. Listen to what *they* really want. Do your best to determine whether you could have a path forward together.

Different situations require different levels of negotiation:

- For simple pickup play or a single encounter, you can negotiate a few straightforward activities and discuss just the details and risks of those specific things.
- With regular partners, or someone you are hoping will become a

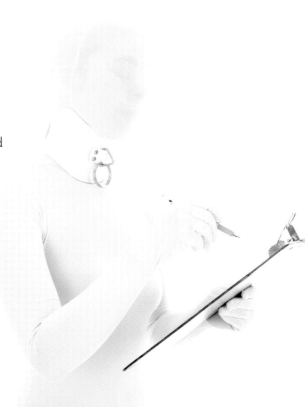

regular partner, you will need more detail in your negotiations so that you understand each other more deeply. This allows you to explore further and with more flexibility as you gain experience with each other.

Below is a general, high-level list of things that are important to understand and discuss. This is a good general start, but you need to research the risks of the specific activities you are interested in and include that information in your negotiation.

This is a *general* list. It does not include many details that are important to a *rope* scene. When you are negotiating a rope scene, you should still follow this framework, or something like it, and you also need to include details specific to rope and any other activities you want to include in the scene. For example, if you plan to tie someone's arms behind their back, you need to know if they have done that before, if it went well, and if they are aware of any medical or physiological issues that would prevent them from doing so now. Those scenario-specific questions are not included in this general list. Rope-specific details will be discussed in the *Reducing Risk* chapter (p. 49).

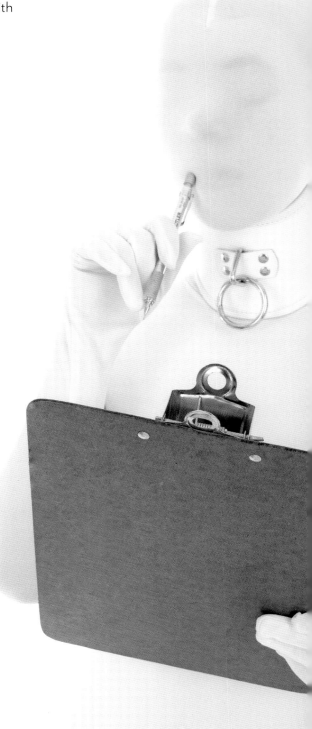

## Important Elements of Negotiation: Who Will be Involved, What are their Roles and Expected Forms of Address?

*Who will be involved?*
Anyone who will be a part of the scene needs to be present at the negotiation. Each person must speak for themselves.
*What roles do you each want to play?*
There are so many fun options!
    Top, bottom, Dom, sub, Switch, pet, housemaid...
    Will there be any power exchange? D/s? M/s? What might that look like?

*What do you want people to call you?*
- Honorifics (Sir, Miss, Mistress, Master)?
- Pet names/terms of affection (pet, kitten, toy, doll)?
- Degrading terms (slut, whore, bitch)?

## Approved Activities (i.e., interests and limits)
It is important to help your partner understand your hot buttons (the things that you love), your soft limits (things that are not to be done for now, but perhaps in the future), and hard limits (things that are an absolute *no*, so don't ask).

Be very clear about what activities are okay for this particular scene. Make no assumptions.

Agree on how intense the scene should be, the mood, and how each participant would like to behave.

- **Mood:** Instructional, intense, dark, light, sensual, violent, gentle, sterile, degrading, humiliating, animalistic, fun-loving, serious, personable, distant, goofy, etc.
- **Intensity Level (pain or sensation):** None, light, moderate, heavy.
- **Deportment:** Obedient vs. bratty, demanding, stern, aggressive, nurturing, professorial, etc.

How does the bottom prefer to be untied — should you emphasize sensuality or speed?

How does the bottom feel about rope marks, and their location — do they need to be able to cover them for work?

Can the Top overpower the bottom and "force" them to do something? Can the bottom "turn the tables" and try to capture the Top instead? Neither is recommended for scenes early in the process of getting to know one another, but these options can be amazing once more knowledge and experience is gained.

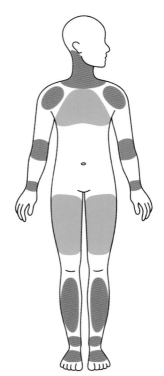

*Front*

### Sensation Play

You can do non-impact sensation play almost anywhere on a person's body. (There are limits depending on what you want to do, so do your research.) Impact play, however, can go more than skin deep if it is intense. If you want to hit hard, you need to avoid places where doing so poses a higher risk of physical harm.

When doing impact play:

- Only strike big muscles and big muscle groups: Pectorals, upper back, ass, thighs, hamstrings, calves, bottom of the feet.
  This rule can be bent when engaging in impact that is surface level. Canes, whips, and other stingy implements are unlikely to contain enough power to injure internal organs. But be reasonable, use common sense, and discuss it first. For example, ask your partner about whether having *surface* level impact on the low back is within their risk profile or if they prefer to avoid it altogether.
- Never strike the kidneys (lower back between the rib cage and pelvic bone) — Strong blows to the kidney will be painful and may result in serious injury.

In the illustrations to the right:

- 🔘 Green areas are normally low risk to impact at reasonable levels (get feedback from your bottom).
- ⚪ White areas are fine for sensation play, but not heavy impact.
- 🔘 Red areas are higher risk and should be avoided.

For example, you can punch someone on the butt quite hard without risking much more than a bruise, but punching someone too hard in the stomach can cause severe injury. As always, talk with your partner first and gradually increase intensity over time. Going too light is better than going too hard and ending up with an injury.

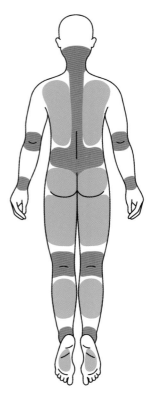

*Back*

### Marks

Some bottoms love marks, from rope or from sensation play or both. They see them as badges of honor. But some people do not want to have marks after a scene for a wide variety of reasons. Or perhaps they can have them in one place, but not another. Discuss this.

### Sexual Activity

Be very clear if any kind of sexual activity is permitted, and thoroughly define "sexual activity" with your partner. *Make no assumptions.* "What do you mean by that?" and "Can you give me an example of what you mean?" are critical questions when it comes to this subject.

- What constitutes sexual touch/activity to you?
- What level of sexual activity are you each looking for?
- Would the Top/bottom like to orgasm in the scene?
- Is the bottom able to orgasm while in scene or is this something that is not common for them?
- Does the bottom enjoy multiple orgasms? What should happen after orgasm? Immediate release? Continued teasing?

   Not only do you need to be clear about what is and what is not okay to do, it is also helpful to provide guidance on things on the approved list: e.g., "I love huge anal plugs, but you need to work them in slowly. Don't have me gagged when you are putting them in because I will need to tell you when to keep pushing and when to pause. Also, after orgasm get it out of me quickly or it will switch from good pain to bad pain."

## Term

When will you do this? For how long? Consent in a scene is finite with a specific start and end time.

   Make it clear to your partner that it is okay for them to back out of *any* activity at *any* time for *any* reason. Reminding each person of this fact can be critically important to creating an emotionally safe environment.

## Risk Management and Safety

Once you know what activities you are interested in, discuss any potential risks and make sure everyone understands and accepts them. Change your plans if you uncover any potential risks that cause particular concern.

### Learning to Read Your Partner

Communication is *mostly* nonverbal. Your scene will go more smoothly if you can read your partner's nonverbal cues. This may come with experience, and you can also just ask.

   Try to get an idea of what your partner's nonverbal communication might look like before becoming responsible for their physical safety. Tops, ask your bottom to show or describe to you how they might look when they are feeling good. What will they look like when they don't feel good?

   If they don't know, then for your first few scenes, keep a watch out. Try to learn what their nonverbal cues are for when they're enjoying themselves, and when they are not. Then inform them so they have that knowledge for the future!

Paying attention to these signals will help you keep things at the right level; your partner might never even need to use their safe words.

**Safe Words/Gestures/Actions**

Every language on Earth already has a wide array of safe words — "Stop," "No," "I'm done" — all of which are great! Words should always be taken to mean what they usually mean *unless you have specifically agreed otherwise*. If you are planning a "non-con" (short for consensually non-consensual) scene, you might want these words to be ignored because you want to be able to say things like "No, no! Stop! You MONSTER!!" And in those cases, everyone involved needs to know what is actually being communicated, so there are no misunderstandings, consent violations, or worse. This is where "safe words" come in!

Safe words, gestures, or actions can be helpful when:
- The bottom will be gagged and unable to speak.
- The bottom is known to go nonverbal when they are in subspace or have a hard time saying the word "no" for whatever reason.

In private scenes, you can pick anything you want for a safe word, and if you are playing at a party there may be a universal safe word so that the people around you will also understand when things need to stop and can intervene if necessary.

Here are several common safe words/gestures/actions:
- The words *Red*, *Yellow*, and *Green*:
  - Red: The scene is over. I'm done. Let me out, check in, and move to aftercare.
  - Yellow: Stop any action and check in. The scene may continue after a check-in, or perhaps be modified or stopped, but talk first.
  - Green: Keep going, I'm loving this!
  - Beige: I am a brat and I want to piss off my Top by implying that I am bored. Hit me harder!
- Grunting/banging/beeping three times in a row, particularly if combined with tilting the head from side to side while making the noise. This can be helpful when gagged.
- Give the bottom something noisy (a chain, steel ball, a bell, etc.) to drop. Again, this is useful if the person will be gagged or if they tend to sink deeply into sub space.
- These last two are usually treated as "yellow." The action stops, the bottom is ungagged and the Top checks in with them before they jointly decide what to do next.

It can be disappointing when things do not go well and it is okay to be disappointed. However, it is not as important as taking care of each other. Ultimately addressing these needs and showing that you care for each other is far more important than feeling a little disappointed for a few minutes. Because hopefully, if you handle the situation well, you will get a chance to play again some other time.

## Physical and Medical

You need to understand if any participant has any physical or medical conditions that may take certain activities off the table.

- "Do you have any current or past injuries that have resulted in areas of sensitivity or any flexibility or mobility challenges?"
  - If a person has had any joint, bone or muscle issues, it may impact their ability to assume a given position or to stay in that position for any length of time.
  - E.g. "I have a nerve injury so, I can't have my hands tied behind my back." or "I have a rotator cuff issue, I can't lift anyone into a suspension right now.", etc...
- "Do you any medical conditions that might make you react to stress or emotion in a heighted or unexpected way?" (e.g. Diabetes, heart conditions, high or low blood pressure ... )
- "Do you have medical insurance?"
  - If your partner sustains an injury while in your rope, who is on the hook, financially?
- "What medications are you taking?"
  - Insulin – You need to know where their emergency glucagon kit is and have it within reach during the scene in case they go low. Confirm they have had food (with protein) and water recently before the scene.
  - Blood thinners – Find out why. There are some things that are much riskier if a person is on blood thinners. Rope suspension, for example. Also, these can have conflicts with other medications. Aspirin, ibuprofen & naproxen also tend to thin the blood a little as well, so people on blood thinners are often told to avoid them and use acetaminophen instead. But confirm with them.
  - Asthma – You need to know how they typically manage it and where they keep their management tools, inhaler, etc. in case they have an episode when you are in a scene.
- "Do you have any STIs we need to plan around?"
  - Ask gently and with understanding. Do not imply that someone with an STI is dirty by asking if they are 'clean'. Asking questions in a judgmental way can discourage people from answering honestly. Remember, honesty is crucial in negotiation!
  - Having an STI doesn't mean you can't play. You just need to know so you can properly plan.
  - Use barrier methods as a matter of routine! "I use safer sex techniques." Just set that as a standard expectation going in, nothing personal, this is just what you do. Condoms, nitrile gloves, dental dams, Lorals.com wearable dental dams!
  - Get screened for STIs annually and in between each sexual partner You can't know if you don't test and knowledge is power. It is important to understand that not every STI is included in a routine screening. If you are concerned about something specific, ask your medical provider if it is included on your screening.

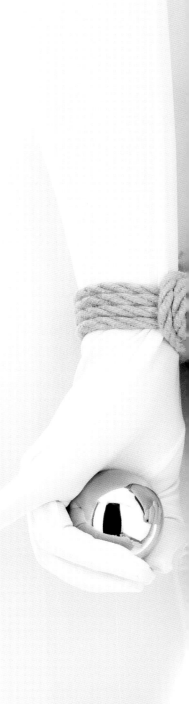

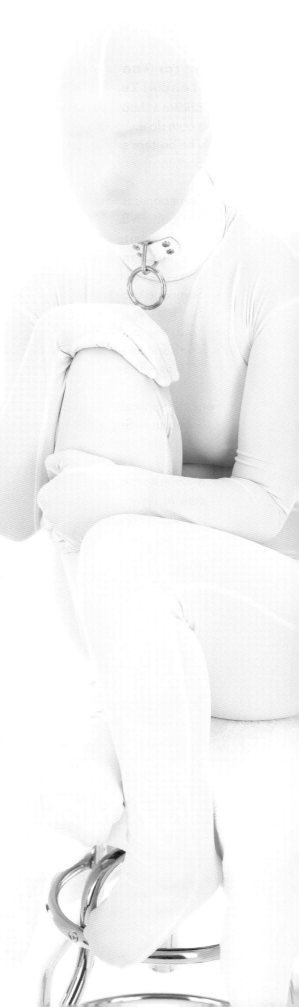

- If anyone is positive for an STI, do some research to ensure that your transmission prevention methods are based on the latest medical research and not on assumption.

## Psychological

Care of the mind is just as important as care of the body.

### Triggers

We usually use the word "trigger" to mean something bad, but it is more complex than that. Triggers can work in different ways for different people. They can be positive or negative. Some things that one person might find negative or angering, might make a different person feel more submissive. But talk about it first, start slow, and move forward with care.

This may be more of a consideration if you engage in verbal humiliation or name calling in a scene, but actions can also be triggers.

Common verbal triggers include negative comments on appearance, intelligence, competence ("you can't even…"), and gendered language. For example: "You can call me a cock-hungry whore, that can be hot, but don't EVER call me an airheaded slut."

If your partner is sensitive about being called names, you need to know and respect that. If they have a history of trauma or abuse and would like to use BDSM as a way of processing that past, very real, pain, you need to know that. If you are not comfortable with or capable of helping someone work through mental or emotional anguish in the context of BDSM, say so. If you are someone's play partner, it is both impossible and unethical for you to provide them with mental healthcare. Kink should never be used as a replacement for mental health services.

### Trauma

"Given what we are planning, do you have any past trauma that might get triggered?"

Some trauma survivors engage in kink as a form of therapy. For example, they might be reliving a specific event, but are doing so in an environment where they are in control and can stop it at any time. You need to know if this is the case. It will be very frightening or unsettling if a trauma reaction happens when you are not expecting it. But if you have discussed it first and agreed on how you should react, you can handle such a reaction with sensitivity, care, and grace should it occur.

If you do not feel able to handle something like that if it were to occur, then change the plan to steer clear of any such issues.

## Plan for The Risks You Uncover and for Other Potential Issues and Problems

There are a thousand weird-ass things that could happen. What will you *both* do if:

- The bottom says they're numb?
- Someone gets nauseous?
- Someone has a panic attack?
- Someone is triggered in some way (flashback/trauma response)?
- The bottom faints?
- The Top starts to feel faint?
- The fire alarm or a tornado siren goes off?
- You get a call from a family member?
- Someone knocks on the door?
- Someone goes into diabetic shock or has a heart attack?
- Your neighbor calls the cops because they hear weird noises?
- The Top has a crisis of confidence? Remember, consent apply to Tops as well as bottoms!

For each applicable risk, determine how you will manage it.

- Safe calls — Set them up, make sure everyone knows you have one and when you will need to be free to be able to make/take the call.
- Medical — Make your plans to accommodate all medical needs. Make sure everyone has taken all their prescribed medication. Make sure you have any necessary medical emergency equipment and supplies — inhaler, emergency glucagon kit, etc.
  - Know the emergency services number in that area. It is 911 in North America. In other countries, 999 and 112 are common. If you don't know, find out *before* you start playing.
  - Know the physical address of the location you are playing in case you need to direct medical services to your location.
  - If something happens that requires a medical professional, DON'T HESITATE to call them. This is not a time to be worried about being embarrassed. Trust me, they have seen it all before; whatever you were doing may not even be particularly interesting to them anymore. Don't let someone die because of your shame.
- Safer sex — Have the equipment and supplies that you may need — gloves, condoms, dental dams, etc.
- Emergency release — Have a way to cut someone out of rope immediately on your person. If there are other kinds of bondage — locks, etc. — have the keys and bolt cutters at hand as well.

### Safe Calls

If you are tying in a public or semi-public place like a party or public dungeon, the venue will normally have people in place to make sure everyone abides by the rules and is being safe, and they are right there if anyone needs assistance. These people are often called Dungeon Monitors. If possible, the first few times you play with someone, it is best to do so in such a place so that you have that safety net.

But when you shift to playing in private you take on additional risk. One of the ways to help manage that risk is to have a "safe call" in place. This is true for all parties involved, not just for bottoms.

A safe call is a pre-arranged time where you will contact a trusted person to confirm that you are safe. That person also knows the real physical location where you are going to be and the real legal names of the person/people you are meeting. If the call is not made on time and your safe call contact cannot get ahold of you, they are to call the authorities and send them to your location.

When everyone involved knows that all the other people have someone that is going to be checking up on them, it makes everyone feel safer.

There are many reasons for a safe call. It can help lower the risk of assault and/or imprisonment, but it is also important if the Top becomes indisposed while the bottom is helpless in some way. Medical emergencies happen (heart attack, diabetic shock, seizure, Gerald's Game). If the bottom is unable to reach their phone, having a safe call in place means that emergency services will be on their way by a certain time. So, it's not just to protect you from the person that you're tying with. It can also help prevent bad things — even accidents — from getting worse.

Safe calls can take many forms depending on the relative level of risk. Here is a common approach:

- Before you meet the person in private, meet in public and get to know them. Preferably more than once.If you decide to meet in private, get the real address you will be going to and the person's real name. Have them show you a government-issued ID. Do not meet a person that is not willing to do this. Take a picture of it to give to your safe call contact.
- Before you go to the location of the private scene:
  - Give your safe call contact your play partner's real name and the address of where you will be, along with the picture of their ID. Do not go to a different location without informing your safe call contact first.
  - Consider temporarily sharing your mobile phone location with your safe call contact.
  - Arrange a time when you will call your safe call contact. Usually, a call is preferred over a text message as it is much easier for a nefarious person to pretend to be you over text.
  - Consider having a code word/phrase that you are to use to indicate wellbeing or plan to have your safe call contact ask you a question that only you would know the answer to. For example, you could agree that "things seem to be going well" actually means that you are afraid for your safety and that "Remember to feed Rex!" means that you feel safe. Choose whatever makes sense for you. If you decide to use a question instead, a correct answer indicates that you are safe and well. If you answer incorrectly, you are in danger and need assistance.

> **Important!**
> Having a safe call is *not* a guarantee of safety. It can be an important tool but a lot of horrible things can happen in a short time. So it is best to meet in public and play at larger parties several times to build trust and experience before you play in private.

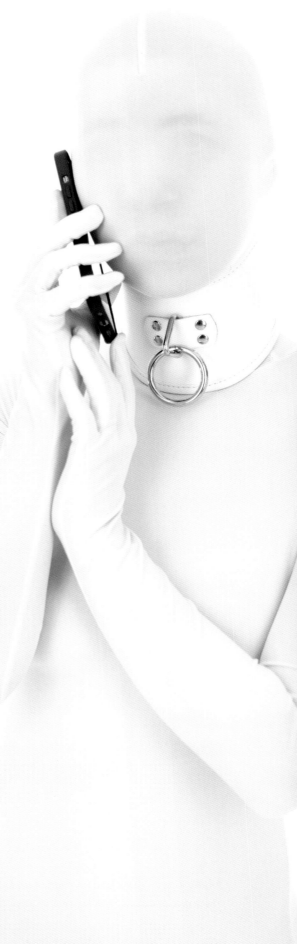

- At the time of the safe call:
  - Call your contact and talk for a short time. Provide the appropriate code. Verify that things are ok.
  - If you do not call on time, your contact should try to call you immediately.
  - **If you do not answer the phone for your safe call, your safe call contact is to call the authorities immediately and send them to your location.**

## Punishments

Important: Punishment is *not* required to play with power exchange.

But if punishments are going to be part of the dynamic, negotiate about what form they will take!

We don't mean "funishment" here. Heavy sensation play can include a wide range of activities that might appear to an outsider to be punishment, but they are done in such a way that all participants get something positive from them. That is not what we mean here. We mean real, negative reinforcement applied by the Top to the bottom to correct an undesired behavior or as the consequence of a failure, etc.

Being punished is a very different psychological space than heavy sensation play. This is a moment in which the Dom/ Master/Mistress may be genuinely displeased or disappointed with their sub/slave and is allowing that displeasure to show. This means that the bottom does not have the emotional safety blanket of knowing they are pleasing their Top. This can leave them profoundly vulnerable in ways that the Top does not intend. Therefore:

If real punishments are going to be part of the dynamic, it is important to discuss them and *negotiate* on this point. Otherwise, it is entirely possible for the Top to select a punishment that may accidentally damage the relationship.

One example: A punishment of withdrawal of affection or attention for a period of time.

If used on the wrong person, they could assume their failure has caused their partner to pull away, which could cause them to question the relationship or send them into a shame or anxiety spiral which could be psychologically damaging and/or could destroy their trust in their Top, and be a possible step toward the end of that relationship.

## Aftercare

A BDSM scene can be an experience unlike any other. Both Top and bottom may experience incredible highs or intense catharsis. Serotonin and endorphins may flow heavily. You can literally experience an altered state of mind. The more intense the scene, the more this may be the case.

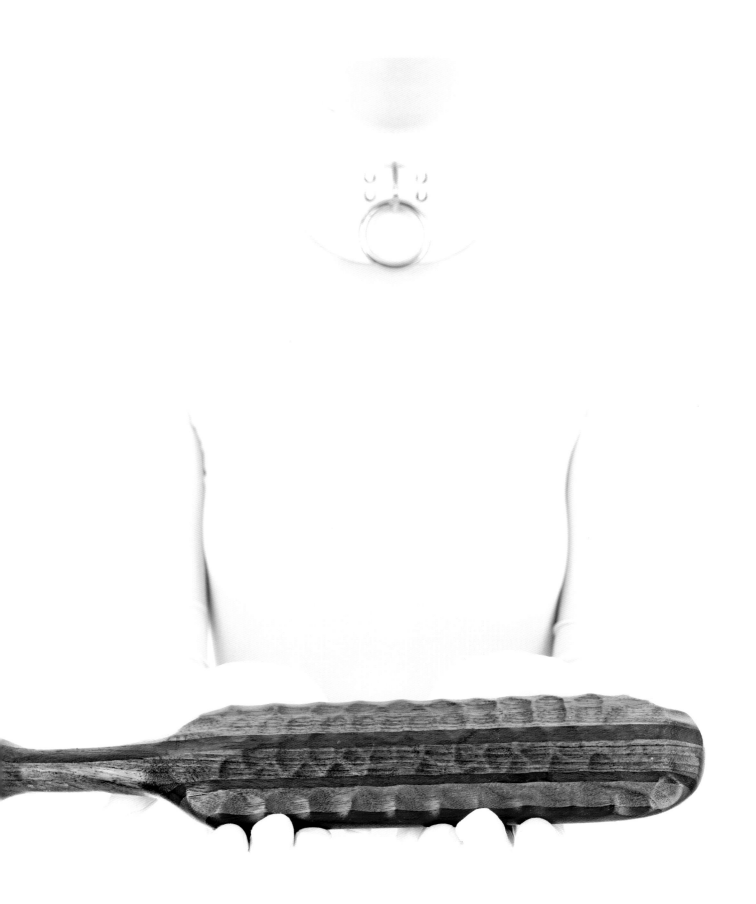

Many kinsters are also makers. The creator of this gorgeous paddle — ElderZee on FetLife — sells it and others through the Etsy.com store TheImpactFairy.

Regardless of how intense the scene, it is important for both the bottom and the Top to take care of each other and help bring each other back to their regular state of being. This is called "providing aftercare." Reassure each other that the experience was a good one, that everything is okay, that they did well, that you care for them, etc. If you ignore this step, one or both of you may have an emotional drop in reaction to the emotional state or to serotonin withdrawal. Some level of drop may happen regardless, but aftercare tends to help.

Aftercare can mean a wide range of different things. Each person will need different things.

One bottom may need to have a cool drink of water, a little snack, and their favorite fuzzy blanket, then want to immediately socialize with others at the party. Another may want to be left in a puddle on the floor for five minutes until they begin moving on their own, at which point they want their Top to help them up and snuggle them for a while.

One Top may need to have their bottom curl up beside them and lay their head on the Top's leg in a gesture of reassurance and affection. Another might get everything they need by caring for the needs of the bottom.

Everyone needs different things. Figure out what you need and share that information.

## Negotiation Tools

It can be helpful to have a paper form to help guide negotiations.
See the *Appendix* (p. 432) for some helpful examples.
You can download printable copies here:
- General Scene and Rope Scene Negotiation Forms: TheDuchy.com/negotiation-forms/
- A BDSM Experience and Curiosity Checklist: TheDuchy.com/bdsm-checklist/

## Negotiation is Not Just for New Partners

If you're tying an existing partner, you still need to negotiate. You can shortcut a lot because you know each other much better, but here are still a few core questions that should always be asked:
- Has anything changed since last time?
- Is everything on the approved list from last time still on the table?
- How are you feeling today? What kind of mood do you crave in the scene?
- Any person-specific topic: "Is your piercing still healing?"

# Setting Up and Conducting the Scene

## Preparation

### Set up the Play Space

- Gather the gear, toys, and materials needed for the scene itself.
- Inspect the things you plan to use. Ensure they are in good condition and are clean.
- Gather safer sex supplies, if applicable.
- Be sure appropriate emergency gear, materials, or medication are within reach.
- Set up appropriate cleanup materials so that this is easy to manage when you are done.
- Set up a space and gather the items needed for aftercare. Doing this now makes for a smooth transition after the scene.

### Check in Just Before the Scene

We are all human. Check in with yourself and with your partner(s) immediately before the scene.

- Do you really want to do *this* scene at *this* time?
- Do they? Do you? Make sure. Confirm. Don't rely on negotiations held days, or even hours, earlier.
- Make it clear that you respect them and their needs more than any plans you made.

### Physical Preparation

Take care of your physical needs before your scene:

- Hydrate.
- Eat normally — have something about an hour before.
- Use the restroom!
- Check in with yourself to confirm you are in the right headspace to scene.

If the scene is to have a D/s component, it can be helpful to give instructions to your partner beforehand, telling them how you want them to prepare.

Consider wearing clothes that enhance the feeling of the roles you both intend to play. Perhaps the submissive should be naked, perhaps in slutty or revealing clothing, perhaps in a corset and heels, or a collar and harness.

This can apply to the Dominant as well. Perhaps you want a classic Fem-Dom look, or a tough look with heavy leather and big boots, or an urbane sophisticate whose suit hides all sorts of kinky secrets. Wear whatever will make you feel how you want to feel.

### Get in the Headspace

It can be helpful to have a preparation ritual to get both of you in the right headspace. Maybe you do it at a particular time; maybe you take a bath, read your favorite BDSM book, polish your floggers, watch some inspiring porn, take a look over this book, whatever it is that puts you in the right mood.

### During the Scene

You made a plan; generally try to follow that plan. But be flexible enough to flow with your partner's and your own internal reactions. Keep strong communication. Check in on how they are doing from time to time. We will discuss a few ways of doing that in the *Risk Prevention and Treatment* section (p. 53). Remember that most communication is nonverbal. Look for their signals and use them to guide you to be lighter or heavier, more gentle or stronger, etc. Verbally verify if you have any questions.

### Don't Add to the Plan

Critical: Don't add anything you had not discussed before the scene.

You can change the plan to make things *lighter* or to *remove* a planned element, but never *add* anything that was not discussed and agreed to before the scene.

People can enter an altered state of mind when in a scene. They are loving what they are feeling so much they would agree to anything. But agreement in such a state is not real consent. If they did not agree to it before the scene, do not do it during, even if they beg you to. It will take strength, but they will respect that strength the day after when they realize you protected them from themselves.

Afterward, at a different time when you are negotiating for a different scene, you can ask them if they want to put those things on the table. Maybe they will trust you enough to try more things with you after they've seen you keep your word and know that you will put their safety first.

### If Something goes Wrong

Unintentionally having things go awry is not inherently bad. It doesn't mean that anyone is a bad person or was careless. What matters is what you do afterwards as a response to that.

Respond quickly and calmly. Stay in control. Do what you said you would do when planning. If needed, gracefully end the scene. Release any elements of bondage and begin caring for whoever needs help. What they will need will be different in each case; use common sense and your preparation to help guide your care.

Demonstrate that you can be relied upon when things go wrong.

## After the Scene
### Coming Down and Aftercare

- Aftercare – Make sure everyone is feeling okay and back to a normal state of mind. Do as you discussed while planning. Take care of each other.
- Physical care – Address any strain or injury.

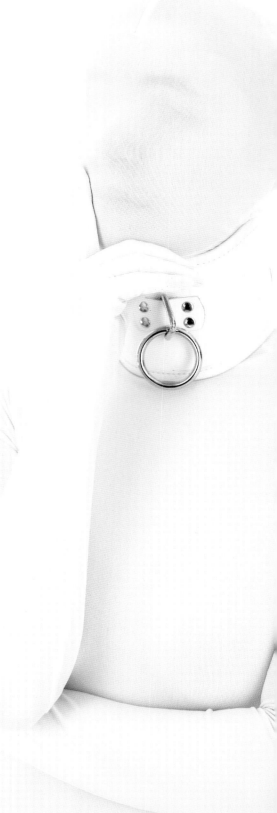

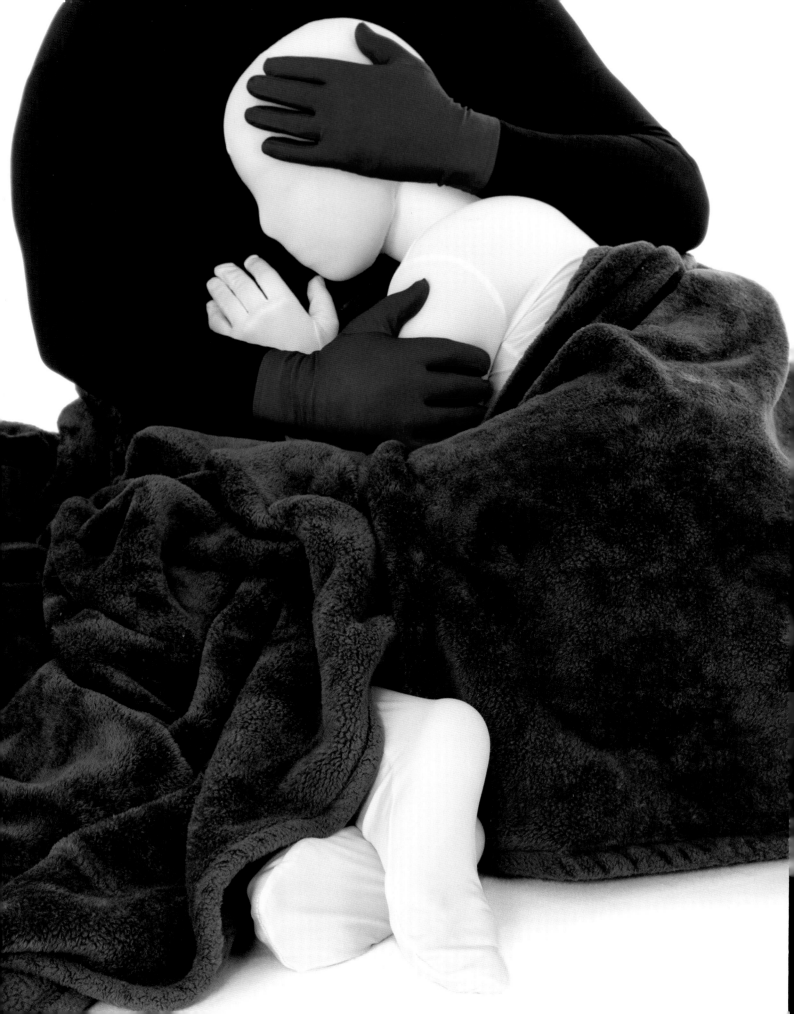

- "It looks like you have some rope marks. Hand me that lotion, let's massage those for a while."
- "Wow you were in that position a long time. Here is some water. Drink more water tonight and it may help to take your preferred pain killer to reduce potential muscle soreness tomorrow." (See the sidebar for some critical information about this.)

## Later

You have been through an experience. You will be mentally and emotionally processing that experience, perhaps for several days. You also may have had various hormones and neurotransmitters rushing through your system due to what you experienced.

It is entirely normal to experience heightened emotions for a few days or to feel what we call "drop" ("Top drop", "sub drop"). This is when you feel a little depressed. This is a common reaction to the highs that you felt. It is easy for some people to confuse this mostly physiological process with regret. If you are playing with someone new, make sure they understand that this might happen and that it is a normal physiological reaction that will pass. Invite them to contact you to discuss it if they wish.

After you have had time to process, try to have a debriefing conversation together.

- Discuss experiences, observations, and reactions.
  - Assume positive intent.
  - Be honest and clear, have a mindset of receptivity and growth.
  - "What would have made that even better?"
  - "Is there anything that didn't work as well for you?"
  - "How did you feel when I... ?"
  - "You seemed to react in a (x) way when I did (y); what was running through your mind at that point?"
  - Use "I feel" and "I felt" statements when describing your own feelings, thoughts and experiences.
- Note lessons learned, positive and negative.
- Decide if you want to continue to play with that person.
- Update your notes on that person so you don't forget what you learned about them, how their body works, and their reactions to the things you tried. Use that to improve next time.

# Appendices — Negotiation Checklist

Check in the *Appendices* for a *Negotiation Form* and a *BDSM Checklist* to get you started. The latest version of these forms can be found at:

## Scene Negotiation Forms

TheDuchy.com/negotiation-forms/

## A BDSM Experience and Curiosity Checklist

TheDuchy.com/bdsm-checklist/

---

**Medication Mindfulness**
**DO NOT just hand them a pain killer and tell them to take it.** It is the responsibility of every person to know their own medical condition, including any potential negative interactions with other medications they may be taking. Over-the-counter pain medications can help reduce inflammation and soreness that may be felt from micro-tears in muscle fibers that may happen if muscles have been stretched or put under stress beyond what they normally experience. But not everyone can take just any type of pain killer. There are many situations where any given pain killer may negatively interact with other medications. It is critical that everyone follow all medical directives and limitations associated with their other medication. For example: Aspirin, ibuprofen and naproxen tend to thin the blood a little (acetaminophen does not), which is important if a person is on prescription blood thinners.

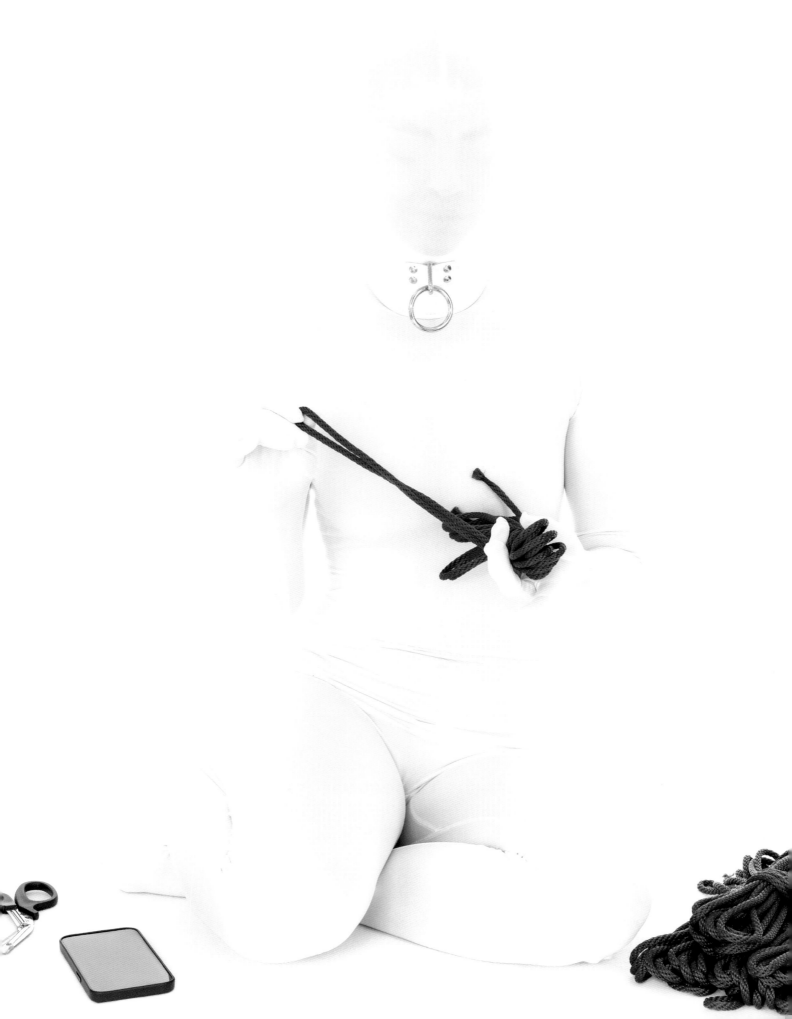

# 2
# Reducing Risk

If you have not yet read Chapter 1, go and do so. It contains a lot of risk and safety information you need that we do not repeat in this chapter. Chapter 1 contains information that's important regardless of the type of scene. This chapter is focused on rope specifically, but you need *both* to get the full picture.

If you intend to put rope on anyone who has a pulse (including yourself), read *this entire chapter*.

If you only intend to put rope only on inanimate objects, you can skip to the next chapter.

> Rope *bottoms*: If something goes wrong, YOU will be the one injured. READ THIS CHAPTER.

Understanding risk is a crucial part of engaging in bondage ethically. If you do not know the potential outcomes of the activities you engage in, then you are not informed, and cannot give *informed* consent.

There are risks associated with rope bondage. You need to understand what they are, how to reduce them, and what to do if something goes wrong. And something *will* go wrong eventually, because:

### Rope Bondage is Not Safe

Rope bondage is some of the most dangerous and injury-prone bondage that you can do. Many BDSM practitioners consider it "edge play." The majority of serious injuries or deaths that occur in a BDSM context involve rope or breath play (controlling when another person is allowed to breathe).

*Using rope on another person without understanding the risks and how to manage them is irresponsible and dangerous.*

- If the Top doesn't know what they are doing, a rope can be positioned improperly, compressing and injuring nerves or blood vessels.
- If the bottom does not know how to detect issues, they may not immediately notice when they are experiencing crucial indicators that something is wrong.
- If the bottom is not communicating with their Top — letting them know their physical limitations, or that they are sensing an issue — the Top cannot react and address the issue.

- Improperly placed ropes can cause severe nerve damage in a very short period of time — minutes, even seconds in some cases. Nerve damage can take weeks or months to heal, and in severe cases, may never fully heal, resulting in a permanent loss of sensation or function.
- If blood flow is cut off for too long or happens in a person with complicating factors, clots can form. A blood clot in the blood stream (an embolism) can cause heart attack, stroke, or even death.
- If a rope bottom falls while in bondage, they could break a limb, dislocate a joint, strike their head, or worse.

So, it bears repeating. **Rope bondage is *not* safe.** Take this seriously.

## YOU are Responsible for Your Own Safety

**Top or bottom, YOU are responsible** for managing your own risk and doing what you can to protect yourself from harm. You need to accept responsibility for your own safety and advocate for yourself.

Read everything in this chapter more than once. Throughout this chapter and the rest of this book, we teach many methods to reduce risk. If you learn, practice, and apply those things, the risk of using these ties will usually be minimal — rope marks, perhaps occasional rope burn, some muscle soreness if the bottom was in a challenging position for a while — but do remember that rope bondage can never be made 100% safe.

Every body is different, every mind is different, every person's physical capability and psychological needs are different, every location and situation is different — so every encounter has its own unique risks. Those risks need to be understood and controlled to a level that is acceptable for everyone involved.

### Bottoms

You need to understand risk and safety considerations just as much — if not more than — Tops, so that you can advocate for yourself. You cannot give informed consent if you are not actually informed and knowledgeable.

If you are doing decorative rope or are otherwise using ties that are not too tight and do not render you truly helpless, the risk is quite low.

The risks dramatically increase if:
- You are truly helpless and unable to free yourself.
- The rope is too tight on a sensitive area or becomes too tight through movement, change in position, or struggle.
- Your body is held in a challenging position too long.

If something goes wrong, you can be injured, perhaps severely, perhaps with lifelong impacts.

So: **Bottoms, read *all* of this chapter. You need to understand it.** It will help you make better decisions about who to trust when you put your safety into another person's hands.

**Tops**

If you are a Top, you are the one who has the *ability* to take action. Your partner cannot. They can tell you things, but if they are bound, it is *your* responsibility to *act*. Your partner has put their trust in you. They rightfully expect you to take care of them. You have a *duty of care*. Learn everything in this chapter — the stuff for Tops and the stuff for the bottoms — and then keep on learning. Don't get over-confident. Play within your level of skill; proceed at a responsible pace.

Learning about risks and safety needs to be an ongoing activity.

This book should not be your only source of information. Information on bondage and rope safety is constantly evolving. This section contains lots of great information and tips that have stood the test of time, but new ideas are constantly being developed and tested; the best of them make their way into the community zeitgeist. By the time you read this, there may be better ways of dealing with some of these things. So, stay active; commit yourself to continual learning!

Disclaimer:

I am not a doctor. *Nothing in this book is medical advice.* **Your doctor outranks this book.**

This is information that has been collected and shared by kinksters around the world and represents what are currently considered common/best practice within the community.

## Injury Prevention Rule #1

# Proceed at a Responsible Pace

One of the best ways to prevent injury is to play within your skill level and your physical capabilities.

## Learn → Practice → Play

When you first learn a new skill, you are not yet ready to use it in a scene. You need to practice outside of a scene first. Once you have a solid grasp on the new skill and are confident that you can use it correctly, you can begin to incorporate it into play.

## One Thing at a Time. Focus

When incorporating new skills into practice, only introduce one new element at a time. This can apply to techniques, levels of risk, and positional difficulty. Doing so allows the Top to focus on executing the new skill or technique with intention and safety at the front of their mind while reducing the number of new variables that they have to keep track of. This also allows the bottom to slowly adjust to and understand the way that they react to the new element that has been introduced. This is especially important if something doesn't work quite right. Introducing one new variable at a time makes pinpointing issues much easier.

## Be Patient, Build Slowly

As a Top, you may desperately want to put your partner into a strict strappado (p. 392) with the elbows tied tightly together behind their back and spank them silly, or as a bottom you may crave to experience that sort of scene. *But that is something you build up to, not something you start with.* It is very rare for a person to be able to touch their elbows behind their back and even more rare for them to be able to stay in that position for any length of time. Doing so without serious flexibility and strength training brings a high risk of muscle and joint injury. Also, if you put the ropes in the wrong location, you could easily cause a compression injury to the nerves that run close the elbows.

The ties in this book are generally low risk if used in conventional ways. Use them to get used to handling rope or to get used to the feeling of rope on your body. Take it slow and easy, work with each other, and practice each new technique before you incorporate it into play.

Enjoy the journey!

## Special Acknowledgement and Thanks

The information in the *Spectrum of Risks, Risk Prevention and Treatment,* and *Nerves and Circulation* sections is based heavily on the work of the amazing team at RopeStudy.com. They worked with many respected riggers around the world, with medical professionals and skilled graphics artists to create a clear, comprehensive, and succinct guide to reducing risks in rope bondage. With their permission, we have used that work to guide the creation of these sections in this book. We owe many thanks to maiitsohyazhi and bound_light and the knowledgeable people that provided them with information, suggestions and resources. You can visit ropestudy.com/nerves to find a list of the sources and people they consulted. These sections have also been further updated with input from Grey's Anatomy, Johns Hopkins and several other sources.

# The Spectrum of Risks

In the milder forms of rope bondage — where things are not too tight and/or where your partner can still adjust their position somewhat — the risks are normally quite low.

By contrast, any form where your partner is truly helpless, or in which the bondage is very tight or is anchored in such a way that it may become tighter if they move or struggle, the risk is higher.

There are many possible risks and concerns, running from mild to severe. Here are some of the most common:

**Mild** ⟶ **Severe**

- Rope marks
- Bruising
- Rope burn
- Musculoskeletal stress or damage
- Stains, sprains, etc.
- Breathing issues
- Positional asphyxia
- Fainting
- Injuries sustained during a fall
- Breaks or dislocations
- Compression injuries

Some kinds of damage heal very slowly and can therefore accumulate over time. Nerve damage is one of these, as are certain injuries to muscles, joints, ligaments, and tendons. Small amounts of damage that you might not even feel at first may not be fully healed when the next injury occurs and thus, damage can build over time to something more serious.

# Risk Prevention and Treatment

What can you do to try and avoid these common risks?

What actions should you take immediately if one of these injuries occurs?

The intention of this section is to help people that have no medical training to be able to provide immediate assistance *without causing more harm.*

Again, we are not medical professionals, and this is not medical advice. These guidelines are based on the best information we had at the time of writing, based on the experiences of the rope community, our research, consultations with people that do have medical training, and advice from reputable online sources like Johns Hopkins and the Mayo Clinic.

*In the event of an injury, the best course of action is to seek medical assistance from a qualified provider.*

We also recommend that everyone who is interested in bondage take a basic first aid and CPR course. They are good skills to have. Hopefully you will never need them.

# Rope Marks

Light to moderate pressure marks made by rope are a common side effect of rope bondage.

If the rope is tighter, the person likes to struggle, or their skin is more sensitive, severe rope marks can occur. These can take the form of bruising under the bands of rope. Marks can be caused by skin getting pinched between ropes, resulting in petechial hemorrhaging (ruptures of capillaries close to the surface of the skin).

### Prevention

Rope marks *will* occur. Petechial hemorrhaging is also common, but the risk of it can be reduced by running your fingers under each band of rope, so the ropes lay on top of the skin more evenly and are less likely to pinch. That said, petechial hemorrhaging is difficult to avoid altogether.

### Treatment

Light rope marks typically go away by themselves after a few hours, but you can sometimes speed the process with moisturizer and a light massage. Petechial hemorrhaging may take a few days to heal.

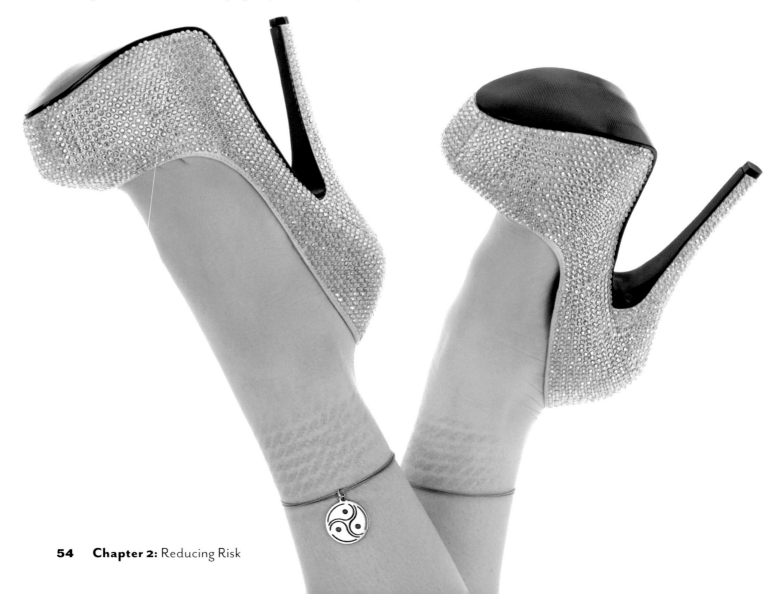

# Rope Burn

Friction from a rope can abrade the skin or burn off the outer layers. Severe versions can break the skin. This risk applies to both Top and bottom.

### Prevention

Move the rope slowly and deliberately. Use the techniques shown in *Protect Your Partner from Rope Burn* (p. 165).

### Treatment

Topical pain-relieving treatments (such as Bengay) can be helpful. If the skin is broken, clean the wound with cool water, treat with an antibiotic cream or ointment and cover with loose gauze. If the wound is deeper than just the top layer of skin, covers a large area, or appears as if it may be charred or infected, seek medical attention.

# Bruising

Like any bruise, bruises from rope can take several days to heal.

### Prevention

Move in a controlled way. Help your partner move in a controlled way. When a person is bound, they are not able to catch themselves if they trip, faint, or fall in some other way. If they need to move around the space while tied, help them to move safely.

### Treatment

You can reduce the effects of a bruise if you take a few actions quickly: Elevate the affected area and rest it. Ice the affected area for 20 minutes and repeat a few times for the first day or two. If there is swelling, add a compression bandage and consider ibuprofen or other anti-inflammatory pain medication if necessary.

For more significant bruising, see the RICE treatment on the next page.

If the bruise is accompanied by intense pain or significant swelling, seek medical attention; there may be something else going on. If the bruise has not faded and is still sensitive after two weeks or you notice other issues in the days after the injury, consult a medical professional.

# Musculoskeletal Stress or Damage

This typically happens if a person is contorted into a position that is not typical for them, if they are held in a position for longer than their body can handle, or as the result of an unexpected movement like a fall. The knees, shoulders, and back are particularly vulnerable.

It may be several hours or even the next day before such an injury is felt. These injuries also can be cumulative. A small injury today adds to a small one last week that hasn't yet healed, which added to one before that — you see the problem.

### Prevention

During negotiation, discuss the bottom's physical capabilities. Use techniques that allow you to work within your partner's comfort zone. For example, if your partner cannot assume a **Box Tie Position** (p. 398), don't try to force them into one; use the **Adjustable Box Tie** technique (p. 405) instead. Both Top and bottom need to build experience with regards to what works and what doesn't for that particular bottom.

Tops: During a scene, move in a careful and controlled manner. Help the bottom to do so as well.

Bottoms: If you want to be tied in a certain position, work on being able to assume that position when you are not tied. Strength and flexibility training can help you to work towards a desired position safely.

### Treatment

If there is intense pain along with immediate and significant swelling, seek medical attention immediately. If a limb or muscle stops working, or you hear a popping sound like a joint coming out of place, seek medical attention immediately.

If an injury is less severe, treat it the same way you would normally treat a bruise, strain, or sprain, using the well-known RICE method.

As always: Listen to your body. Seek medical attention if you believe you might need it.

## Fainting and Related Injuries

Loss of consciousness can happen unexpectedly and for a variety of reasons. Dehydration, low blood sugar, standing in one position for too long, standing up suddenly after sitting or lying down for a while, low blood pressure, difficulty breathing, breathing too fast or hard, blood flow issues, being too hot — the list goes on.

When a person faints while in rope, particularly if they are attached to something, they can injure themselves as they fall. As their entire body becomes 'dead weight', immense pressure can be applied to areas of the body that would be otherwise protected when a person is conscious and capable of adjusting their position.

### Prevention

Hydrate and eat a small snack roughly an hour before playing — preferably something high in protein.

Be watchful of early warning signs. If a person goes pale, starts sweating heavily, says they are feeling weak or dizzy or nauseated, reports a tightness in the chest, reports difficulty breathing, or seems to be short of breath, they might be on the verge of fainting.

### Treatment

*If they are feeling faint, but have not fainted:*
Stop what you are doing and help them gently to sit on a chair or lay on

### RICE — Rest, Ice, Compression, Elevation

**Rest** — Pain is your body's way of telling you something is wrong. Stop, change or take a break from the activity that caused the pain. But don't avoid all physical activity. Protect the area that is in pain. Give the body time to recover.

**Ice** — Cold reduces pain by reducing swelling and numbing the area slightly. Ice immediately. Cover an ice pack with a light towel and apply to the area for 15-20 minutes. Repeat every two to three hours while you're awake for the first 24-48 hours after the injury.

**Compression** — To help stop swelling, compress the area with an elastic bandage until the swelling stops. You want it snug, but not too tight or you may impact circulation. Begin wrapping at the end farthest from your heart. Loosen the wrap if the pain increases, the area becomes numb, turns blue or cool, or if swelling occurs below the wrapped area.

**Elevation** — Raise the injured area above the level of your heart when you can, especially at night. For example, if you have pain in your knee or ankle, prop your leg up on a pillow while you sleep. This helps reduce swelling. You may find it helpful to use a nonsteroidal anti-inflammatory medications (like ibuprofen or naproxen) along with the RICE treatment.

## Fainting

**Immediate Actions**

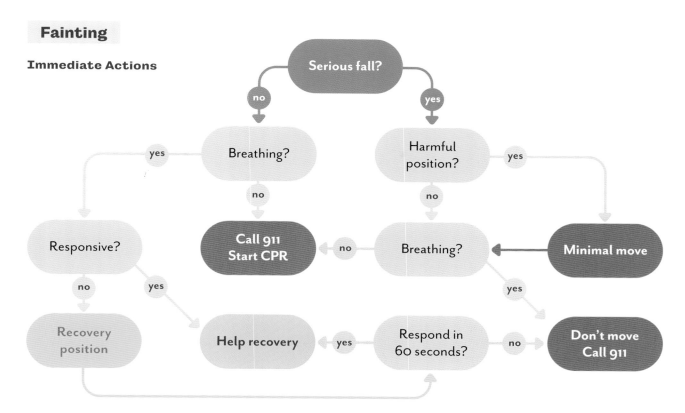

the ground. Remove any rope and/or clothing that might be impacting breathing or blood flow. If sitting, have them put their head between their knees. If laying down, have them lay on their back with their knees elevated about 12 inches or on their side with their knees bent. Offer them water or juice and then a snack when they seem like they're able to eat.

*If they did faint, but did not fall and sustain other injuries:*
Check for responsiveness by tapping them gently on the shoulder and asking them loudly if they are okay. They should recover within one minute. Do all of the same things you did for *If they are feeling faint.* Stay with them until they have fully recovered.

   If they do not respond within one minute, call emergency services. 911 in North America. 999 and 112 are common in other countries. If you don't know the emergency number for the country you're in, find out before you start playing.

*If they are not breathing or they are breathing, but remain unresponsive after one minute:*
If there are people present, point to a specific person and, using a commanding voice, say, "You! Call 911" (or other local emergency number). If no one is with you, call the emergency number yourself and put the phone on speaker. If you are trained, begin CPR. Follow the instructions of the emergency operator.

*If they fell or suffered some injury and are not responsive:*
Do not move them unless doing so is absolutely necessary to prevent further injury or harm. Call 911 or your local emergency number.

# Breathing Issues/ Positional Asphyxiation

Believe it or not, **humans need to be able to breathe**. As the saying goes: You only have about three minutes to live, but the timer gets reset every time you take a breath.

### Prevention

*Restriction*: A person can breathe by moving either their diaphragm or their chest or both. If you put a tight band of rope on the soft waist, you can make it difficult for them to move their diaphragm. They then need to breathe by moving their chest instead (this results in a "heaving chest" which some people find very hot), but this can be difficult for some. Restricting both the chest and the diaphragm at the same time makes breathing much more difficult and increases the risk significantly. This is why it is important that you *do not* tie both the waist and chest tightly.

*Positional issues:* It is also possible to immobilize one or both of a person's breathing mechanisms by putting them into extreme positions. For example, if you tie them into a tight ball or a hog tie. Such challenging positions can make breathing extremely difficult. When attempting these positions, it is critically important to work well within the rope bottom's physical capabilities and closely monitor them. Someone unable to breathe is unable to speak to let you know there is a problem! Cases like this are where it can be helpful to give them something heavy or loud to drop if they need help.

*Asthma:* During negotiation, ask if your partner has asthma or any other breathing issues. Have their inhaler or other emergency tools immediately within reach. During the scene, take care to manage their breathing rate. If they are starting to breathe heavily, calm things down until they catch their breath.

### Treatment

React immediately the moment you detect any issue with breathing. Loosen the ropes quickly. If the bottom is in distress, cut them free. If they need an inhaler, give it to them as soon as they are able to take in breath (meaning if they are unable to draw a breath due to restriction or position, cut them free first, then give them the inhaler. If they *can* breathe and just need the inhaler, give it to them first, then untie them).

# Injuries Sustained During a Fall

When doing floor-level bondage ("floor work", i.e. non-suspension) like the ties in this book, it is still possible for a person to fall. For example: If they are seated in a precarious position, they may tip and fall, unable to catch themselves. If a person is standing with their ankles and arms tied and they begin to fall over, it would be very difficult for them to catch their balance. If they are attached to an overhead point — not suspended from it, just tied to it — and something goes wrong, they could fall before they know what is happening. They might faint. A fall can happen from a standing position or off a piece of furniture or down an architectural feature like steps.

### Prevention

Be conscious of falling or tripping hazards. Keep a close watch on someone in a position where falling is possible. Keep your play area free from tripping hazards the best you can. Bottoms, be careful when in rope; particularly if moving around the space when tied. Tops, help your bottoms move safely.

### Treatment

*Small falls:* Check for injury and treat that injury. Bruising, swelling, perhaps bleeding or abrasion, as long as they are not serious, should be treated just as you normally would.

*Serious falls:* Any broken bones, severe pain, strikes to the head, loss of consciousness, or any indication that there may have been damage to the spine (immediate onset of pain in the neck or back, any immediate numbness that the person didn't have before, any paralysis or incontinence) indicate that something serious has happened.

If the person is responsive and alert, they can guide your response to the injury. For example, a broken arm is serious, but it may not require that an ambulance be called. The person may instead prefer that a friend drive them to the nearest Urgent Care facility — but keep in mind that just because they think they feel okay in the moment, this does not mean they have not suffered a serious injury. Shock is common. They should still be checked out by a medical professional.

If they are not responsive or alert: Take immediate emergency action.

- If they are breathing, do not to move them unless absolutely necessary to prevent further harm, e.g. the position they are in is preventing them from being able to breathe or impairing circulation. If they are excessively bleeding, you may need to move them to put pressure on the wound. If you do need to move them, only do so the minimum amount required to resolve the issue. Don't cut or remove the rope. Doing so risks moving them; just leave it there unless it is impacting breathing or blood flow.
- Call 911. If there are others present, point to a specific person and, using a commanding voice, say, "You! Call 911" (or other local emergency number). This allows you to take the next actions while they deal with the call.
- Check to see if they are responsive and breathing.
- If they are not breathing, begin CPR if you are trained.
- If the person becomes responsive, try to keep the person from moving. Tell them that help is on its way. Talk to them to help keep them calm.

# Compression Injuries

When rope presses too deeply into a person, it can disrupt the flow of blood or damage nerves. This can happen if the rope itself is too tight or if too much pressure is being added to a person's body using rope.

*Compressing blood vessels* in such a way that impacts circulation is typically not a major concern (p. 62-63). Unless a person has a complicating condition related to blood (ask them about this), the flow of blood can usually be reduced or even cut off for quite a while without issue; 30 minutes or so. That said, it is not comfortable, so fix this issue as soon as you can; you just normally don't need to drop everything to deal with it on an emergency basis.

*Compressing nerves,* on the other hand, is something that must be dealt with *immediately*. This typically presents as a change in a person's sense of touch (perhaps the skin on some of their fingers goes numb or feels strange in some other way) or as a loss of strength or control of some part of the body (for example, "wrist drop", when a person cannot lift their hand). Nerve compression can result in nerve damage in a very short period of time — minutes or even seconds, depending on type and severity. Nerve damage can take months or years to heal, and it some cases it may *never* fully heal.

### Prevention

Don't tie too tightly; you should always be able to get two fingers under any band of rope. Pay close attention to the Nerve Compression section (p. 65) and learn where nerves are more vulnerable to compression. Particularly risky areas include the wrist, the outside of the upper arm and elbow, the armpit, and the inside of the leg. In the tutorials themselves, we will discuss specific risks of that specific technique, along with methods to reduce those risks by managing how tightly the rope is tied or the placement of rope — or both.

Remember that changing the bottom's position after the tie is complete can change the tightness. What was an acceptable tightness in one position may be too tight if you then move the person into a different position. It is best to have your partner get into the general position you want them in as you are tying them.

Learn tests for touch sensitivity and motor function changes. Teach your partner how to do those tests themselves and have them build them into habits. There's more on this in *Major Indicators of Compression* (p. 72).

### Treatment

*Pre-injury:*

If you or your partner detect that an issue may be occurring — for example, the bottom's thumb or forefinger start to go numb — take action immediately.

Move the band of ropes causing the compression; even 1 inch or so can make a difference. If the issue does not resolve in 15 seconds, remove that element of the bondage.

Build quick releases, or "outs", into your bondage. For example, use a **Slipped Somerville Bowline** (p. 196) as part of a **Box Tie** (p. 397) so you can release the wrists in just seconds, thereby relieving the pressure on the upper arms.

If the issue seems severe, and you cannot release them quickly, cut the ropes off. If you need to cut ropes, be sure your bottom won't fall and injure themselves in a different way!

*If an injury occurs:*
If there is intense pain, seek medical attention immediately.

If a lower-severity injury occurs, there is little that can be done at home to fix it.

Anecdotes suggest that if you know the specific site of the issue, it can be helpful to rest it for a few hours then resume gentle movement of it the next day or so. DO NOT try to stretch or massage it to try to get things back in place. That doesn't work with nerves and can cause further damage. Keep in mind that the location of the injury may not be the location where the symptom is felt. For example, when the radial nerve in the upper arm is compressed, it is often felt as numbness in the thumb or forefinger. Read *Major Indicators of Compression* (p. 72) for more information.

Keep in mind that nerve damage can be cumulative. A little today on top of unhealed damage from the week before will just keep building.

If you are still feeling symptoms after 2-3 days, consult a medical professional.

# Nerves and Circulation

One of the most important risks to understand in rope bondage is how the pressure of rope on the body — or the positions that a body might be held in during a tie — can impact and even damage nerves and blood vessels.

**Nerve damage is insidious**. It can happen almost instantly or can build gradually over time, with multiple small injuries building to something more serious. It can take months to heal, or years, or it may never fully heal. **Therefore, it is important that everyone involved recognize that this risk is always present, and that even if both Top and bottom do what they can to reduce the risk, nerve injury may still occur.**

Both Tops and bottoms need to learn as much as they can about:
• The various types of nerve injuries possible during rope bondage.
• How best to mitigate the risks.
• How to recognize when something is wrong.
• How to respond to issues and injuries, should they occur.

It's also important that bottoms learn as much as they can about their own bodies and capabilities and help Tops understand how to tie them in ways that meet the bottoms' specific needs while reducing the risk to a level that both are comfortable assuming.

## Blood Flow and Circulation Loss
### The Brain
One very important (and hopefully obvious) thing: Never cut off the flow of blood to the brain. Never put pressure across the front of the neck for any length of time. The carotid arteries and jugular veins that run through the front of the neck are sensitive; messing with them is highly risky.

Yes, erotic choking is something that some people do, but it is highly risky edge play. Using rope to do so adds even more danger to an already dangerous activity. There is nuance here, but this is a *foundations* book and choking is beyond the scope of what we will discuss here.

### Flow of Blood Through the Front of the Neck

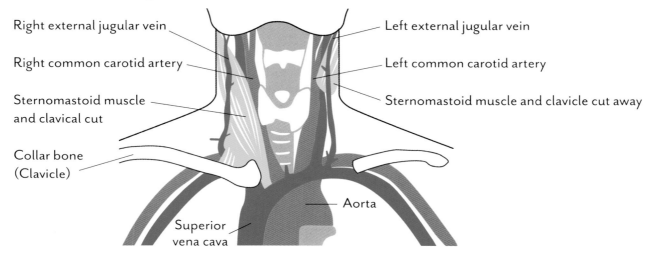

Right external jugular vein

Right common carotid artery

Sternomastoid muscle and clavical cut

Collar bone (Clavicle)

Left external jugular vein

Left common carotid artery

Sternomastoid muscle and clavicle cut away

Aorta

Superior vena cava

### Elsewhere
In other parts of the body, circulation loss over a short period of time isn't generally a major concern. However, you should keep an eye on any changes to the color of the skin. When tied in such a way that blood flow is being impacted, the skin may change color (or may not; each body is different):

• If the skin becomes darker (a shade of red, even dark red or purple): This is common in rope bondage and is not usually a concern over short periods of time (30 minutes) unless there is a complicating medical factor (like pre-existing circulation issues, e.g. diabetes, peripheral vascular disease, Raynaud's syndrome, etc.). Getting darker means that blood is collecting in that location because it is not able to flow out as easily as it normally does (impaired venous return).

- If the skin becomes *paler:* This can mean that blood is not able to flow into the area like it should (impaired arterial flow). This is a much more serious situation and should be addressed immediately. This is less common, however, because arteries normally run more deeply in the body and are not compressed as easily.

While there is not normally a lot of risk if a limb is without circulation for 30 minutes or more, in the bondage world, most people want to limit risk as much as they can and will not allow blood flow to remain restricted for more than 15 to 20 minutes. They will also often take immediate steps to improve circulation by dressing ropes, moving wraps, or changing positions. In some cases, circulation loss for a period of time is unavoidable, but keep it to that reasonable time limit.

### Regularly Test for Restricted Blood Flow

- Check your partner's skin color and temperature before and during the scene. Know what is normal *for your partner,* so you can tell what is not normal.
- If the skin goes paler, adjust the bondage to loosen the restriction to that area.

## Circulation Issues Can Mask Nerve Issues

*Important:* When circulation is reduced, it is easier to miss important warning signs of other issues. A common result of this is nerve damage.

For example, loss of sensation could be due to loss of blood flow or it could be the result of a compressed nerve. If it is due to circulation, it will not normally cause any long-term issues as long as it is addressed within 20 minutes or so. But if it was really a nerve issue — or there was both a circulation and a nerve issue at the same time — the nerve part of the problem could result in a long-term injury in just a few minutes, or even less depending on the specific circumstances.

*Bottoms:* Learn how to do sensitivity checks and make it a habit to do them.

*Tops:* If your bottom alerts you to a change in sensation, you need to check for nerve compression and resolve any you find. If you determine that the issue was circulatory *and* you *both **jointly*** decide to continue with the scene, you can choose to do that, but the burden is then on you, the Top, to closely and continually monitor for additional/new nerve compression.

*Bottoms:* If you agree to allow the scene to continue in such a circumstance, you need to recognize the additional risk you are taking.

## How Can You Tell the Difference Between Circulation Loss and Nerve Compression?

Here are some tests that both Tops and bottoms can do to help distinguish between circulation loss and nerve compression. But understand that these tests are not 100% reliable!

Each body is different and it's possible you might do these tests and completely believe that the issue is circulatory and still end up with some type of nerve damage. That said, they're the best we have, and are worth doing regularly.

|  | Circulation loss | Nerve compression |
| --- | --- | --- |
| **Speed of sensation loss** | Gradual | Gradual or sudden |
| **Area of sensation loss** | Whole limb | Partial limb/fingers |
| **Mobility** | No loss of mobility | Loss of mobility |
| **Capillary nail refill** | Slow refill | Normal refill |

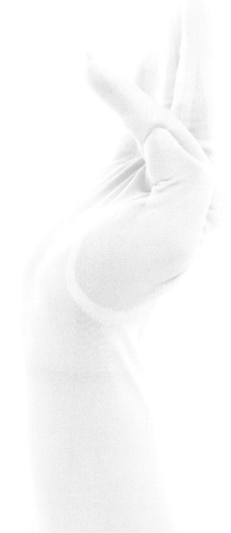

- **Speed of the sensation loss:** With circulation issues, loss of sensation usually appears gradually and in stages (slight tingling, clumsy fingers, more intense pain, complete numbness) but this may vary from person to person. With nerve compression, loss of sensation can be gradual or sudden. Therefore, if there is a sudden loss of sensation ("my left thumb just went numb"), assume nerve compression. If it was gradual, look to other indicators to determine which it is.

- **Area of sensation loss:** With circulation issues, loss of sensation tends to affect the entire limb or entire hand/foot. Loss of sensation due to nerve compression tends to affect the specific areas that receive sensory input from that nerve. It is important for the bottom to do sensory tests (p. 72) from time to time and report any issues. For example, sensation on the top of the thumb and forefinger is supplied by the radial nerve, so if most of a person's hand feels normal, but they suddenly have numbness in just their thumb and forefinger, there is nerve compression somewhere along the path of the radial nerve. Continue reading for more details on this and other nerves.

- **Loss of mobility:** Certain nerves are responsible for enabling the body to move in certain ways. Sudden inability to move the hands or feet in particular ways when a person can normally do so can indicate severe nerve compression. It is important to do mobility tests (p. 73) before the scene so that you know if there are any pre-existing issues. (If a person cannot twist their wrist like they are opening a doorknob under normal circumstances, you cannot use that as a test during the scene.)

- **Capillary nail refill:** Press on the nail of a finger or toe until it turns white. Release pressure and see how quickly color returns to the nail. If it takes longer than a second or two, the issue is more likely to be circulation loss. Again, it is important to do this test before your scene with someone so you know what is normal for them on that day. If a person already has circulation issues, this test is not going to be helpful.

# Nerve Compression

In case you skipped the opening of the section, we will repeat this:

**Nerve damage is insidious.** It can happen almost instantly, or can build gradually over time, with multiple small injuries building to something more serious. It can take months to heal, or years, or it may never fully heal. Therefore, it is important that everyone involved recognize that this risk is *always* present, and that even if both Top and bottom do what they can to reduce the risk, nerve injury may still occur.

## Nerve Functions and Common Indicators of Compression

Nerves do two major things:
- Provide *sensation* to a particular part of the body.
- Provide *motor functions* ("mobility") to a particular part of the body.

Nerve compression can result in the following (but not always):
- Tingling or burning sensation.
- Numbness or loss of sensation.
- Weakness or loss of mobility.

One or more of these sensations may occur at the same time. It is also possible that you will not feel anything unusual before the damage is already done.

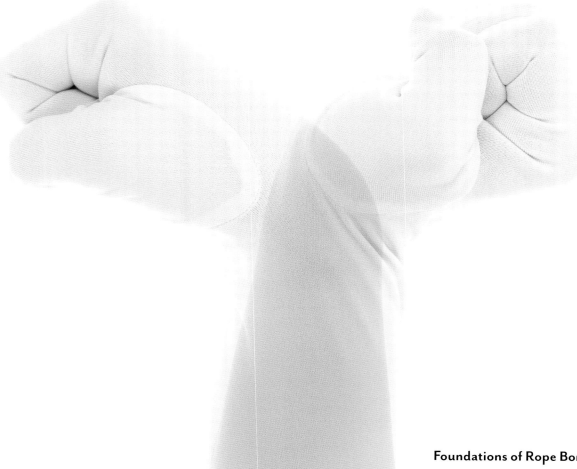

## Common Causes of Compression or Injury

When doing rope, there seem to be three common ways nerves might be injured:

- **Direct mechanical impact on the nerves:** The rope is positioned on or very close to the nerve, and it presses on the nerve directly, causing compression or shearing, resulting in injury.
- **Indirect stress on the nerves:** The location of the rope (even when not directly over a nerve) and/or the position of the body (especially in ties that require significant stretching, twisting, etc. for which the bottom is not trained) impacts the nerve indirectly, resulting in injury.
- **Anoxia/ischemia of the nerves:** The blood supply to the nerve is restricted and can impact both sensory and motor nerve function. This is one way circulation issues can result in nerve issues.

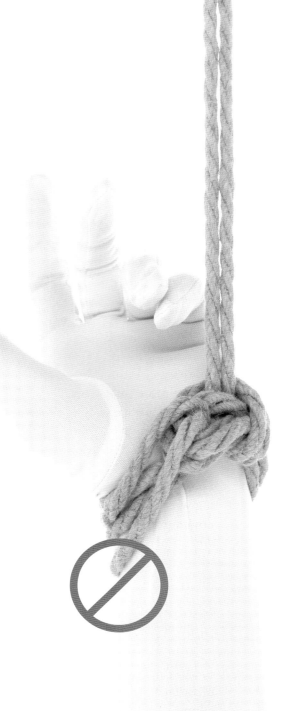

The risk of nerve injury may be greater for those with "loose" skin or with large amounts of subcutaneous tissue, which is typically comprised mainly of fat cells. In situations like this, the skin and the nerves and tissue beneath the skin may move in such a way as to apply shearing forces which may more easily injure the nerve. Take extra precautions to make sure the cuff is tensioned evenly and appropriately for the body part being tied, and that the band is wide enough to appropriately distribute the forces that may be applied to it. For more on this, see *Body Type Considerations* (p. 324).

Also, all bodies are different. Some people are more prone to nerve compression injury than others. You can test for this before you tie. Use your fingers to lightly massage or gently press on commonly vulnerable nerves. Note their sensitivity and location and use that information as you are tying.

## Prevention Through Tying Well

While being intentional about *where* rope is placed is important, it is just as important to be intentional about *how* the rope is applied. In this book, tips and procedures designed to reduce risk will be shown alongside specific ties. However, each situation and person is unique, so here are some guidelines to keep in mind when applying rope:

- **The more vulnerable the location, the greater the risk.**
  Certain nerves are more vulnerable in some anatomical locations than in others. Learn which areas are particularly vulnerable and tie in ways that avoid or minimize compression in those areas. Apply this knowledge and adjust when tying on different people. Finally, incorporate your understanding of the anatomy of your bottom into the other areas of risk management (negotiation, circulation issues, medical concerns, etc.).
- **The longer the rope is on the body, the greater the risk.**
  One implication is that "more intense" or "more risky" rope should be shorter in duration. Another implication is that the Top's control and efficiency are an important safety factor.

- **The greater the tension of the rope, the greater the risk.**
  Managing tension is a critical part of maintaining control over your rope and the situation in which the rope is being used. The tension of a particular tie should be "sufficiently tight" for specific circumstances in which it is applied to a person, and not tighter. Several variables contribute to what is considered "sufficiently tight", including the tie itself, the purpose it serves, the body on which it is being tied, and the intentions of the rigger. A general rule to follow when beginning is to apply enough tension to prevent the rope from moving, shifting, or changing tension throughout the scene. This is why rope work that involves full suspension is significantly riskier than floor work.

- **The narrower the band, the greater the risk.**
  The smaller the area across which a force is distributed, the more pressure that force will exert. Using a wider band of rope will distribute the same amount of force across a wider area, therefore reducing the pressure exerted on any particular part of the body. This is only true if the tension of all of the wraps is the same.

- **The more uneven the tension in the band, the greater the risk.**
  Any twisting or overlapping of the lines can create a similar effect by increasing the pressure applied under those points while also warping the tension of the other lines.

## Repetitive Injury

It is worth noting that repetitive injury, to one degree or another, is common amongst experienced rope bottoms. Repetitive injury occurs when a nerve (or group of nerves) is repeatedly stressed over the course of several different rope sessions — no single one of which caused noticeable injury at the time. The damage caused by "microtrauma" or "micro-injury", can add up over time. Then during one particular session it may become noticeable, bringing to light the extent of an injury that had been building over time.

Repetitive injuries can occur even when the rope is "tied well" every time. As we said before, **rope is not safe**. Repetitive injury is a risk of partaking in rope bondage and is not necessarily anyone's "fault" if appropriate precautions were taken and effective communication was practiced.

Mitigating cumulative nerve injuries can be done through consistent and proactive musculoskeletal and nervous system care. Monitoring and slowly building the strength and mobility of critical joints (shoulders, knees, ankles) can assist in injury prevention. Before doing so, seek the advice of a licensed physical therapist or rehabilitation specialist.

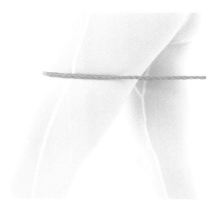

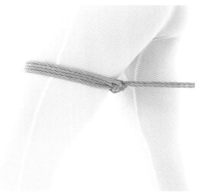

Single Strand (top) and a 4-Strand Cuff Band. Ten pounds of force digs in much deeper when it's just a single strand.

# Major Areas of Greater Risk
**Nerve Paths**

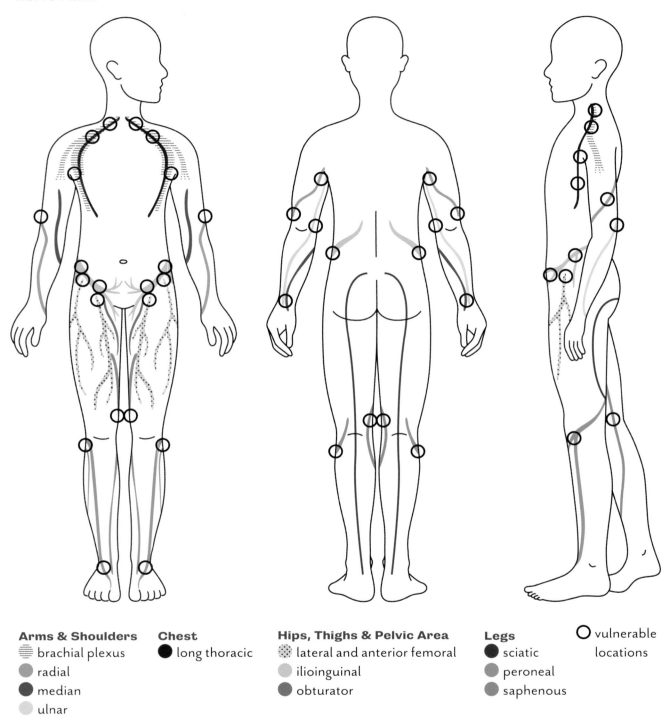

**Arms & Shoulders**
- brachial plexus
- radial
- median
- ulnar

**Chest**
- long thoracic

**Hips, Thighs & Pelvic Area**
- lateral and anterior femoral
- ilioinguinal
- obturator

**Legs**
- sciatic
- peroneal
- saphenous

○ vulnerable locations

These are the nerves that are more likely to be impacted by common forms of rope bondage. These are the general location of those nerves for most people. But each body is unique; paths might be different for any given person. It is worth your time to learn about the concerns, needs, limits, and experiences of each person you want to put in rope. Depending on your partner and what you choose to do with them, you may encounter things not on this list. If your partner reports anything weird, anything not normal for them that occurred during or after your encounter, don't ignore it. Research what might have caused it and what can help in recovery and avoiding re-injury.

**Sensory Innervation**

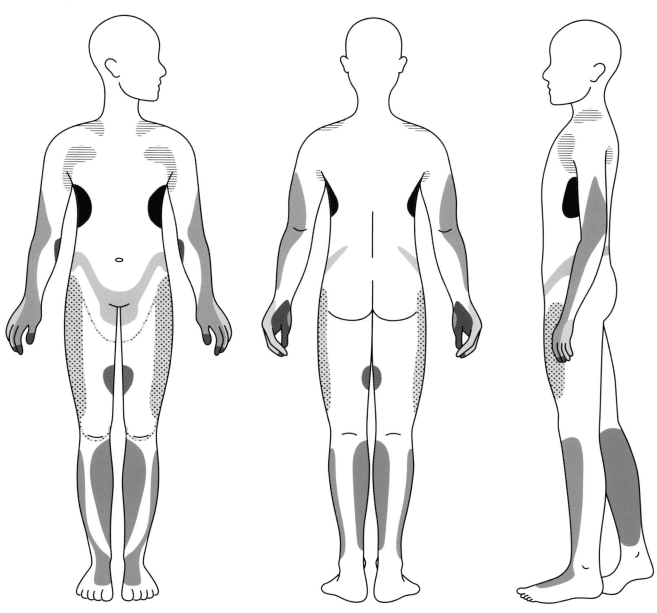

## Some General Advice

Avoid tying tightly on or near joints. Not only are joints more sensitive parts of the body, but nerves are typically more exposed in these areas.

Apply rope on the parts of the limb or body on which there is more muscle, as muscles tend to protect nerves from compression. This is not true for every location on the body, however; there are instances in which muscles can *contribute* to compression rather than prevent it. Familiarize yourself with the nerves, the locations in which they are most vulnerable, and the consequences of compressing them.

## A Closer Look at the Arm:
## Locations, Indications, and Implications

Many nerve-related injuries occur in the arms.

**Major Nerves in the Arm:**

**Brachial Plexus**

The brachial plexus is a network of nerves that runs from the spinal cord, through the neck and shoulder region and into the arm and hand.

- **More vulnerable locations:** The front of the chest (the "dip" near the corner of the neck and shoulders), across the front of the shoulder, and through/under the armpit.
- **Rope placement:** Placing rope so that it puts pressure on these areas can cause nerve compression. In particular:
  - Thin bands under significant tension too close to the neck or running from the back of the neck to the front of the armpit.
  - Thick rope knots, joins, or bulges in or immediately in front of the armpit.
  - Shoulder bands with knots near the front of the neck.
- **Special consideration:** Compression in this area can occur through body position as well as rope placement. Holding a person's arms behind their back puts strain across the front of the shoulders. Simply assuming this position can compress the brachial plexus in some people.

  Assuming a **Box Tie Position** (p. 398) without applying rope can help a bottom determine if they may experience brachial plexus compression when holding this kind of position.
- **Results of compression:** Compression of the brachial plexus often feels the same as compression of the radial, ulnar, or median nerves (tingling, numbness, loss of motor control in the hand). If you have tried several different ties and they all seem to result in your partner reporting compression symptoms, the issue may actually be compression of the brachial plexus.

**Radial Nerve**

- **More vulnerable locations:** The radial nerve runs around the back of the upper arm to the forearm. On most people the area of greatest vulnerability lies on the outer side and back of the upper arm, near where the deltoid meets the triceps. It is also possible to compress the radial nerve at the wrist.
- **Rope placement:** Compression of the radial nerve is most commonly seen in ties that include a band that runs around the entire upper body to include the upper arms, especially if the arms are behind the back as in a **Box Tie**. With such ties, it is easy to accidently run the band right over the most vulnerable spot. Even a little pressure in such a situation can result in nerve compression. To reduce this risk, it can help to keep the rope away from the range between the lower half to lower third of the upper arm. Also, it is important to remind

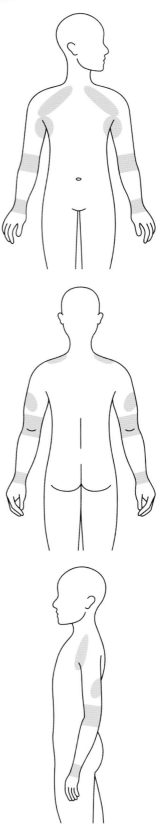

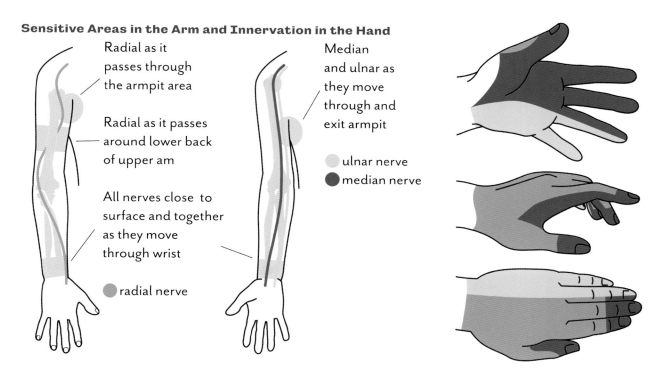

**Sensitive Areas in the Arm and Innervation in the Hand**

Radial as it passes through the armpit area

Radial as it passes around lower back of upper am

All nerves close to surface and together as they move through wrist

● radial nerve

Median and ulnar as they move through and exit armpit

○ ulnar nerve
● median nerve

your partner to do their sensory and mobility tests and report issues immediately so you can adjust the position of the rope.

• **Results of compression:** Loss of sensation along a portion of the back of the hand (see the diagram above), abnormal sensations that can resemble tingling or pricking, and a loss of motor control in the hand are all symptoms of radial nerve compression. "Wrist drop" is a result of radial nerve palsy — impairment of the nerve's ability to process signals from the brain — symptoms of which include the inability to hold one's hand in line with the arm and the inability to extend the hand and fingers.

### Ulnar Nerve

• **More vulnerable locations:** The ulnar nerve runs along the side of the arm that is closest to the body. It is most vulnerable to external compression behind the elbow (your 'funny bone'), under the armpit, and at the wrist.

• **Rope placement:** Compression of this nerve is most likely to occur when tight or loaded rope is placed close to the elbow or around the wrist.

• **Results of compression:** Symptoms of ulnar nerve compression can include loss of sensation in the ring finger and pinky finger, tingling or abnormal sensation in these areas, and the loss of motor control and grip strength.

### Median Nerve

• **More vulnerable locations:** The median nerve follows a similar path as the ulnar nerve; traveling through the underarm area, alongside the body, extending through the wrist into the hand. It is most vulnerable to compression under the arms and as it moves through the wrist.

**Sensory Tests**

Run your thumbnail against the sides and bottoms of your fingers, one-by-one.

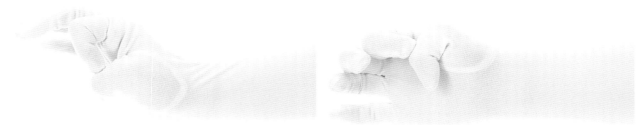

Run the fingernail of your forefinger against the side and back of your thumb.

- **Rope placement** – Compression of the median nerve is most likely to occur due to tight or loaded rope near the wrist.
- **Results of compression** – Symptoms of median nerve compression can include loss of sensation in the tips of the index, middle, and ring fingers, abnormal sensation in these areas, and the inability to make a tight fist. Repetitive compression of the median nerve can result in carpal tunnel syndrome.

## Major Indicators of Compression

### Sensory

Abnormal sensation, known as "paresthesia," is a very common symptom of nerve compression that you have experienced if you have ever had a limb 'fall asleep.' Paresthesia can present as a decrease in sensation, numbness, tingling (pins and needles), burning, or just feeling 'strange.' When these symptoms are experienced in the hand, the exact location can provide some information regarding which nerve is being impinged. The compression or injury can be at any point along the path of that nerve.

### Motor

Impaired ability to flex, extend, or otherwise move specific parts of the body can be an indicator of nerve compression as well. When it comes to these nerves, here are a few motions that can indicate impingement:

- **Radial Nerve** — Difficulty extending the hand backwards in a 'stop' motion.
- **Ulnar Nerve** — Difficulty extending the ring and pinky fingers (referred to as an 'ulnar claw').
- **Median Nerve** — Difficulty flexing the index and middle fingers (e.g., when making a fist).

**Motor/Mobililty Tests**

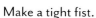

Make a tight fist.

Extend that fist upward.

Flex that fist downward.

Extend your finger straight out.

**Regularly Test for Peripheral Nerve Compression in the Arm**
Do this both before the scene and periodically throughout.

*Tops:*
- Have the bottom grip two of your fingers and squeeze them as hard as they can so you can feel the strength of their grip. If their grip strength weakens noticeably, they may be having motor issues.
- Have your partner do the sensory and mobility tests below before the scene so you know what is normal for that person. Having an understanding of baseline strength and sensory ability is critical to detecting change. Periodically during the scene, instruct your bottom to do their sensory and mobility checks. If the bottom reports or you detect any changes in their sensation or motor skills, immediately direct your attention to addressing the issue.

*Bottoms:*
- Regularly test your skin sensitivity and motor function throughout the scene.
- *Sensory Tests* — To test for numbness or changes in sensation, run your thumbnail gently against the skin of each of your fingers. Do the same with the fingernail of your first finger along your thumb. Ensure that you are using your nail to complete this action rather than the soft part of your finger.
- *Motor/Mobility Tests* — Flex all of your fingers into a tight fist, flex your fist downward as if knocking on a door, extend your fist backward, and extend all of the fingers away from the palm. This series of movements tests the motor function of the ulnar, median, and radial nerves.

### Nerves Elsewhere in the Body

The nerves in the arms, shoulders, and neck are the most likely to be impacted by the types of ties in this book and they are the most commonly discussed in the rope bondage world. But there are other sensitive nerves throughout the body that can be impacted as you explore beyond what you find here. Check out TheDuchy.com/nerves and TheDuchy.com/risk-management for more information.

Here are a few key examples so you know what to look up, based on your plans:

- Tight rope around the rib cage may impact the long thoracic nerve.
- Too much pressure on the crease of the leg and hip may impact the lateral femoral cutaneous nerve or the ilioinguinal and iliohypogastric nerve, which can also be impacted by pressure at the top of the hip bone.
- Tight rope around the upper thigh can impact the obturator nerve.
- Rope around the lower thigh or behind the knee can impact the saphenous nerve.
- Tight rope around the legs near the knee or tightly around the ankle can impact the peroneal nerve.
- Tying a person's legs up to their body (as in a **Malasana** tie (p. 389) to an extreme degree or for a long time can impact the sciatic nerve.

### Responding to Injury

At the *first sign* of a potential nerve compression issue, work to relieve any sources of compression as quickly as possible. This may include:

- Adjusting the position of the rope on the body. Sometimes moving a band of rope up or down even just an inch or two is all that is required to alleviate the issue.
- Shifting the physical position of the bottom to relieve the pressure on particular part of a tie. The bottom may be able to do this themselves or may need help to do so.
- Removing the rope from the affected location.

If none of these actions results in immediate and noticeable relief (within 15 seconds), end the rope session and remove all rope completely.

Time is a critical factor where nerve compression is concerned. The sooner the issue is addressed, the more likely that any injury will be minor and will heal relatively quickly. *Every minute of delay can greatly increase the damage.*

#### Assess Severity of the Injury

- If the injury involves abnormal sensation but no loss of motor function, and if normal sensation returns within a few hours, then the damage is likely mild and will heal without medical intervention. Avoid additional compression of the entire affected area until the nerves are completely healed. Most people completely recover from mild nerve injuries within 6-8 weeks. Keep in mind that symptoms

### Speed is Crucial

If you do not immediately know where the source of a nerve impingement is, don't waste time trying to figure it out. If moving any band of rope on the upper or lower parts of the arm doesn't resolve the issue within 15 seconds, remove the tie. Nerve compression may have been caused by the position of the body or something else entirely. Any detective work regarding which specific nerve may have been impinged, and how, is best done when the potential cause has been removed. Use the new information you have learned to plan for future scenes and exploration.

may dissipate before the nerve itself is completely healed.

- If the injury involves loss of mobility or strength, consider implementing the first-aid treatment described below and monitor the area closely for signs of change. If mobility does not improve within 24-48 hours, consult a medical professional.
- If the symptoms are severe, seek professional help immediately.

**Response and Treatment**

- Remove all sources of compression while maintaining as much control as possible to lower the risk of more injury. Avoid moving the bottom beyond what is necessary to remove the rope.
- Do not stretch or massage the injured area or the potential source location of the injury. Doing so may injure the nerve further. Remember, the site where sensation or mobility issues are being experienced may not be the same as the location of the injury.
- Rest the area for several days following the most recent injury. Depending on the location and severity, it may be necessary to immobilize the area using a splint.
- After a day or two of rest, conservatively explore the range of motion of the affected limbs or joints. If abnormal sensation or loss of motor function are still present after two or more days of rest, seek advice and treatment from a licensed physical therapist.
- There is evidence supporting the role of B vitamins in nerve regeneration and remyelination of nerve cells after injury. Vitamin B12, in particular, appears to directly support nerve cell survival and repair with the combination of vitamins B1, B6, and B12 showing positive effects as well.

If sensory or motor symptoms do not improve within 24-48 hours — or if pain and/or other symptoms accompany the injury — see a medical doctor as soon as possible. Do not use this book as a substitute for medical attention. The advice of a licensed medical professional always outranks the information presented in this text.

When consulting with a medical professional about an injury sustained from rope bondage, be completely honest about the origin of the injury. Keeping relevant information from a healthcare provider may impact the quality of care that you receive.

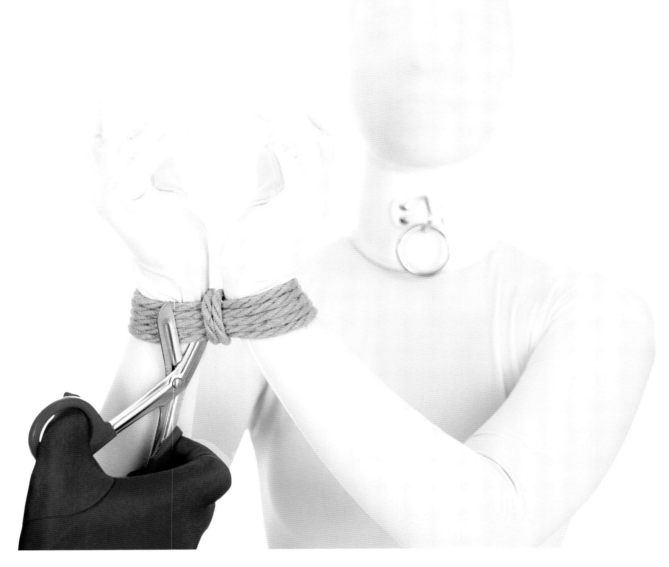

# Have Multiple "Outs"

You always need to be prepared to get someone out of rope instantly, if needed. This means having some means of cutting the rope in your pocket, on your belt, or another place immediately within reach.

Important: There are many ways to plan ahead and avoid getting into a situation where you might need to cut the rope, including:

- Play within your skill level and the skill level of your partner.
- Negotiate thoroughly, clarify everything.
- Make sure all your physical and medical needs are met before playing.
- Build experience with a person over time. Start easy and move to more complex things once you are both more comfortable with each other.
- Tie well. Don't tie too tightly. Avoid areas of greater risk of compression.
- If putting someone in a challenging position or one with a higher risk of nerve compression, use techniques that allow for quick release like the Slipped Somerville Bowline (p. 196) and the Quick-Release Hojo Cuff (p. 226).
- Use shorter ropes to give you more options or "outs" in emergencies.

If you follow and practice these guidelines and other safety concepts in this book, you will be less likely to get into a situation where you need to cut a rope. You can build the skills and experience to quickly and calmly untie a person. This is usually better unless the situation is an emergency.

The key to maintaining control over rope is tension. Once a blade of any kind cuts through your rope, you do not have control over the tension and you do not have control over your rope. In some cases, maintaining control matters less than removing the rope as quickly as possible. However, by being diligent with negotiation, communication, and building in "outs", you can save yourself from having to cut rope in most cases — and you can maintain control over the rope and the scene.

But emergency situations can and will *still* happen, no matter how good you are or how well you prepare!

Despite best efforts, a medical emergency may arise. An accident of some type can occur. The bottom may have a panic attack. The fire alarm may go off. A nosey neighbor or relative might knock on your door. There are many situations that may require that you are able to quickly release your partner.

*If it is an emergency, do not hesitate. Act quickly.* Assess the situation and get them free as quickly as you can safely do so. If that means holding their weight while you or a bystander cuts the rope — do it.

When in doubt, cut them out.

Always have a tool within reach to quickly and *safely* cut rope! I personally always have EMT shears in my bag and put them right beside me when I am rigging, but I also have a backup rescue hook on my belt. The situation will dictate which one I reach for.

- Recommended – High quality, heavy-duty emergency EMT shears are the most reliable, lowest risk option for most people. They are designed to cut seatbelts, leather boots, and more in an emergency. Their shape and blunted tips are important features that reduce risk when being used. However, they are bulkier than rescue hooks (below) and may be difficult to use in some positions. Be wary of cheap ones that dull quickly, or be prepared to replace them after a few uses.

- Also good, but with risks – Rescue hooks. These are fast and nimble. I personally wear one on my belt at all times. It is important to understand that they work well when rope is under tension, but not as well if the rope is slack. You may need to add tension to the rope in some cases to help them cut. Also, there have been cases of people using them incorrectly and causing a secondary injury. If you choose this option, research how to use them properly and practice doing so.

- Not recommended, but used sometimes – Knives. Some people use knives, but we recommend against this. These are the highest risk option. It is far easier to slip and make a bad situation worse when using a knife. If you insist on using one, at lease choose a "rescue knife" that has a blade only on one side AND has a squared off or blunted tip.

- Do not use tools that are not designed for emergency use near a human. Anything with a sharp point, such as scissors or knives, should not be used in an emergency.

## Be Prepared!

It is very important to practice cutting rope. Sacrifice a piece of rope and test out how it cuts with your chosen cutting tool. Try cutting it under tension and when slack, try cutting a bundle of ropes as well as just a single strand.

Does your tool cut cleanly and quickly? How hard is it to cut? How long does it take? Do you have to "chew" at the ropes with it, or have to make multiple passes?

If you get anything other than a smooth, clean, controlled cut, choose another tool.

**Recommended:**

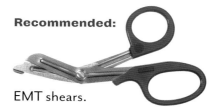

EMT shears.

**Good, but with Risks:**

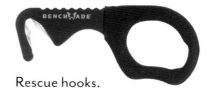

Rescue hooks.

**Not Recommended:**

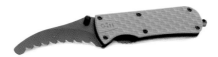

Single sided rescue blade.

**Do Not Use:**

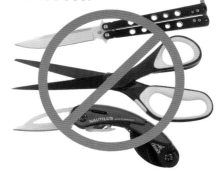

# Rope Hygiene

Bodies are not clean. Rope goes on bodies.
Extrapolate from there.

Rope can (and should) be cleaned but cannot be fully sanitized. If rope comes into contact with bodily fluids other than sweat — for example, if it's run between the teeth or between the legs, through/around the genitals or across the anus — there is no guarantee that you will be able to remove all traces of those fluids or materials.

What if a piece of rope was around someone's foot and they had athlete's foot and then that same piece of rope is placed in your mouth? Ick.

Consider STI transmission. The risk here is relatively low compared to other forms, but it can still be a risk.

If you would like to reduce the risk in this area, use a barrier method between your partner and your rope. Alternatively, if a Top plays with a particular person routinely, they may reserve a particular piece of rope for that person.

Many rope bottoms take on this responsibility themselves for their own health and hygiene. They carry their own rope kit that is "fluid bonded" and will only ever be used on them. If plans call for rope to touch their genitals or mouth, they use their own personal rope.

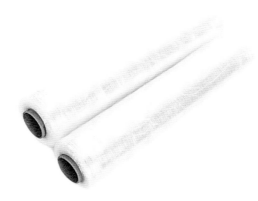

# Quick References

A quick reference list of important high-level points.

## Considerations for Tops (Bottoms Read This Too)

### *You* are Responsible

Once your partner is bound, only you can act. It is *your responsibility* to act when you detect or are informed of an issue. You have a duty of care. It is your partner's responsibility to tell you if they detect an issue, but you need to be proactively looking for them, too.

Your partner is entrusting you with their safety. This is a major exchange of power.

*Never* play when you are not at your best, whether from drugs, alcohol, or lack of sleep.

### Leave Your Ego at the Door

Do not attempt anything in a scene that you have not practiced and mastered outside of a scene.

You can gain theoretical knowledge in a short amount of time, but you still need practice to internalize that knowledge and develop muscle memory, to make it second nature and to become competent before you use it in a scene.

Master the basics and then get personal training from an experienced person before you try advanced bondage techniques, etc.

## Know Your Partner

Communication is critical.

You must give your partner the permission and confidence to tell you things.

Honestly and clearly talk about what you want to do.

Ask what your partner wants and be sure to build these elements into your plan as well.

Make sure they know they can stop any activity at any time, and you will not be mad at them or disappointed with them; that *they* are more important than any plans you may have for a scene.

Agree on safe words, actions, signals. Remember, in a power-exchange context (D/s, M/s) it can be hard for a sub or slave to say "no" when they want to please you. Be aware of this potential hurdle if you are in a power exchange dynamic and talk about it with your partner beforehand. *Order* them to tell you if they sense an issue that could result in injury, physical or otherwise. Reassure them that telling you is the right thing to do and is required.

It can be helpful to set up safe words/gestures/actions (p. 36).

Know your bottom's physical condition and health issues, including:

- Physical injuries and medical history that may impact a person's physical capabilities.
- Bone issues, diabetes, asthma, breathing/cardiac issues, fibromyalgia — anything that can impact a person's ability to breathe, messes with their blood pressure when under stress, or changes what you might expect about a person's reactions.
- Flexibility — be realistic about your partner's capabilities.
- Skin temperature — learn what is normal for your bottom before the scene, so you know what is not normal during the scene.

Understand any mental or emotional triggers that may be touched on by what you have planned, as well as any limits or guidance your partner may have about where they like rope to be placed and where they do not.

## Emergencies — Plan for the Worst Case

Shit happens. Be prepared:

- Have multiple ways to get your partner free quickly and safely.
- Plan ahead, and use ties that can be released quickly in an emergency.
- Have EMT shears or an EMT hook within reach.
- Have a method of calling for help, whether that is a fully charged phone or another person nearby.

### Before You Start

- Check the condition of your rope before you use it.
- Make sure any other gear, equipment, or items that you plan to use are clean and in good working order before you use them.
- Make sure both you and your bottom have your basic needs cared for (food, water, restroom, meds) before starting a scene.

### During the Scene:
### Respect and Care for Your Bottom

You have no power until the bottom grants it to you. RESPECT THAT. Protect that trust.

- Respect your bottom's limits scrupulously. You do not want to be known as the person that violates trust.
- Never leave someone in bondage alone.
- Be constantly aware of the bottom's breathing. Too fast or slow could mean excitement or signal trouble.
- Check in with your partner in ways that do not interfere with their experience.
- Have an aftercare routine. The scene is not over until the bottom is completely untied and back to their normal state of mind.
- Help them out of the rope. Do this slowly, carefully stretching the muscles that have been under tension.

### Aftercare

This is a time of reconnection and a time to bring your bottom back to themselves.

This can be critical to a person's mental well-being. Some people really sink into a different place when in bondage and they need to be reclaimed.

Aftercare needs are different for different people. Some bottoms explicitly want to be left alone to wallow in the sensations after a scene, while others crave physical closeness. Ask your partner what they need for aftercare as part of your negotiations.

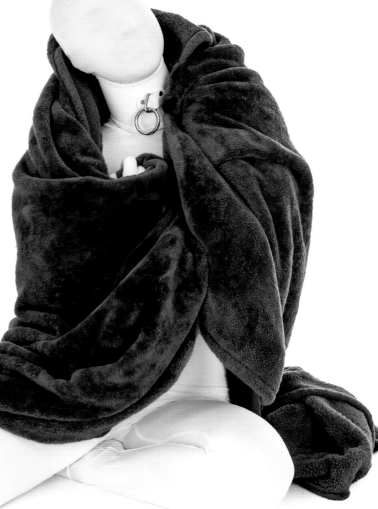

# Considerations for Bottoms (Tops Read This Too)

## Rules Apply to You Too

Anything you expect from a Top, you should expect from yourself. You also need to be courteous, respectful, clear, honest, fully participate in negotiation, don't be creepy, etc. If you expect people to respect you, you need to respect other people. It's a rule for general life, yes, and it applies just as much here.

## Your Needs and Desires Matter

You are a person with your own mind and body; your own physical, emotional, and mental needs and limitations. It is crucial that you are honest with yourself and your Top. Talk about these things; your Top can't know what you don't tell them.

Discuss your hot buttons and your hard and soft limits:

- What you crave or actively desire to do.
- What you are willing to do.
- What you prefer not to do but might be willing to try (soft limits).
- What you do not want to do under any circumstances (hard limits).

Your answers should match with what you are feeling the day of the scene, change the plan if necessary.

If you don't have a lot of detail in the above conversation yet, that's okay! In fact, it's more than okay because you are communicating honestly with yourself and whoever you choose to play with. Take your time when exploring new things, check in with yourself, learn through careful exploration and experience.

Discuss your physical capabilities, flexibility, strength and any limitations.

Physical qualities such as your age, physical condition, flexibility, and weight are not definitive, deciding factors that determine you can enjoy rope. But they are not irrelevant either. They may impact the type of rope scene you can safely do, or the intensity of that scene. You may need accommodations to do some things, and you may not be able to do some things. It all comes down to knowing yourself, your limits and how your body reacts in rope. A Top may have techniques that will help with a given goal, or they may not. It is the combination of both you and your Top's capabilities — both physical and skill-based — that determine if a given type of scene is possible.

Discuss medical issues that may impact what you want to do. Know your limits! These include:

- Physical injuries and previous surgeries that may impact what you can do.
- Bone issues, diabetes, asthma, breathing/cardiac issues, high or low blood pressure, fibromyalgia, being on powerful blood thinners, etc.
- Any mental or emotional triggers you may have that may be touched on by the scene you are negotiating.

## It is Crucial that you Evaluate your Own Risk and Communicate with your Top

If you do not communicate the relevant details about your medical, physical, emotional, and mental state before you begin, your Top will be unable to properly plan for your safety. If you are not comfortable disclosing those details to a particular Top, you should not scene with them.

If you do not communicate issues that are occurring while in a scene, your Top will be unable to address those issues.

If anything is feeling numb/tingling/cold/weird or if you are feeling "bad pain", tell your Top *immediately*.

If you are starting to become fatigued, let them know!

If you want to stop — no matter the reason — tell them!

Don't be afraid to speak up even if you only *think* something weird might be happening. Communicate honestly and early and your Top will have a better chance of fixing things before they become a problem.

Here is a helpful way of thinking about this:

### Immediate Actions

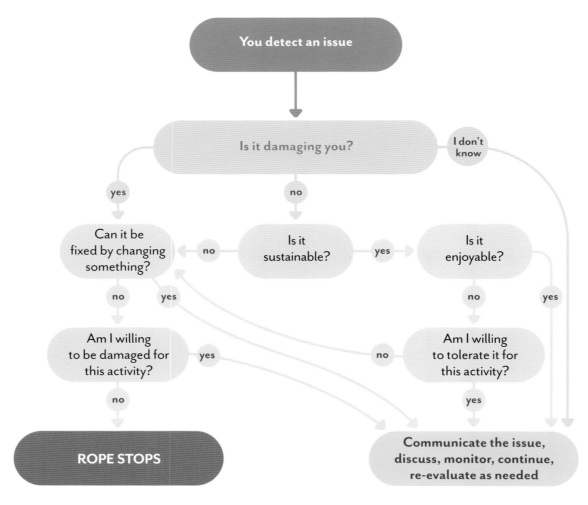

If you find yourself working through a decision like this, **share that decision making with your Top!** They need to know what you are thinking so they, too, can have input. If you decide that an activity is worth injuring yourself, but your Top does not agree, moving forward with that activity could be a violation of the *Top's* consent. **Make all risk-taking decisions** *explicit* and *together*!

## Other Important Considerations

Make sure you have a connection with your Top and feel you can trust them; by giving them this control, you *are* trusting them with a lot, perhaps even your life.

If your Rope Top is less experienced, limit the scene to less risky options. They may not yet understand how to control trailing rope ends and you could get hit by flailing ends, so protect your face and eyes! Don't watch them tying.

Going without clothing can make tying easier, if you are comfortable doing so. If you do wear clothing, wear something snug that doesn't reduce your range of motion. Slippery fabrics can cause the rope to move in unexpected ways; avoid them. When it comes to jewelry, minimize or remove anything that might become tangled in rope or be pressed into the skin. Alert your Top to anything that cannot be removed or that you choose to leave in place.

To maximize your safety and comfort while in scene, work on strength and flexibility training outside of play time. Pay special attention to the health and mobility of joints that you would like to put into stressful or unusual positions when in bondage.

Warm up before a scene. Stretch. Be careful not to stretch yourself too far, though. This could make overstretching and/or straining more likely. If there is a particular position you want to be tied in, practice assuming that position while not in bondage.

Accept the aftercare your Top offers, unless you know yourself well enough to know that you do not need it. Ask your Top if they have any aftercare needs, too! Let them know when you feel that your needs have been met and you are ready to end the aftercare session.

## Self-bondage Rules

- Never tie yourself up in a way that you cannot escape.
- Make sure your phone is charged and within reach.
- Always have a way to cut the rope in an emergency.
- Listen to (and respond to) your body.
- Set up a safe call for yourself. If something goes wrong and you cannot release yourself or reach your phone, you know someone will be checking on you.

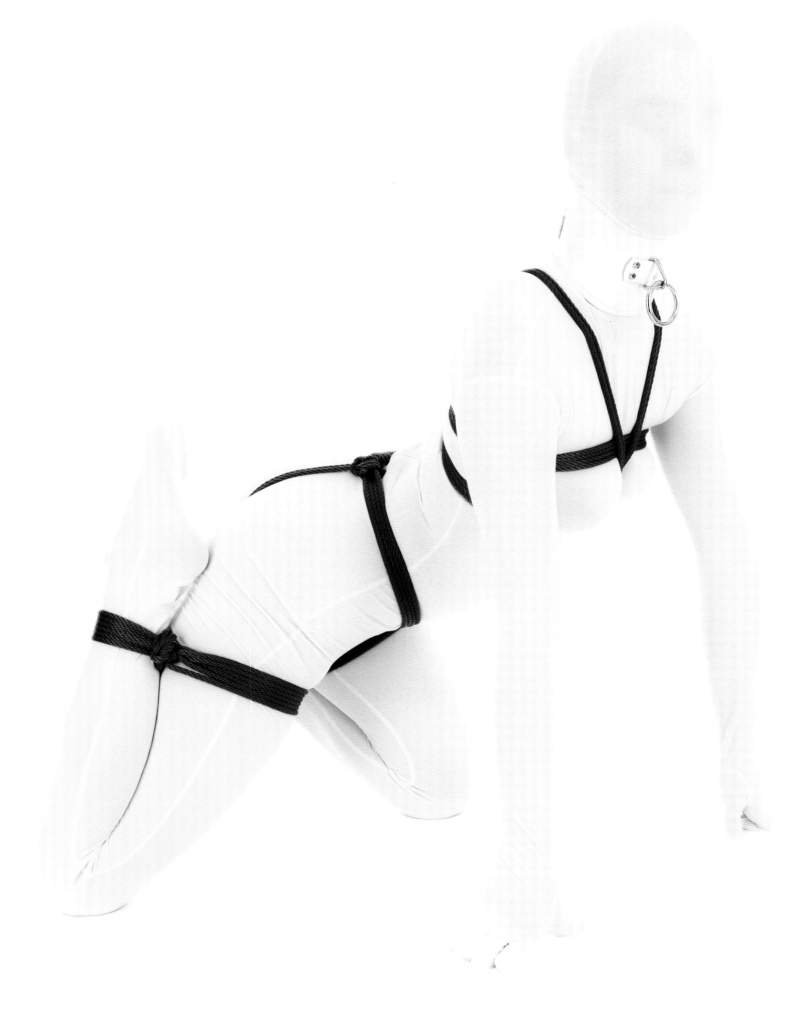

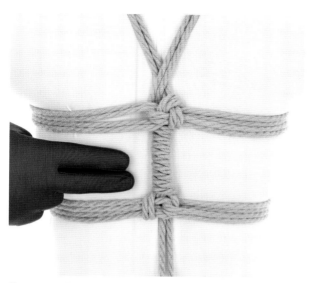

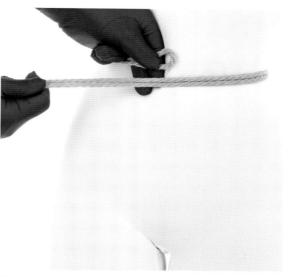

**Stem** — The vertical portion of rope that connects and stabilizes a rope harness. For example, the vertical line that runs between the upper and lower chest strap of a **Shinju** (p. 345).

**Forward tension** — This refers to the situation when a tie is executed with the rope continuing to travel in the same general direction.

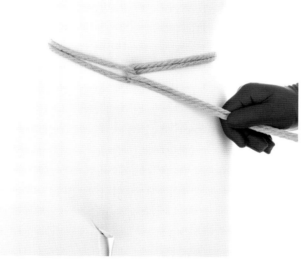

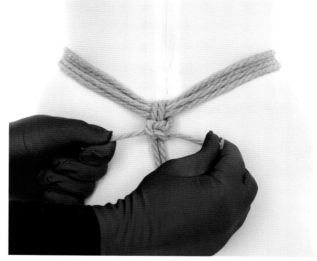

**Reverse tension** — This refers to the situation when a tie is executed with the rope changing the direction in which it is traveling at some point in time. This adds friction and creates a node that can be used as part of the structure of the tie. It also allows for the rigger to exert more control over their tie while rigging.

**Lock off the rope** — This means to tie the working end into the bondage so that the bondage will not come loose. This can be done in any way that will work in that situation. Typically, this is done by adding a **Half Hitch** or two, or a **Square Knot**, but there are other options covered in *How to "Lock Off"* (p. 168) and in *Using Up Rope* (p. 279).

# Finding the Bight (The Middle of the Rope)

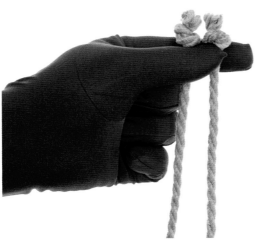

**1.** Hold the ends of the rope in one hand.

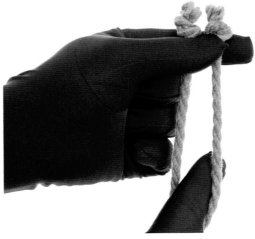

**2.** Put a finger of your other hand between them and...

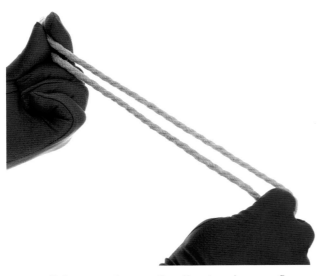

**3.** ...pull the strands equally, allowing them to flow around your finger...

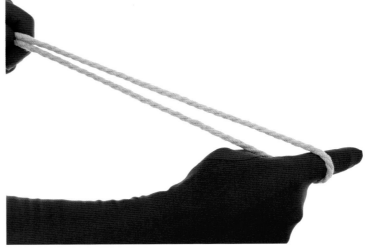

**4.** ...until you get to the end. This is the middle of the rope, called the bight or the primary bight.

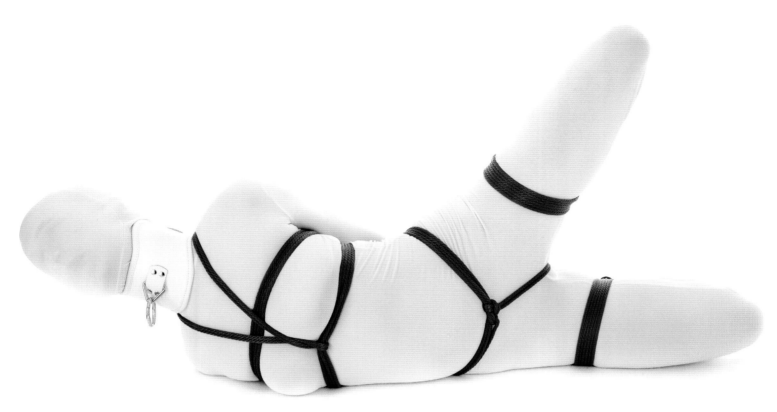

# Layering Bondage

Most bondage scenes or scenarios are made up of more than one element. Perhaps you have a chest harness and a waist harness and rope cuffs on both wrists and both ankles, and all these elements are attached to each other, or to a bed or chair. You can add layer after layer of bondage to make a scene more interesting or more restrictive.

Layering bondage is where you can begin to exercise your creativity and create intricate-looking scenes.

For lots of fun examples and inspiration, check out the *Building Great Scenes Using Multiple Ties* chapter (p. 383).

# Western vs. Eastern Style

Western style and eastern style are two main styles of rope bondage; each has various sub-styles and fusion styles. The primary difference is in which part of the rope you start with when beginning a tie.

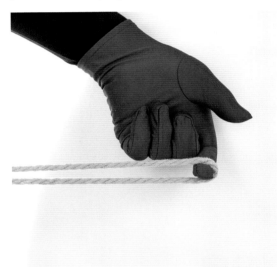

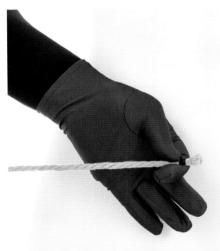

**Eastern style or Japanese style** — Starts with the bight of a rope folded in two. Often is also concerned with the esthetic appeal of a tie. Most of the techniques in this book are eastern style.

**Western style** — Starts from the end of the rope and ties with one line. Think of cowboys tying up cattle in the old west.

Most common ties are of the eastern style as this method allows the rigger to lay down two strands at once. This is helpful because we often want at least four strands for a cuff or strap to distribute force across a wider area and reduce the risk of injury. Tying with two strands at once also allows us to do so more quickly.

# Collapsing vs. Non-collapsing Loops

Collapsing loop — Sometimes also called a noose. This is a loop that will get smaller and tighter when the tail is pulled. Example: **A Lark's Head Knot** (p. 243). *A collapsing loop should never be used on a human; it must be converted into a non-collapsing loop.*

   Non-collapsing loop — Sometimes also called a stable loop. This is a loop of rope that will not get smaller or tighten when the tail is pulled. One common way to convert a collapsing loop to a non-collapsing one is to add a **Half Hitch** (p. 132).

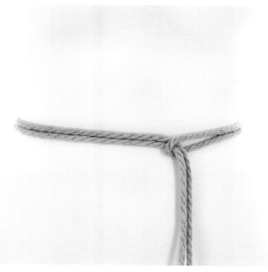

**1.** If you run the tail of a rope through the bight, you have created a **Lark's Head Knot** around the waist.

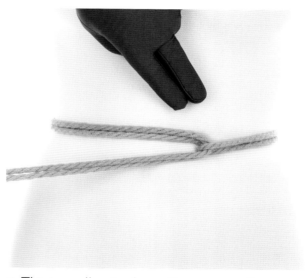

**2.** This is a collapsing loop. *Never use a collapsing loop directly on a person.*

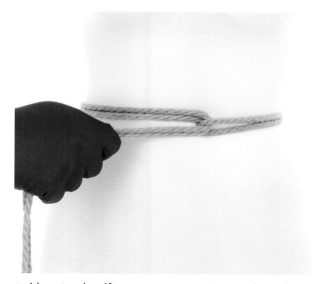

**3.** Here is why: If you reverse tension on the tail like I am doing here, then....

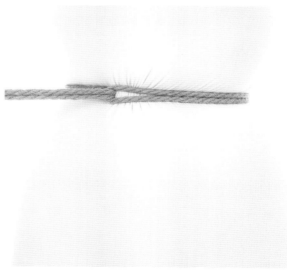

**4.** ...pull on the tail, it will collapse — get tighter. This is dangerous. *continues...*

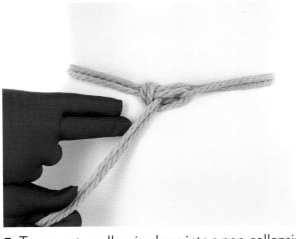

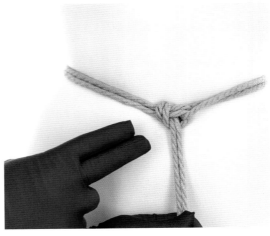

**5.** To convert a collapsing loop into a non-collapsing loop, add a **Half Hitch**. This is just a new loop around the existing lines.

**6.** Tighten the **Half Hitch**.

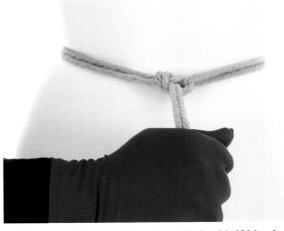

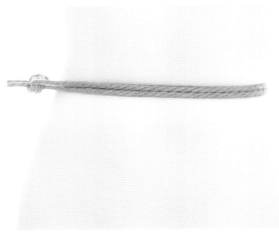

**7.** This time if you pull on the tail, the **Half Hitch** grabs all the strands it goes around and pulls them all together.

**8.** This way the loop can no longer collapse.

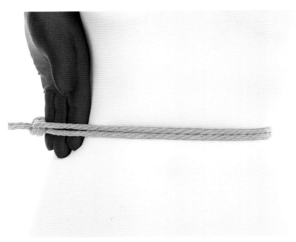

**9.** Instead of getting tighter, the loop stays the same size, no matter how hard I pull.

# Your Toy Bag

Your toy bag will reflect you and the things you like to do. But there are a few items that should always be included.

## Recommended

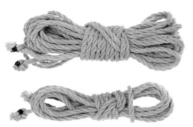 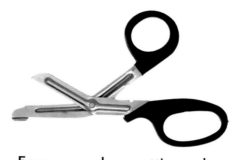 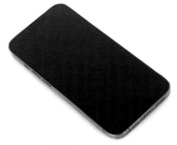

**General-use rope** — Of course! Have enough to do what you have planned and perhaps a little more just in case inspiration strikes!

**Emergency release cutting tool** — This should be EMT shears and/or EMT cutting hook.

**Phone** — Another important piece of emergency equipment. If needed, you can look up first aid or call for help. Make sure it is charged!

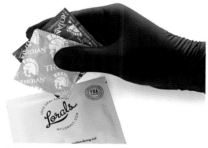 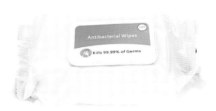 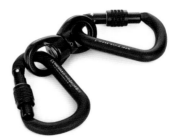

**Safer sex supplies** — Barriers like nitrile gloves, condoms, and dental dams keep everyone safe. Hand sanitizer too.

**Cleaning supplies** — Sanitizing wipes (alcohol/antiseptic) are good for cleaning furniture or equipment.

**Connectors** — Carabiners and panic snaps can be helpful for making quick connections and for other purposes.

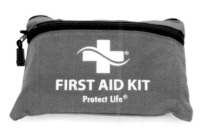 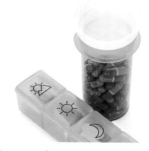 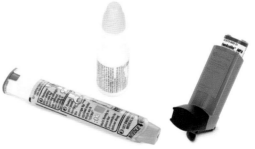

**Basic First Aid kit** — A small kit with a few important pieces:
- Adhesive bandages (various sizes)
- Antibiotic topical ointment
- Anti-inflammatory medication
- Elastic bandage
- Gauze wrap/pads
- Nitrile protective gloves
- Activated cold pack

**Any medication you need** — Make sure that you both are in your best state. You've taken your meds. You have both eaten and had some water recently.

**Emergency medical supplies, if applicable** — Glucagon kit, asthma inhaler, EpiPen, etc. If someone involved in the scene may have an emergency, have what they may need within arm's reach.

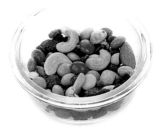

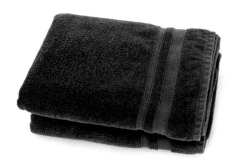

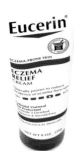

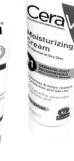

**Healthy snack and water** — To restore hydration and blood sugar after a scene. Straws can be helpful.

**Towel/blanket** — Helpful for laying on furniture or floor for hygiene purposes, and for aftercare.

**Lotion** — Helpful for aftercare massage, if desired. Be sure to have a hypoallergenic kind.

# Optional but Useful

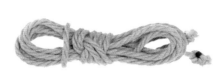

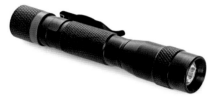

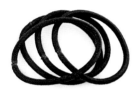

**Fluid-bonded rope** — Your partner's fluid-bonded rope, if appropriate. See *Rope Hygiene* (p. 78).

**Small flashlight** — Play spaces are often dark; a flashlight is less intrusive than a phone.

**Hair ties** — Super helpful to have on hand in case you tie someone with long hair.

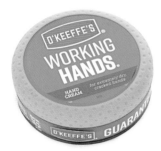

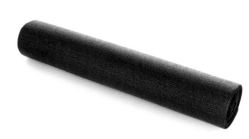

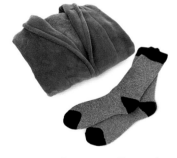

**Hand cream** — Tying can be rough on your hands. Using a good cream after you tie can help.

**Exercise mat** — If you are tying someplace with a hard floor, a mat will provide a softer surface.

**Warming fuzzies** — Something to keep you and your partner warm throughout or after a scene.

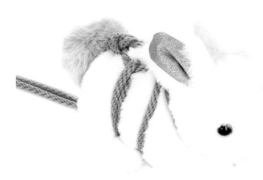

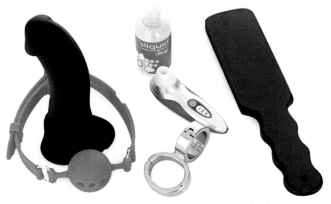

**Person-specific aftercare tools** — If you know a person's favorite comfort item, bring it!

**Toys for other types of play** — Rope isn't the only game in town!

# Rope Itself — Type, Thickness, Length

A very common question is, "What type of rope should I use?" Well, as with most things, there is no one true way. It depends on what you want to use it for.

## Types

There are many types of rope. They all have their own unique look and feel. Natural vs. synthetic fiber, braided vs. twisted, twisted one way vs. the other. There are many options.

When you are just starting out, use something inexpensive that feels good in your hands and on your skin. You don't have to make any big investment in high-quality bondage rope until you know that you really enjoy it. Don't get me wrong, hemp and jute when processed for use in bondage feel great and are a pleasure to tie with, but there is quite a bit of work that goes into that processing, so they do come with a price tag. Many people start with other choices.

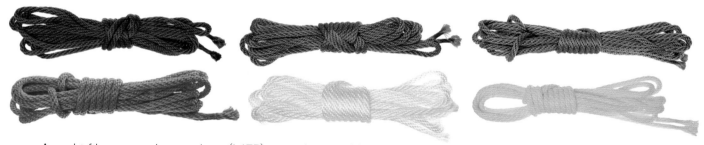

A multi-filament polypropylene (MFP) rope designed for bondage can be a good starting choice. It is less expensive and has decent "tooth" (friction) so that knots and ties will hold well if you make them tight. It also comes in lots of colors. There are a number of good sources for MFP online or you can head over to TheDuchy.com for links to good sources of rope. Nylon is also popular, but is a little more slippery; you will sometimes need to double your knots to make it hold properly.

Maybe you prefer the feel or look of a natural fiber rope like hemp or jute. That's a great choice, too! However, you do want to be more careful where you buy natural fiber rope. If you buy such rope from a hardware store, it will be in a rough and raw state — it will have lots of fibers sticking out of it and it will not have been oiled. Riggers do a few things to their ropes to lower their tendency to give rope burn and to increase the life of the rope. They add small amounts of stable oil to them (jojoba oil is popular, as is mineral oil) and they burn off the extra fibers, and may do other things to break in the rope. If you buy rope from a hardware store, understand that it may be less comfortable to work with. Then again, some people prefer that rougher feeling!

## Rope Types

### What Type of Rope is Best for You?

| | Type | Popularity | Cost[1] | Breaking Strength[2] (lbs) | Roughness[3] | Water? | Suspension? | Comments |
|---|---|---|---|---|---|---|---|---|
| **Natural Fiber** | Hemp | ★★★★ | $$$ | 600 | ★★★ | | ✓ | Very popular with riggers worldwide. Has a classic look and can be used in suspension. Can be dyed, but the colors will be muted or rich, rarely bright. |
| | Jute | ★★★★ | $$$ | 200 | ★★★ | | | Very popular with riggers worldwide. Has a classic look and can be used in suspension. Can be dyed, but the colors will be muted or rich, rarely bright. |
| | Cotton | ★★★ | $ | 350 | ★★ | ✓ | | A common starter rope; inexpensive, light, soft, but still holds knots well. Look for "three-strand twisted". Avoid "solid core" versions. Takes dye well. |
| | Linen/ Flax | ★★ | $$ | 400 | ★★★ | | | Very similar to hemp, but softer and tends to be more consistent in appearance. |
| | Coconut | ★★ | $ | 80 | ★★★★ | | | Extremely rough. More for torment then confinement. Most people just stop struggling altogether after a little time in coconut rope. |
| **Synthetic Fiber** | Nylon | ★★★ | $ | 1450 | ★ | ✓ | | Another common starter rope. Watch out for hardware store nylon/poly blends; if you try to dye them, the poly part won't take the dye. |
| | MFP | ★★★ | $$ | 1100 | ★ | ✓ | ✓ | Works like nylon, but knots tend to hold somewhat better. Comes in lots of colors. Can't be dyed at home. Some like this for suspension anchor lines. |
| | POSH | ★★ | $$$ | 1200 | ★★ | ✓ | ✓ | Looks and handles similarly to hemp. Popular for suspension support lines as it is much stronger than natural hemp. |
| | Hempex | ★ | $ | 1100 | ★★★ | ✓ | ✓ | Another synthetic hemp substitute. Not as popular as POSH, but still good. |

Rope can be grouped into two main families:

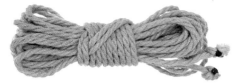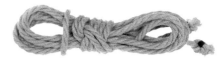

Natural fiber ropes — These generally have better friction or "tooth," so knots grab better and it takes less to get them to hold securely. They also don't stretch as much and have more consistent stretch characteristics. Dye can work in unusual ways with these ropes and it can be hard to get bright colors.
*Common Types:* Hemp, Jute, Cotton

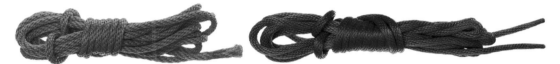

Synthetic fiber ropes — These usually have a smoother, more supple feel. They are stronger and can be more easily cleaned. They often have less tooth than natural fiber ropes, so you may need to double some kinds of knots. They can be found in many colors. They can be a little inconsistent/unpredictable with how they stretch, so they are less commonly used for harnesses when doing suspension, but POSH and Hempex (and, to a lesser extent, MFP) are commonly used for suspension lines.
*Common types:* Nylon, MFP, POSH, Hempex

## What type of rope is best for you?

You're going to have to try a few types and see what you like! If you join a rope group, you can ask people what types they have and if you can see what they feel like.

The table on the facing page breaks down different kinds of ropes that are more popular for bondage and their various qualities so you can decide for yourself. If you do not see a particular type, it means it is not as commonly used. Perhaps it is too rough (sisal, manila), too weak, too expensive (silk, bamboo, alpaca), or too stiff and uncomfortable (regular polypropylene) for rope bondage. You will find people that do use these less common types, but as this is a foundations book, we will stick to the more popular options.

**Footnotes (table)**
**1 Cost** — The higher cost shown for hemp and jute is if you buy it from a rope bondage supplier and it has already been processed with oils and had excess fibers removed, etc. If you buy it raw and process it yourself, the cost of the rope is much lower.
**2 Breaking Strength** — These numbers (rounded down) are guidelines only and assume lab conditions with new ¼-inch rope. There is tremendous variation in these numbers from different manufacturers, so always check the specs from the source you are considering. Note: For liability reasons, it is quite common for bondage rope producers to not publish breaking strength numbers for natural fiber ropes. Sources for the numbers in the table: rwrope.com, ropeandcord.com, engineeringtoolbox.com
**3 Roughness** — This is a proxy for how it will feel on the skin and for how well knots will hold. Rope that is more rough (has more "tooth") will tend to hold knots better. Too much roughness and it will tend to jam — which is why manila rope is not on this list.

# Rope Construction

The choice of twisted or braided rope is a personal preference, but they do look and behave differently. Twisted rope has more bumps in it which tends to increase the friction and make knots hold nicely. Braided rope is smoother and some feel it is more sensuous. Generally, riggers tend not to mix different types of rope in a single scene as it looks odd, aesthetically speaking.

    * For bondage purposes, avoid rope that has a core. A core adds strength, but it holds the rope more rigidly in shape. The rope can not flatten as much, which means that force is more concentrated in a narrower area instead of being spread more evenly across the skin; this increases the risk of injury to nerves or blood vessels.

    ** Paracord — Braided nylon sheath over twisted nylon thread making up the core. Not common, but has use in certain types of specialty bondage not covered in this book, like microbondage and Hojōjutsu.

## Twisted Strand Rope Construction

Many people love the look and feel of traditional rope, which is twisted strand rope made of natural fibers. Here are the names of the various parts of a twisted strand rope:

**❶** A twisted strand **rope** is made up of...
**❷** ...three to five **strands** (three is the most common).
**❸** Strands are made up of **yarns**. (In this rope, each strand is composed of 4 yarns.)
**❹** Yarns are made of individual **fibers**.

Each layer is twisted in the opposite direction of the layer before. This interconnects all the fibers, allowing their internal friction to grip each other firmly to make a strong rope.

    One of the reasons we recommend using **The Hook** or **The Scissor** technique to handle rope (p. 156) is because if you use your thumb and forefinger in a pincher-like movement to grab the rope, you might grab just one strand and not the whole rope. If you do that and pull, you can pull the strands apart, "unlaying" them. This is called hyperthreading, and it is not good for your rope. It is difficult to get your rope properly back in order (to "re-lay" it) if it has been pulled apart like this and, even if you do get it to look right, it will never be quite as strong.

    Damage from hyperthreading is one of the things you look for when you are inspecting rope.

Rope can be constructed in a number of common ways. Here are a few examples:

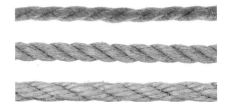

**Twisted strand** — Good for bondage. Twists can go either way. Tends to feel rougher. *Common Types: Hemp, Jute, Cotton.*

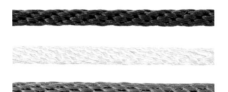

**Braided** (but not solid core) — Good for bondage. Tends to feel smoother. *Common Types: Nylon, MFP (Multi-filament polypropylene).*

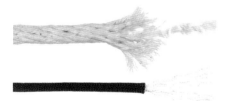

**Solid core** — Not good for bondage.* Braided sheath over twisted nylon thread makes up the core. *Common Types: Solid core Nylon, Cotton sash cord, Paracord***

# Inspecting Rope

Rope is a consumable. It will get used up and will need to be replaced. As it gets used, it gets worn — fibers break, strands or yarns stretch at different rates than others, and it gets nicked, hyperthreaded, subjected to rope burn or kinked. You need to routinely inspect your rope to confirm that it is still in good condition.

- Look over the entire rope for wear. The bight and the ends tend to take the most wear.
- Look for uneven wear/stretched fibers. This can show as a rope that looks like a slight spiral.
- Look for fibers that have been broken or melted by excess friction.

This is critically important, so it bears repeating: Rope is a consumable. Don't treat it like a precious commodity. Replace it when it gets worn. This is *especially* important if that rope is going to be used in suspension.

A retired piece of rope can go on to live a new life in several ways. Longer pieces of rope are often most worn at the bight and at the ends. If you cut those parts out and keep the resulting shorter pieces, they can be a convenient size for wrists or ankles, or for extending rope near the end of a tie if you need just a little more.

If you cannot salvage portions of the rope, you can use it to make impact toys like a flogger! See Flogger Forge on TheDuchy.com (TheDuchy.com/flogger-forge/) for instructions on making any of these impact toys or designing your own!

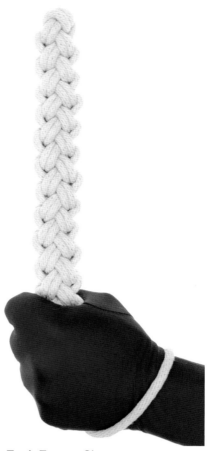

Zoe's Zipper-Slapper.

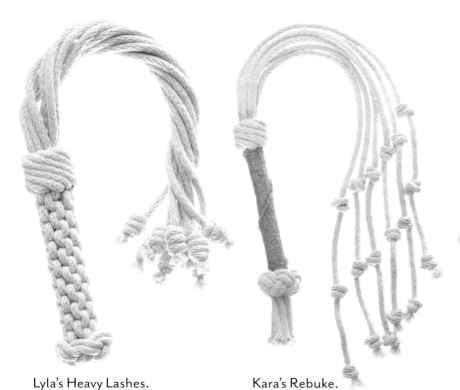

Lyla's Heavy Lashes.    Kara's Rebuke.    Tonyas Twisted Tongue.

## Coloring or Dying Ropes

- MFP or nylon can be purchased in the color you want.
- White nylon can be dyed at home to any range of color, including bright or light colors.
- Cotton can be dyed at home. This can also achieve bright or light colors.
- Hemp or jute can be dyed at home, but the color is duller/more matte. A deep, rich color can be achieved if you put in double the amount of dye.

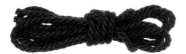

Nylon (1 packet of dye).

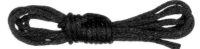

Hemp (2 packets of dye).

Note: If you buy your rope from a hardware store, be aware that polypropylene ("poly") doesn't accept common dyes. If you buy a nylon/poly blend (a very common type of rope), dyeing it will have this effect:

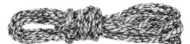

Nylon/Poly-Pro (1 packet).

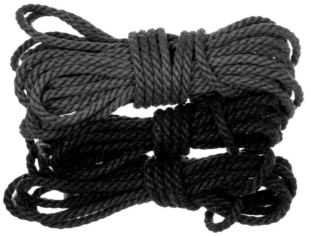

Hemp, dyed by manufacturer.

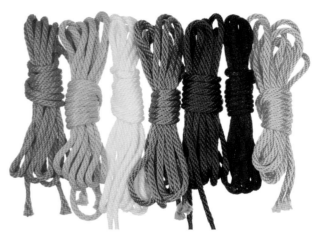

MFP, dyed by manufacturer.

The next questions are usually:
- What thickness (diameter) should I use?
- What lengths of rope should I have, and how many of each?

## Recommended Thickness (Diameter)

As with everything else, there is no one correct way of doing things. That said:

- The most commonly used diameter is ¼-inch, often sold as 6mm. This is the most flexible for the widest variety of bondage situations.
- Many riggers recommend ⁵⁄₁₆-inch for suspension support lines (aka "up lines" or "anchor lines"), although ¼-inch is also common, especially if it is MFP or POSH.
- Some riggers use ⁵⁄₁₆-inch or ⅜-inch diameter when working with bottoms with larger body types. This can help make things more comfortable, but comes with trade offs. See *Body Type Considerations* (p. 324) for more.
- Less commonly, but not unusual, some riggers love ³⁄₁₆-inch for floor work (non-suspension bondage) as it is more intense and the look is different.

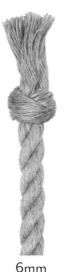
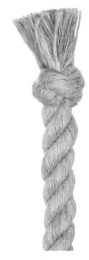

6mm          8mm

# Recommended Lengths

It is important to understand that every person you tie will be a different build and will require a different amount of rope, even for the same tie. A 6-foot body builder will need more rope for a chest or waist harness than a 5-foot person of slimmer build. You will almost never have rope that is exactly the right length to make a tie come out perfectly.

There are techniques for extending rope when you need more for a given tie (p. 274), and there are techniques for "using up" leftover rope (p. 279).

Unless there is a special need, most riggers work with a kit that include these standard lengths:

- 26 to 30 feet — Good for harnesses and long runs. This is sometimes simply called a "rope."
- 15 feet — Good around thighs or knees, as a waist belt, or when you need to extend a rope. This is sometimes referred to as a "half rope."
- 10 feet — Good for wrists or ankles or tying limbs to bedposts, stuff like that. This is sometimes referred to as a "short rope."

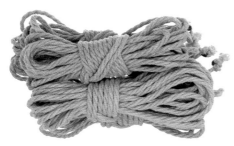 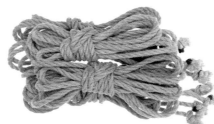 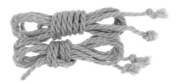

# A Beginner's Rope Kit

My standard kit includes:

- Four or more 30 feet pieces. This gives me two ropes for a chest harness and two for a waist harness.
- Four or more 15 feet pieces. This gives me one for each limb.
- Two or more 10 feet pieces. This is a convenient length for a **Double Column** or for **Extending Rope**.
- Other items listed in *Your Toy Bag* (p. 93).

Many riggers only use two lengths: The 30 feet "rope" and the 15 feet "half rope" above. This gives them less to organize and manage, while still having good flexibility.

Some only carry one length: The 30 feet rope. They never fish for a different length of rope (they are all the same) but they *do* have to plan ahead to manage or use up the tails.

As you practice and experiment, you will figure out what you like.

# Coiling and Storing Rope

There are lots of options for this as well but here are a few of the most common.

### Hanging Your Rope

If you have the space and privacy, consider just hanging your rope over a dowel or closet rod. You will only want to do this if you have a rod that is wider than 1½-inches, so that you don't kink your rope too sharply. This is what I do for the ropes I use every day.

### Creating a Hank, Figure–8 Style

Most people want to keep their ropes in convenient bundles, called hanks.

One of the more useful ways to wrap ropes is in a Figure-8 pattern. By doing this, the hank will be less likely to become tangled.

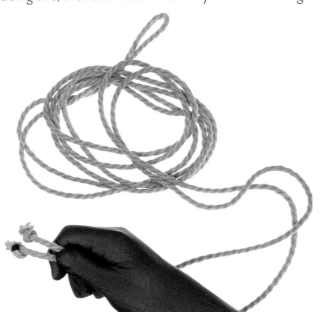

**1.** Find both ends of your rope.

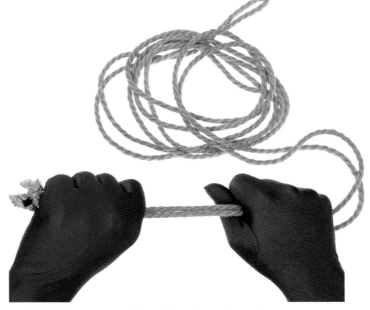

**2.** Hold the rope with both hands in the palms-downward position, about 8-10 inches apart. Have the ends in your left hand.

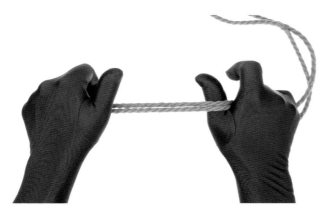

**3.** Put your left thumb on top of the rope and your right thumb under.

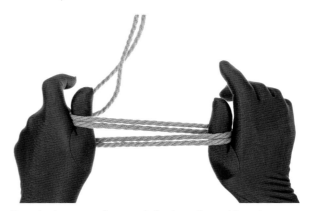

**4.** Reach down with your left thumb and hook the rope.

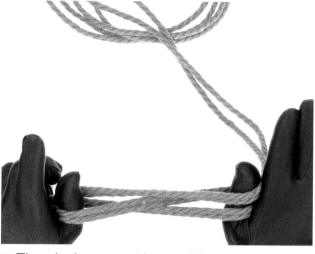

**5.** Then do the same with your right.

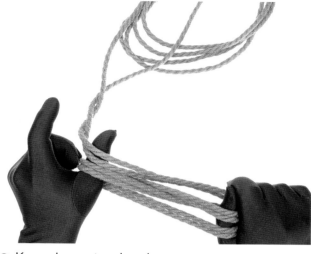

**6.** Keep alternating thumbs...

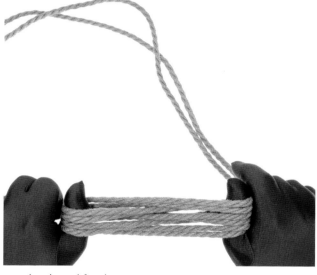

**7.** ...back and forth...

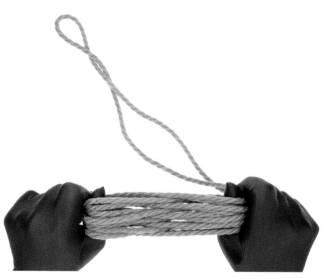

**8.** ...until you are near the end.

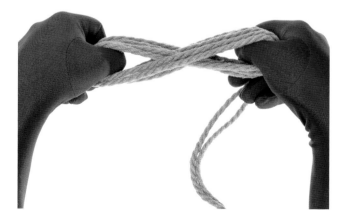

**9.** You should now have a nicely organized Figure-8 pattern like this...

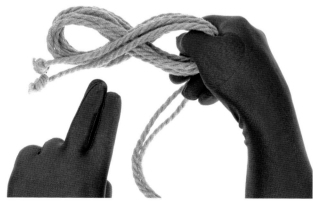

**10.** ...with the end neatly within the pattern.

*continues...*

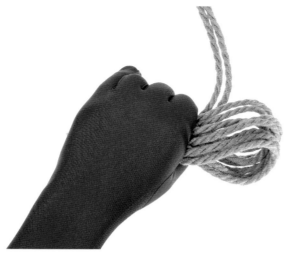

**11.** Shift your grip.

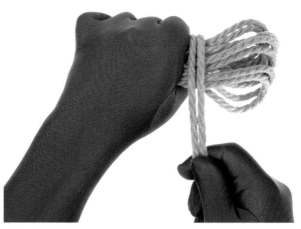

**12.** Begin wrapping the remaining tail around the hank.

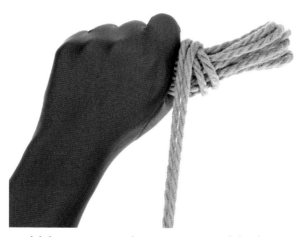

**13.** Make your second wrap over top of the first wrap.

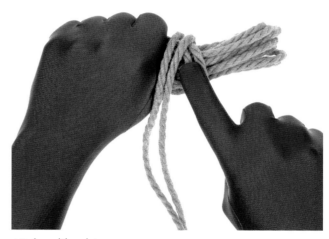

**14.** Just like this.

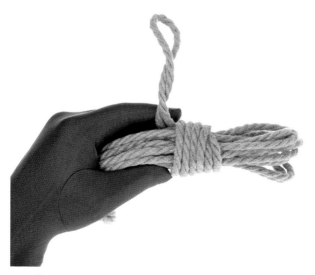

**15.** Continue wrapping until you have 4 inches or so remaining.

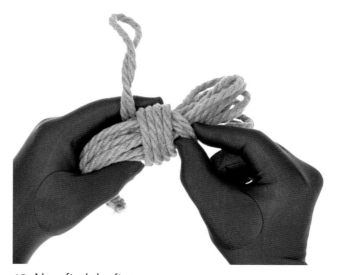

**16.** Now find the first wrap...

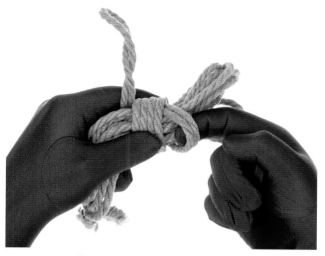

**17.** ...and pull it out just a little.

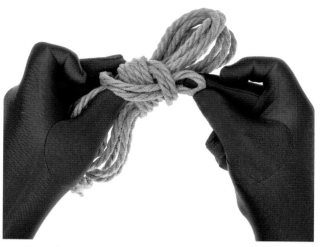

**18.** Run the bight under that first wrap.

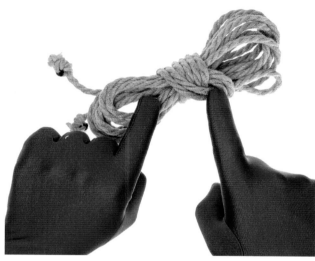

**19.** Now find the other side of that first wrap.

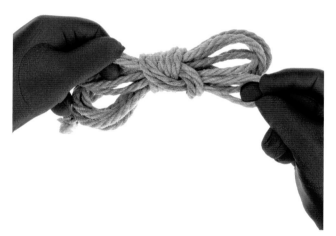

**20.** Pull it and the bight in opposite directions to tighten.

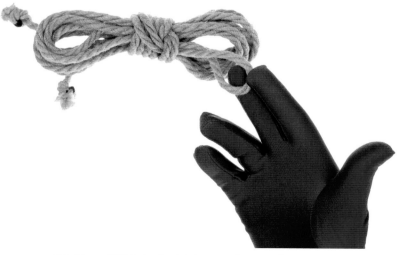

**21.** Done! This is the bight, ready to go!

## Coiling and Storing Rope

### Storing Rope Longer

If you will be storing your rope for longer than a week or two, do one more thing. This helps protect the bight and is better if you are going to store your ropes for a longer time.

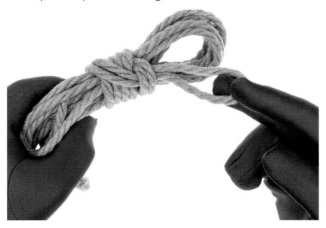

**22.** Continue from where you left off.

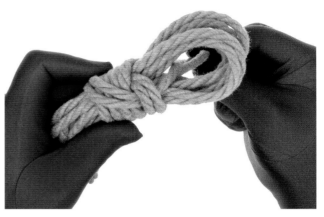

**23.** Run the bight through the coils of the rope.

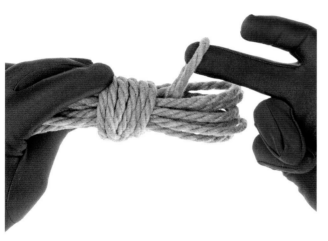

**24.** Like this.

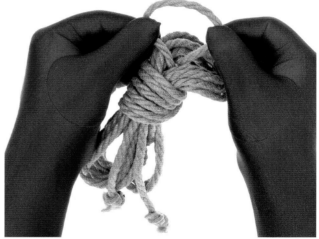

**25.** On the other side of the coil, grab the bight, open it into a loop, then...

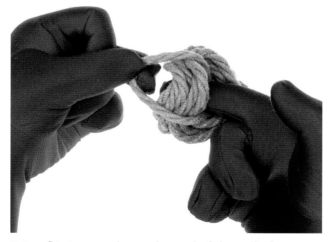

**26.** ...flip it up and over the end of the coil of rope.

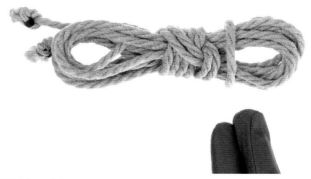

**27.** Like this.

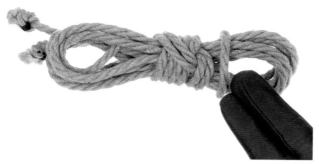

**28.** The bight is barely bent at all. This is better for rope longevity.

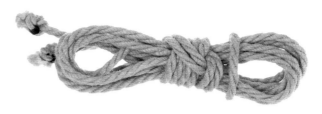

**29.** Your completed hank should look like this from one side...

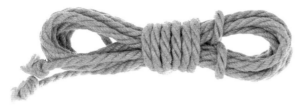

**30.** ...and this from the other.

## Long Term Storage

If you are not going to use your ropes for months at a time or longer, it is better to put them into a simple coil. Doing so means that no part of the rope is bent at too great an angle for too long a period. Your ropes will be in better condition when you come back to them.

- To do this, start at the end, not the bight.
- Then do a simple coil.
- Use a piece of string or twist tie, etc., around the ends to hold the coil together, if desired.
- Store the coil somewhere dark and dry.

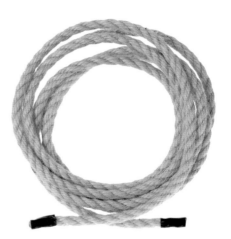

## Coiling and Storing Rope

**When You are Ready to Use Your Rope**

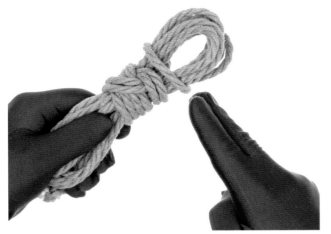

**1.** If your bight is through the hank...

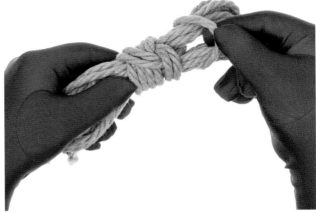

**2.** ...free it first.

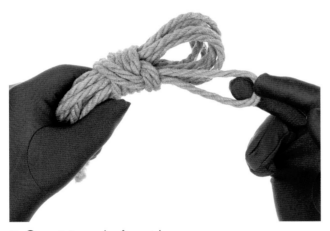

**3.** Once it is on the first side...

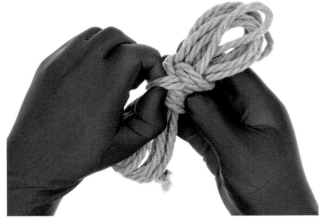

**4.** ...free it from the wrap.

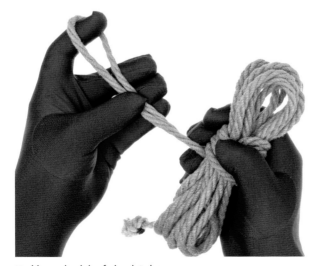

**5.** Keep hold of the bight.

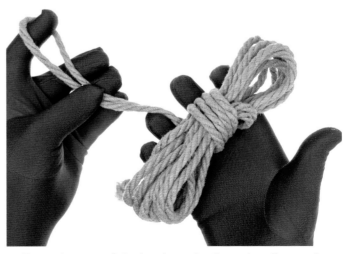

**6.** Drop the rest of the hank on the floor. It will uncoil without tangling and you are ready to tie!

## Chain Stitch

This can be a good choice when you need to wash your ropes. Put your rope into a loose chain stitch and throw it into a laundry bag. This will allow the water and soap better access to the individual strands and will result in better cleaning but will not let it get turned into a tangled mess.

This approach is quite stable but is not good for long-term storage. If you leave your rope stored in this way for even a few days, it tends to be a bit kinky when undone.

(Pauses for the obvious joke.)

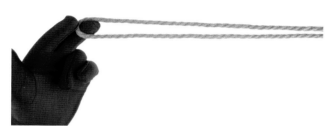

**1.** Begin with your rope folded in half.

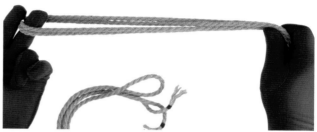

**2.** If your rope is long, perhaps fold it in half again.

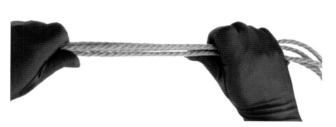

**3.** Hold the bight and...

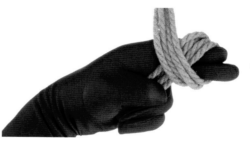

**4.** ...make a small loop over your fingers with the tail.

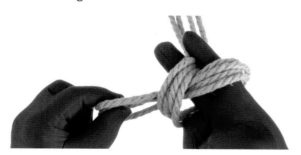

**5.** Reach through that loop and grab the tail.

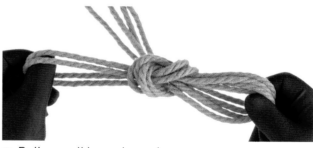

**6.** Pull a small loop through.

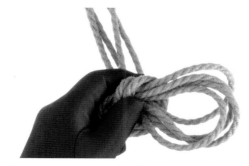

**7.** Like this. Don't make the loop too big.

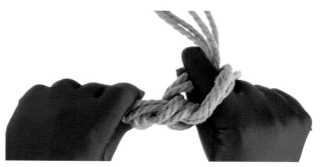

**8.** Reach through that new small loop and grab the tail.

*continues...*

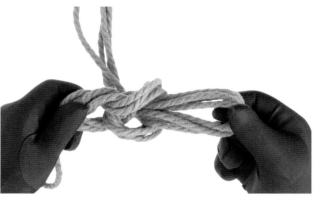

**9.** Pull yet another small loop through.

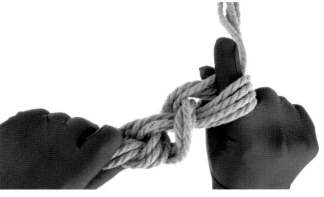

**10.** Repeat until you run out of rope.

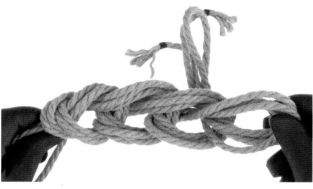

**11.** When you reach the end...

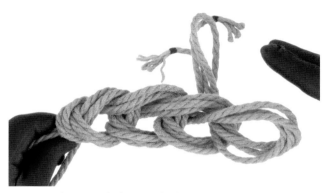

**12.** ...and you only have a little tail left...

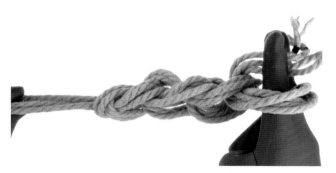

**13.** ...pull the last little bit of the tail all the way though.

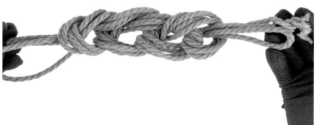

**14.** Like this. This locks it off.

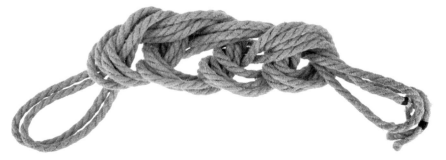

**15.** Done!

**Untying a Chain Stitch**

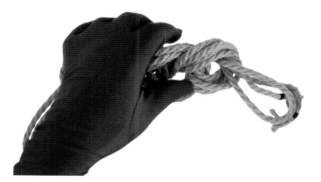

**1.** When you are ready to use the rope...

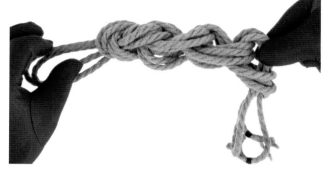

**2.** ...grab the bight...

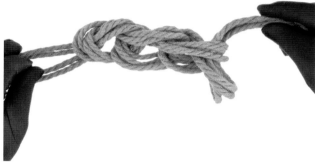

**3.** ...then remove the tail from the last loop.

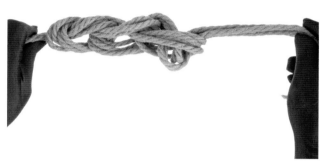

**4.** Pull the tail.

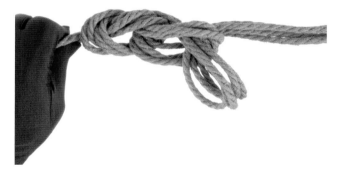

**5.** The whole chain will come undone.

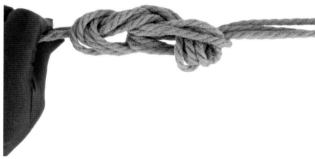

**6.** Keep going.

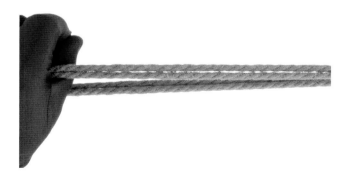

**7.** Keep going!

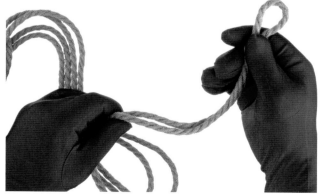

**8.** Grab the bight and you are ready to go!

# Rope Ends

There are many ways to finish off the ends of your rope to keep them from unraveling — from the simple and fast to the decorative. Here are a few of the popular ways. There are *many* more.

For more detailed step-by-step instructions and videos, check out: TheDuchy.com/rope-ends/.

Some people prefer smooth ends with no knots. Others prefer having small knots at the end as it makes it easier to extend rope (p. 274) and can give you more options for locking off a tie (p. 168). The trade-off to knotted ends is that there is a minor speed bump at the end when doing a tail pull. Some riggers put knots in the end of their rope and some don't. Try it yourself and decide what you like!

Here are some examples shown on ¼-inch twisted Hemp, in order of bulk.

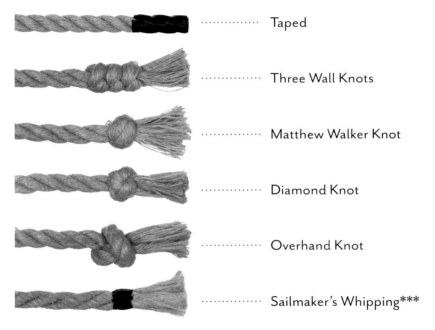

- .............. Taped
- .............. Three Wall Knots
- .............. Matthew Walker Knot
- .............. Diamond Knot
- .............. Overhand Knot
- .............. Sailmaker's Whipping***

*** Whipping is the application of smaller cord, string, or thread to the end of the rope to keep it from unraveling. We include this example as it is a popular option from some suppliers and is popular with some riggers. Techniques for whipping rope are not included in this book.

# Use an Overhand Knot

The simplest knot to end your rope is the **Overhand Knot** (p. 124). The trade-off is that it is more bulky than other choices.

    You want to make that knot in the correct direction so as to maintain the twists of the rope.

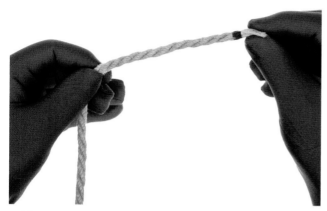

**1.** If using a twisted-strand rope...

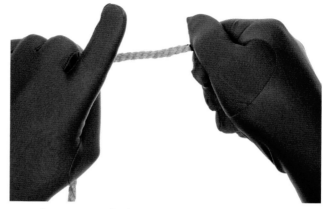

**2.** ...determine which direction you need to twist it in order to tighten the twist.

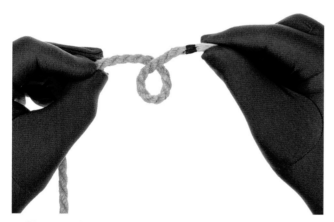

**3.** Twist in that direction until it automatically creates a loop.

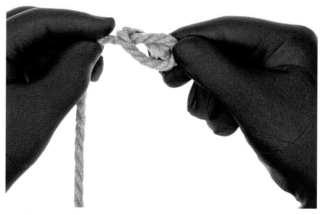

**4.** Tuck the end through that loop.

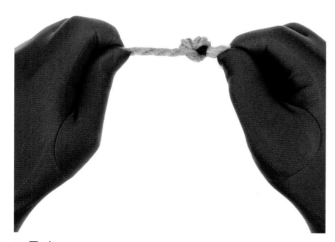

**5.** Tighten..

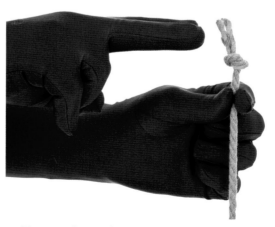

**6.** Trim to about ¾-inch.

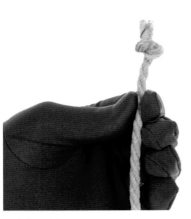

**7.** Like this.

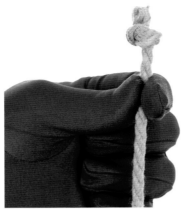

**8.** Done!

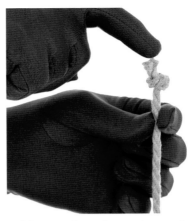

**9.** You can fuzz the end to make it look nicer.

## Tape and/or Melt the Ends

Another simple ending technique is to tape the end before you cut the rope.

If the rope is made of synthetic fiber, you can also gently melt the tip of the end.

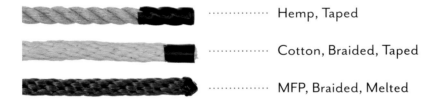

·············· Hemp, Taped

·············· Cotton, Braided, Taped

·············· MFP, Braided, Melted

## Tool Dip

You can use tool dip, but use this trick to get nice ends.

Do the dipping in two stages:

- Cut your rope and immediately dip it about 1 inch.
- Hang your rope with the ends downward.
- Let that first dipping dry. The end might still spread out a little while it is drying.
- Once it is dry, trim a little off the end of the rope to remove the part that spread out. Be sure to leave at least ½-¾ inch of dipped end remaining.
- Then dip that much cleaner end a second time.
- Hang to dry.

# The Matthew Walker Knot for 3-Stranded Rope

One issue with using an **Overhand Knot** is that it is quite bulky. That means that it is more difficult to pull through when doing a tail pull. There are other knots that are a little smaller and more streamlined. The **Matthew Walker Knot** is a great choice for this.

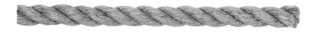

**1.** This is easiest if you start with a freshly-cut rope.

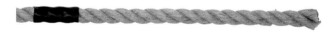
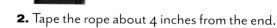

**2.** Tape the rope about 4 inches from the end.

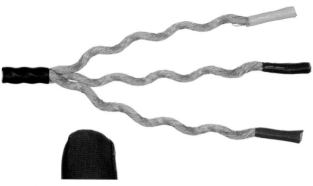

**3.** Unlay the rope.

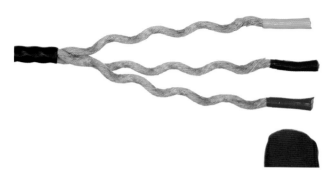

**4.** The first few times you try this, you may want to tape the ends of each strand as well to keep them in order. I am going to color-code them to make it easier to see what is happening.

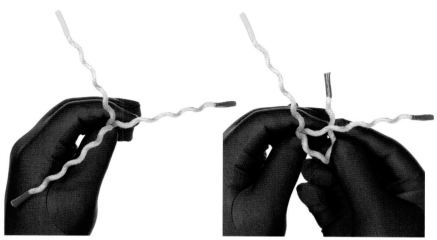
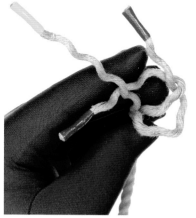

**5.** Look at the knot from above.

**6.** Take each strand and run it under the next strand in order. So... red under blue...

**7.** ...blue under yellow...

*continues...*

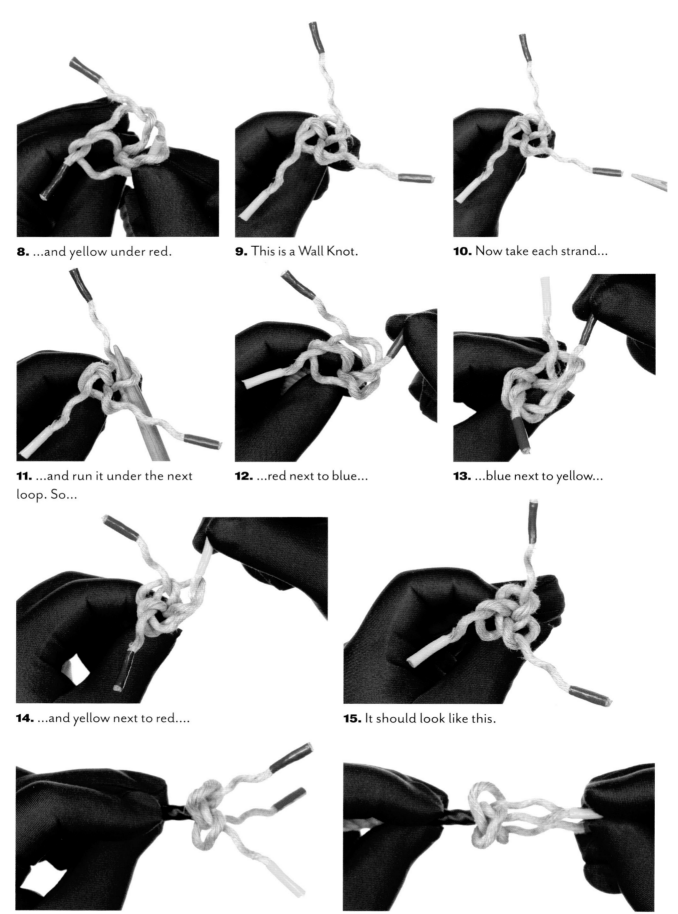

**8.** ...and yellow under red.

**9.** This is a Wall Knot.

**10.** Now take each strand...

**11.** ...and run it under the next loop. So...

**12.** ...red next to blue...

**13.** ...blue next to yellow...

**14.** ...and yellow next to red....

**15.** It should look like this.

**16.** Now turn the knot sideways.

**17.** Gently pull the strands just a little.

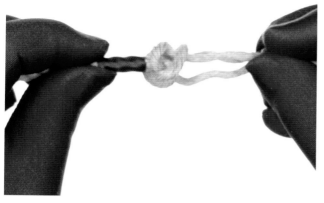

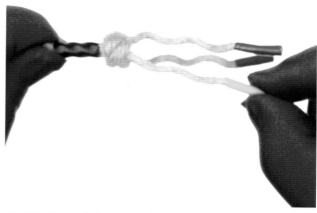

**18.** Work the knot to move the strands down so that they are tight against the tape collar you created in Step 2.

**19.** Work carefully to get the strands to lay neatly. You may need to work with individual strands.

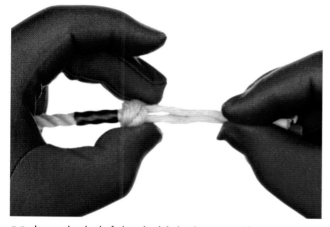

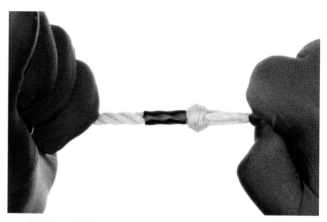

**20.** It can be helpful to hold the knot itself as you do.

**21.** Tighten fully.

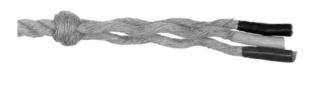

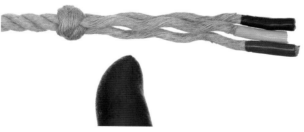

**22.** Remove the tape collar.

**23.** Trim the ends.

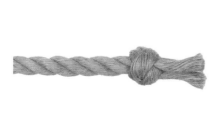

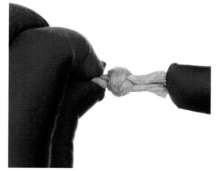

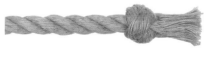

**24.** Leave at least ¾-inch.

**25.** Fluff the ends.

**26.** Done!

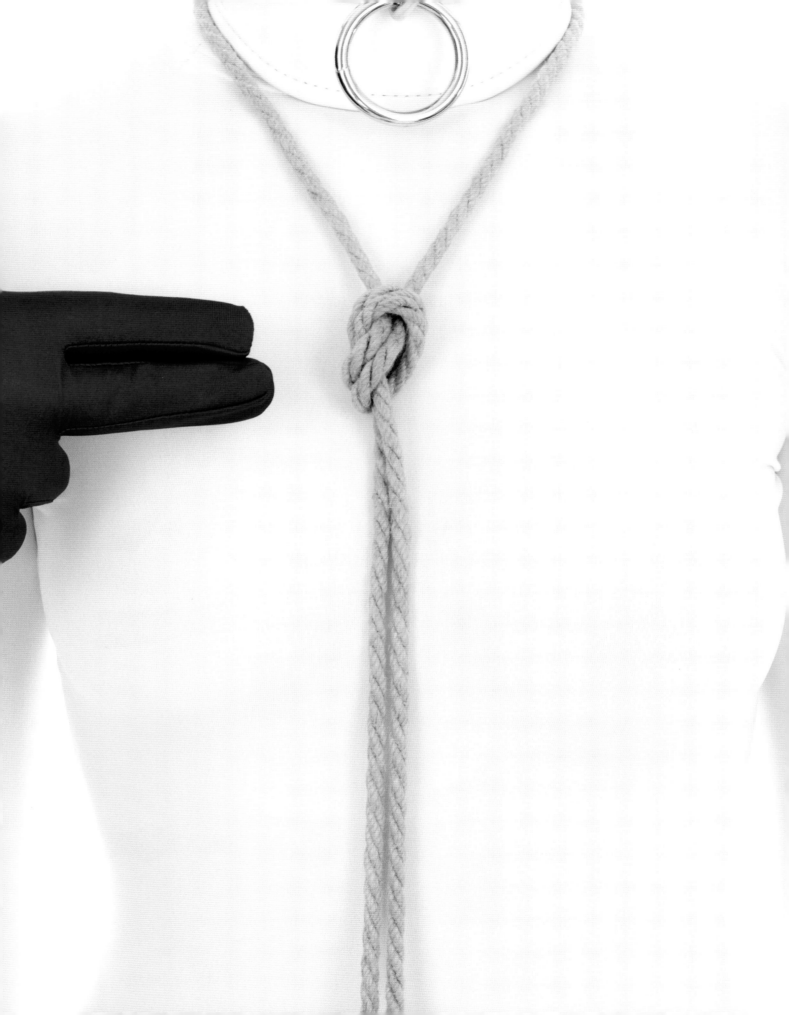

# 4

# The Four Fundamental Knots

Before you get into bondage ties, you need to understand four fundamental knots. You will use these all the time. For example, one of the ties commonly used as a wrist cuff is just a **Lark's Head Knot** with some extra wraps and then locked off with a **Half Hitch**!

Even if you think you understand these knots, don't jump ahead. There may be details or variations that you haven't seen before and are important for you to understand. Almost every tie in this book is assembled using these knots as basic building blocks. Here are the knots you need to master.

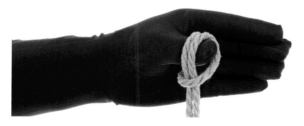

**Lark's Head Knot**

This simple sliding knot is a common building block used to start a tie or add rope.

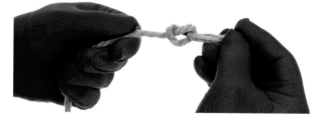

**Overhand Knot**

This knot is commonly used to finish the end of a rope — so it does not fray — or as a stop knot.

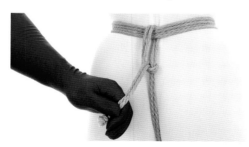

**Half Hitch**

This simple wrap of rope around other ropes is a basic building block of many other knots.

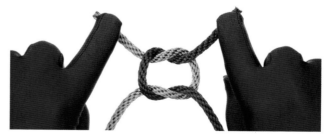

**Square Knot/Surgeon's Knot**

This common knot is used for holding two ends of rope together, for instance to "lock off" a tie.

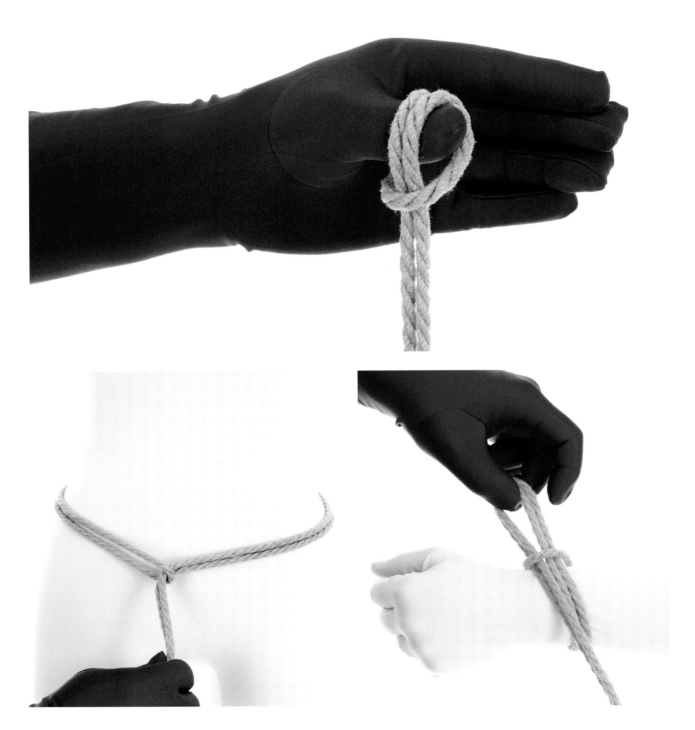

# The Lark's Head

A **Lark's Head** is a simple sliding knot. If used by itself, it forms a collapsing loop. That means that if you pull on the tail, it gets tighter. Because of that, a collapsing loop should never be used directly as a bondage cuff. That said, it is a very common first step in the creation of many other ties.

TheDuchy.com/larks-head-knot/

# Overhand Knot — Core Technique

An **Overhand Knot** is one of the fastest and easiest ways to keep the end of your rope from fraying. For others, see *Rope Ends* (p. 112).

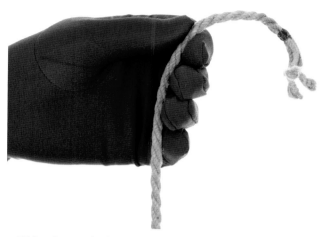

**1.** Take the end of a rope.

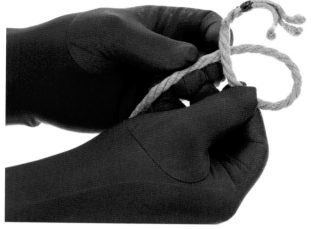

**2.** Form a loop, laying the end on top of itself.

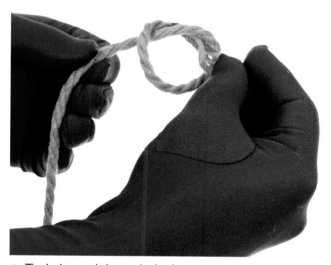

**3.** Tuck the end through the loop.

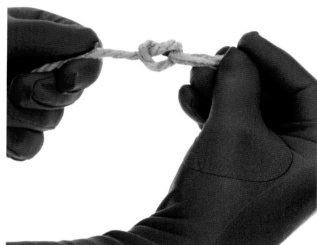

**4.** Tighten.

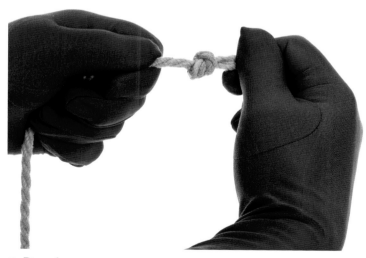

**5.** Done!

# Overhand on a Bight

You can form an **Overhand Knot** on a bight or with two strands.

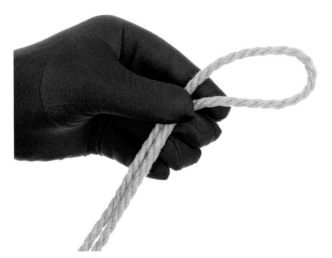

**1.** Start with the bight.

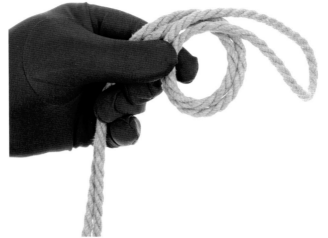

**2.** Loop the bight, laying it on top of itself.

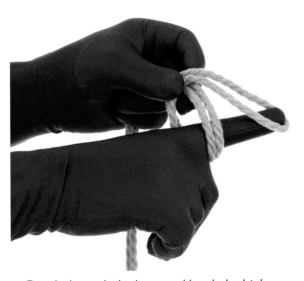

**3.** Reach through the loop and hook the bight.

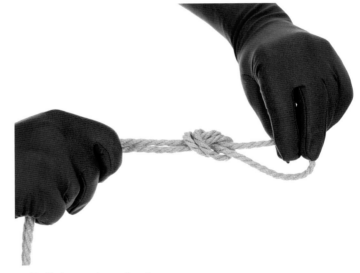

**4.** Pull through and tighten.

# Mark the Bight with an Overhand Knot

This is a helpful technique to make sure you don't lose your bight while rigging. While you are untying, you don't want to take the time to wrap the rope for storage each time you take a piece off. Perhaps you plan to keep tying and will use that rope again before you are done. You also don't want to lose the time necessary to find the bight every time you pick up a rope. This can help!

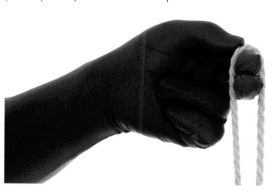

**1.** Let's say you have just taken a rope off your partner and you now have the bight.

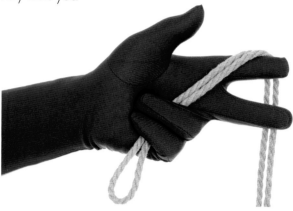

**2.** Hold the bight in one hand. Hold your pointer and middle fingers a little apart.

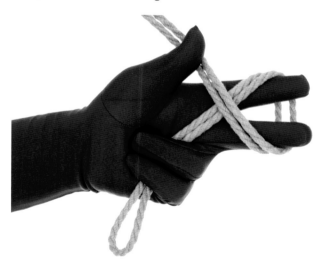

**3.** Loop the rope around your fingers, laying the tail on top of the bight.

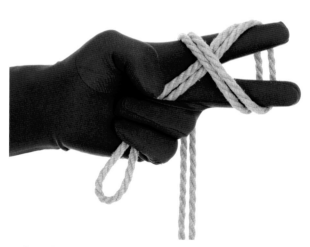

**4.** Lay the tail on the back side of your hand.

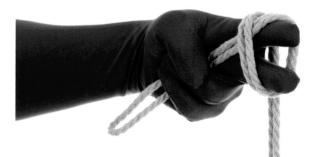

**5.** You can see the tail through the loop.

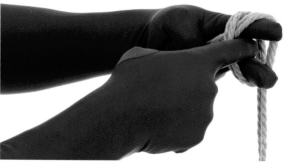

**6.** Reach through the space between your fingers and hook the tail. *continues...*

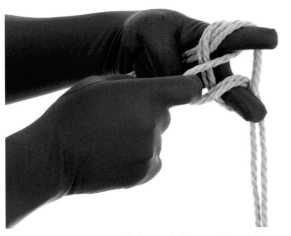

**7.** Pull a small loop of the tail through that loop.

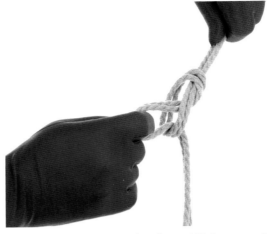

**8.** Keep a firm grip on that loop. With your other hand, shift your grip so you are just holding the bight.

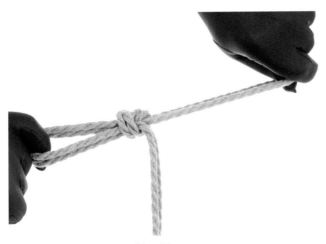

**9.** Pull tight. This is a **Slip Knot**.

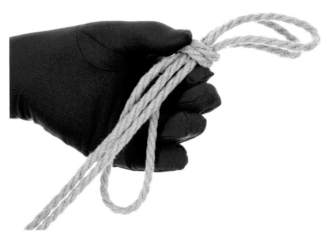

**10.** You can now put this rope down and, when you need it later, you can instantly find the bight.

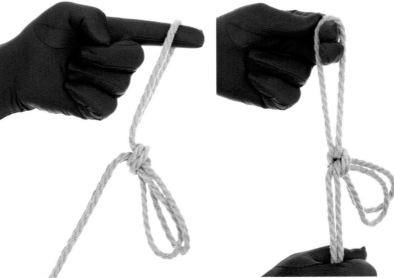

**11.** When you want to use it again, pick it up by the bight.

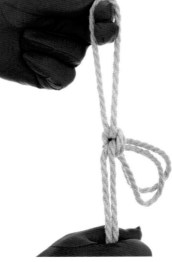

**12.** Pull the tail with one strong move to remove the **Slip Knot**.

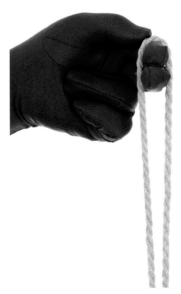

**13.** Bight in hand, the rope is ready to use!

# Tying Overhand Knots Consistently When Rigging

If you are the type of person who wants things to look consistent, then you want to tie your knots using a consistent technique. Here is one that can be helpful.

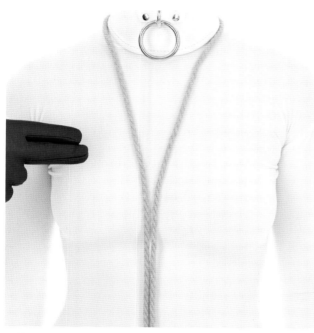

**1.** This technique is used in the **Hishi Karada** (p. 358), which starts with a series of **Overhand Knots**.

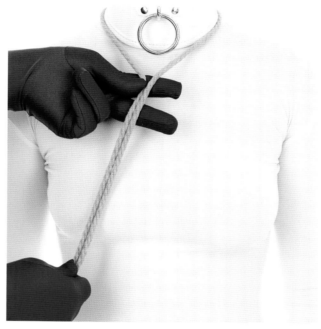

**2.** Place two fingers behind the tail. The fingers should be slightly apart.

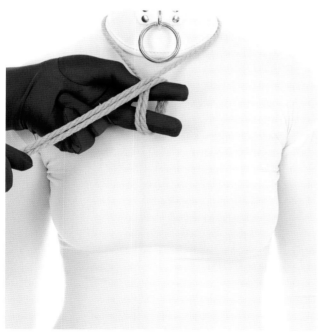

**3.** Loop the tail around your fingers, laying it on top of itself.

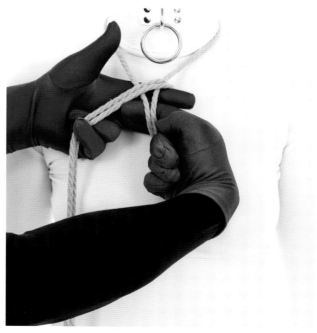

**4.** Reach through that loop with a finger of the other hand... *continues...*

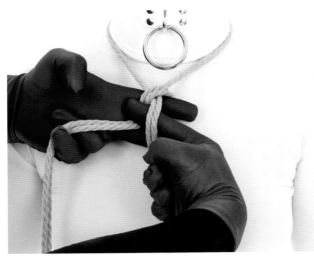

**5.** ...and hook the tail.

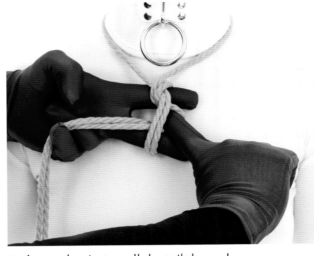

**6.** As you begin to pull the tail through...

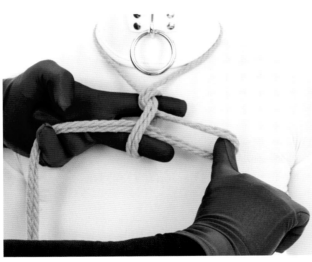

**7.** ...keep the fingers of your other hand spread to keep the loop open so the tail can easily pass through.

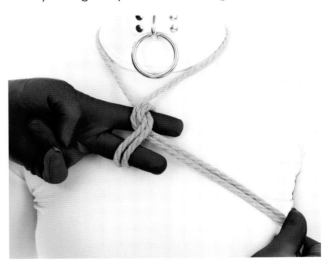

**8.** Pull the tail all the way through.

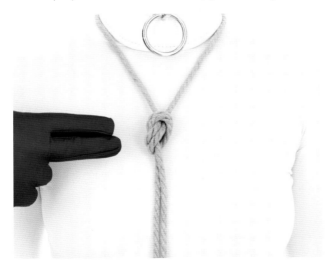

**9.** The form of the **Overhand Knot** is now complete; it just needs to be tightened. You can adjust its location while tightening.

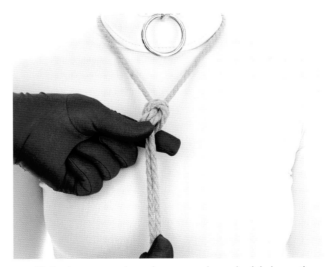

**10.** If the knot needs to be moved up, hold the tail and pull the knot upward.

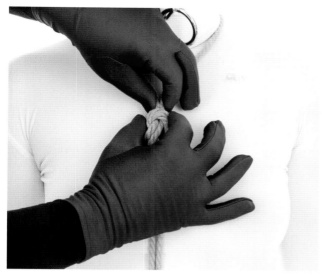

**11.** If the knot needs to be moved down, hold the ropes above the knot and pull the knot downward.

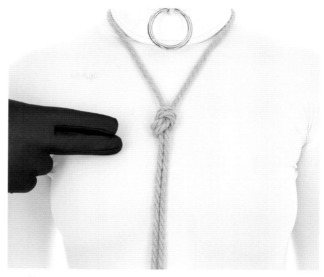

**12.** Done.

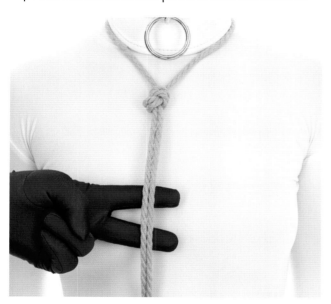

**13.** If you use the same technique every time...

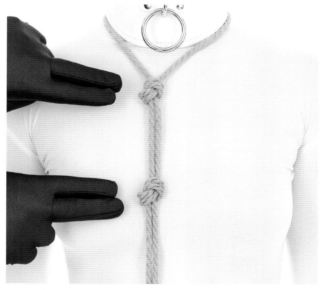

**14.** ...the knots will look the same every time.

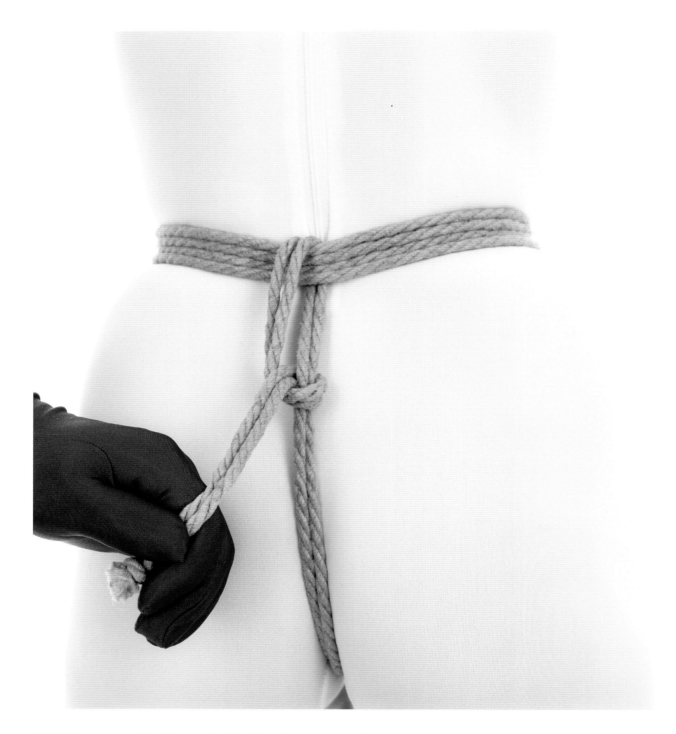

# The Half Hitch

The Half Hitch is just a single wrap of rope around another standing line of rope, used for a variety of purposes such as locking off a band as part of a tie or locking off the end of the rope when the tie is complete. You can also use two Half Hitches to anchor a rope to something.

TheDuchy.com/half-hitches/

# Core Technique + Locking Off/Anchoring to a Band

With practice and muscle memory, you will be able to complete a **Half Hitch** in seconds without thinking about the procedure, but it is helpful to understand the details of the procedure and the reasons for each step while you are learning.

This process can be used to create a **Half Hitch** no matter what direction the tail is coming from.

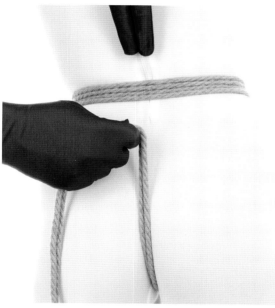

**1.** Run the tail under/around the thing you are anchoring to. Here we are locking off to a band of rope.

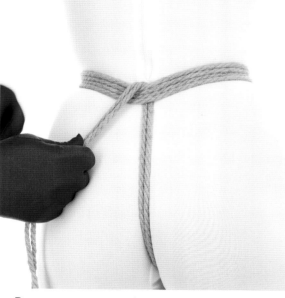

**2.** Reverse tension on the tail, setting the tension on the incoming line.

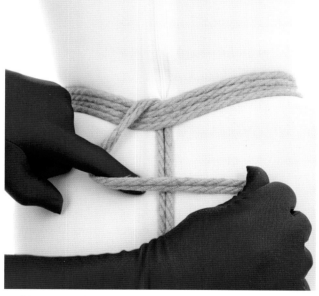

**3.** Place your finger between the tail and the incoming line, then lay the tail on top of the standing line to make this "4" shape.

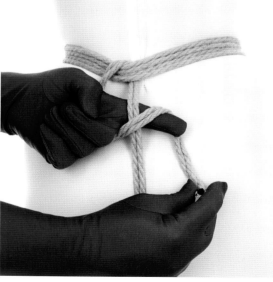

**4.** Slip your finger under the incoming line, then loop the tail over your finger. *continues...*

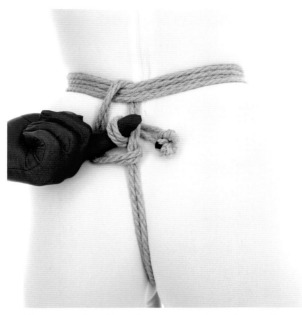

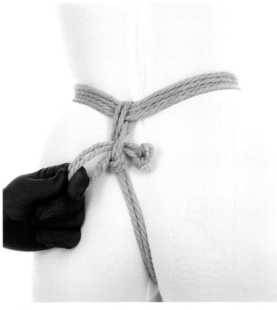

**5.** Turn your hand so that you can bend your finger and use it as a hook to begin pulling the tail through.

**6.** As soon as your finger is out from under the standing line, pull it slightly downward against the twist you are creating. This holds the **Hitch** open for the moment, leaving a large and free passage through which you can more easily pull the tail.

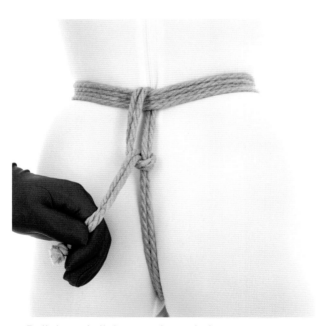

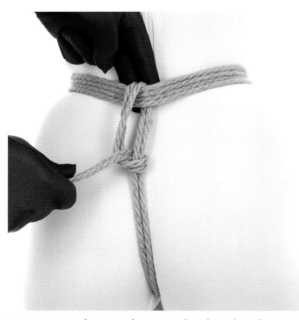

**7.** Pull the tail all the way through; keep tension on it while...

**8.** ...you reach up with your other hand and put pressure on the rope where it goes around the thing you are tying to.

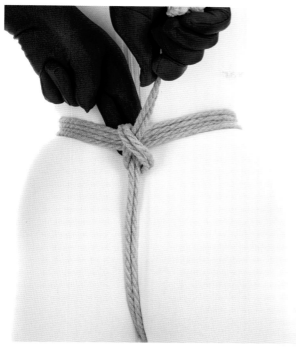

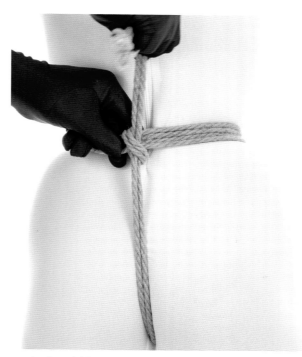

**9.** Keep pressure there so that the line stays in position while you pull the tail up quickly and firmly, "snapping" the knot closed.

**10.** It should be tight against what you are tying to, like this.

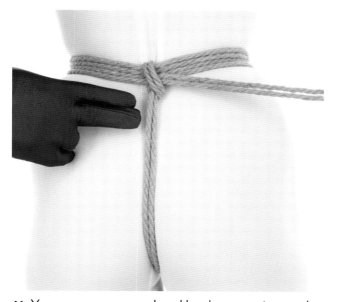

### This Works for all Orientations
This is one of the most common things you will do, so it is important to be able to do it from any angle or orientation. Regardless of the way from which the rope comes in, the procedure for doing the **Half Hitch** is basically the same.

**11.** You can remove your hand but keep tension on the tail for now.

If you are locking off a band or something in the middle of a tie, this may be all you need.

If you are locking the rope to some hard point, you will need to add a second **Half Hitch** to hold the rope firmly in place. Continue onto the next page to see this done on a band. To see it done on a hard point, see *Anchoring a Tail to a Hard Point* (p. 138).

## The Half Hitch

### Two Half Hitches

To completely lock a line off to something else as we are doing in this example, you need to add a second **Half Hitch**. This is called **Two Half Hitches**, oddly enough, and is one of the most common knots used to anchor a rope to something else, be it another line of rope (as in this example) or something else like a hard point. Repeat exactly what you did before:

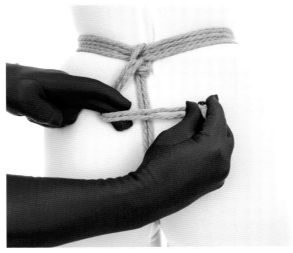

**1.** Make the "4."

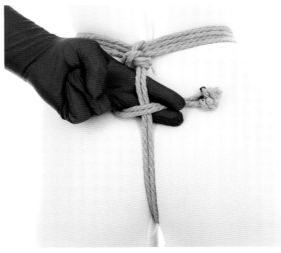

**2.** Reach under the incoming line to grab the tail. This time I am using the scissor technique with my pointer and middle finger, which also works great.

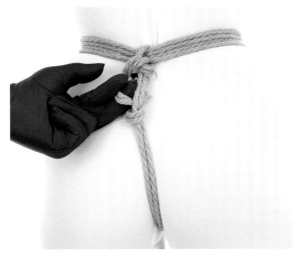

**3.** Pull the tail through...

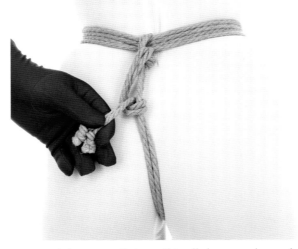

**4.** ...and down until the tail is all the way through.

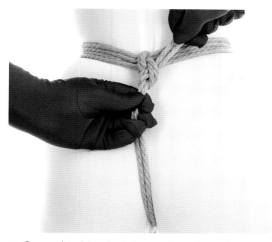

**5.** Snap this **Hitch** tight against the other.

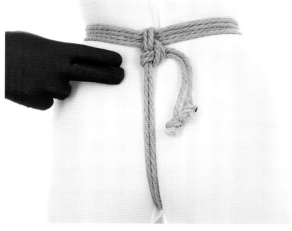

**6.** The **Two Half Hitches Knot** is now complete. But...

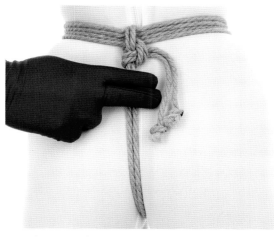

**7.** ...there is a little rope left over. If you leave it dangling, the knot will look unfinished and sloppy!

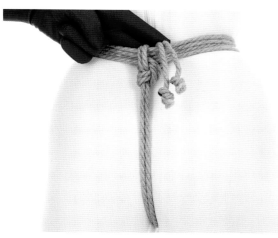

**8.** Get rid of the extra rope in some way. For example, you can wrap it around nearby lines. See *Using Up Extra Rope* (p. 279) for other ideas.

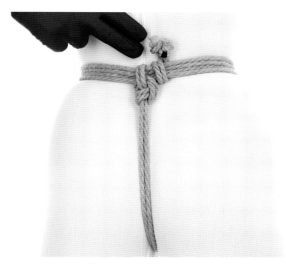

**9.** When you get to the end...

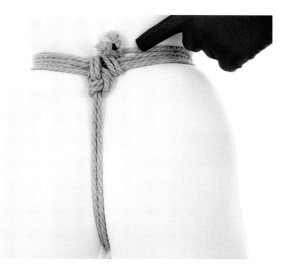

**10.** ...if you have knots in your rope, simply tuck your ends between some strands that are under tension. If you do not, tuck the ends under the previous wrap and pull tight.

# Anchoring a Tail to a Hard Point Using Two Half Hitches

This is one of the fastest and easiest ways to lock a tail off to a hard point. For example, perhaps you want to tie a cuffed wrist or ankle to a bedpost. This is a common application of what was shown in the *Locking off to a Band* example, just shown in a different situation.

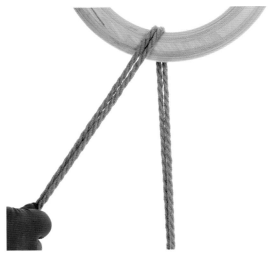

**1.** Grab the tail and run it around your hard point. Pull the tail to adjust the desired position and tension.

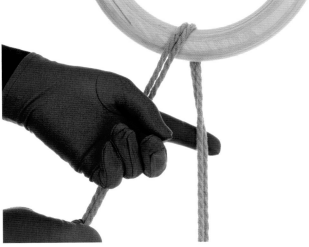

**2.** Do the same as shown in the core technique: Place your finger between the tail and the standing line.

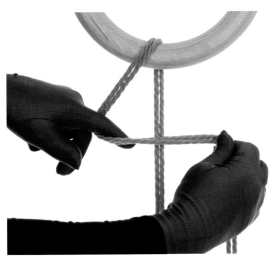

**3.** Hook the tail on that finger and lay it on top of the standing line, making this "4" shape.

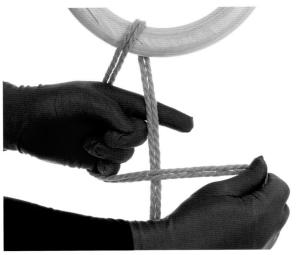

**4.** Put your finger behind the standing line.

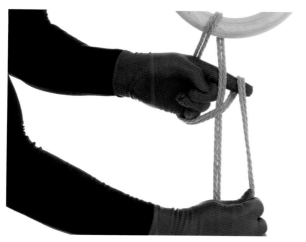

**5.** Loop the tail over your finger.

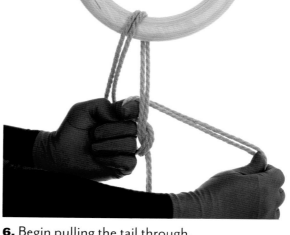

**6.** Begin pulling the tail through.

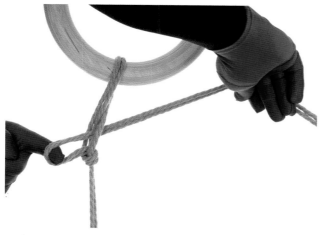

**7.** As soon as your finger is out from under the standing line, pull it slightly downward against the twist you are creating; this holds the **Hitch** open for the moment, leaving a large and free passage through which you can more easily pull the tail.

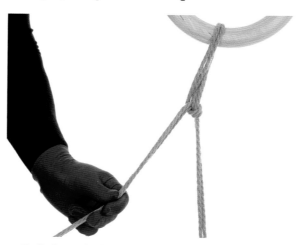

**8.** Pull the tail all the way through and keep tension on it while...

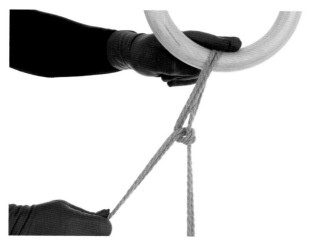

**9.** ...you reach up with your other hand and put pressure on the rope where it goes around the thing you are tying it to.

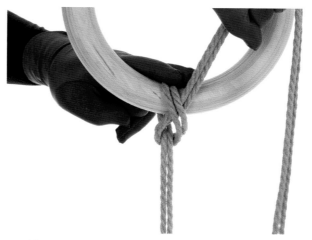

**10.** Keep pressure there so that the line stays in position while you pull the tail quickly and firmly, "snapping" the knot closed. *continues...*

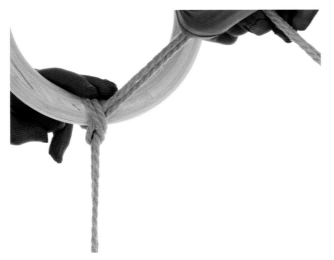

**11.** It should be tight against what you are tying it to, like this.

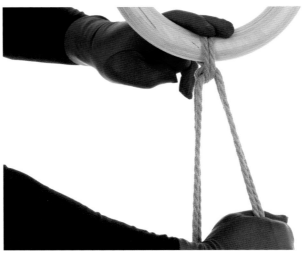

**12.** You need a second **Half Hitch** to finish the lock. Bring the tail back down and repeat what you just did.

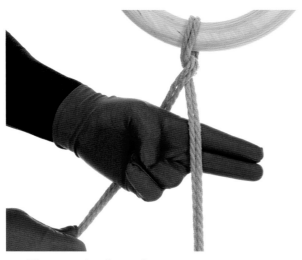

**13.** This time I will use the scissor grip.

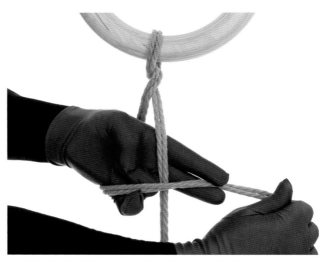

**14.** Make "4" shape and grab the tail with your pointer and middle finger.

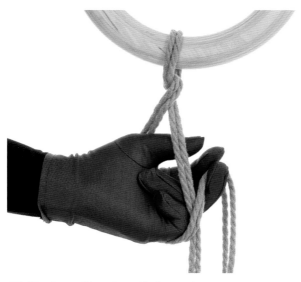

**15.** Begin pulling the tail through.

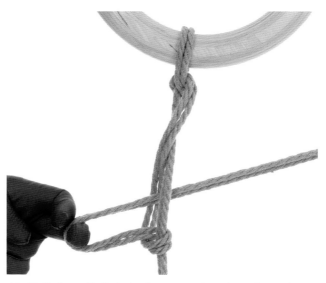

**16.** Pull the tail slightly downward against the twist.

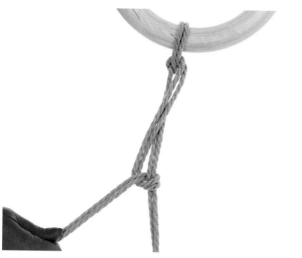

**17.** Fully pull the tail through, keeping tension on it.

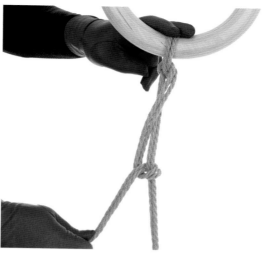

**18.** Put pressure on where the rope meets the hard point you are anchoring to and...

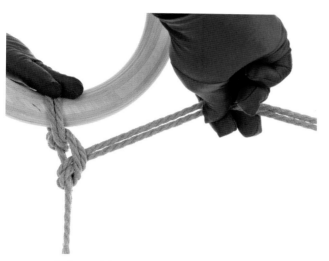

**19.** ...pull the tail firmly to "snap" the knot closed.

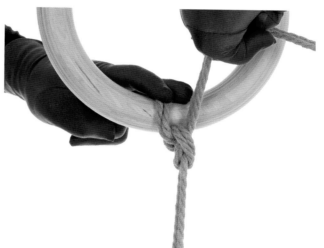

**20.** Make sure the knot is tight.

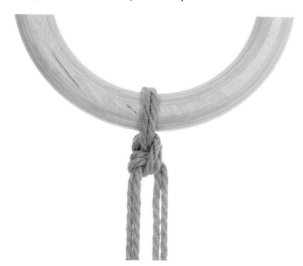

**21.** Done!

# Locking Off a Band

Another use of a **Half Hitch** is to lock or "lock off" a band. This is different than the previous one where you were using a **Half Hitch** to anchor or lock off *to* a band. In this case, the **Half Hitch** is an innate part of the process of creating the band.

Here we have created the wraps for a band of rope around the hips. But this is still a collapsing loop. Any tension on the tail will pull the tail through the secondary bight and tighten around the column. We don't want that. We want any tension on the tail to pull equally on all the strands of the band. Which is why we have to *lock off* the band.

The solution is simple: Just use the tail to make a **Half Hitch** around the strands of the band! Once that is done, any tension on the tail will just cinch the **Half Hitch** more tightly around the strands of the band. The strands of the band will all get pulled equally. This is how we convert a collapsing loop into a non-collapsing loop!

There are two ways to do this:

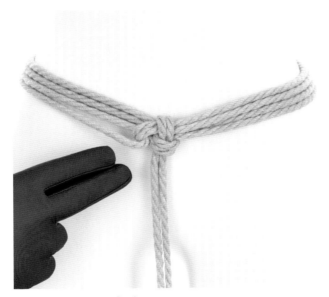

Forward-tension Style

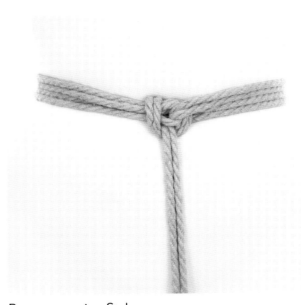

Reverse-tension Style

When locking off a band of rope, you can use a **Half Hitch** on either side of the junction point. If you do it on the side in which the tail is already naturally flowing, it is a "forward-tension" style. If you first reverse the direction of the tail once more and lock off on the other side, it is a "reverse-tension" style.

## Locking Off a Band — Forward-tension Style

This version is less bulky and makes an attractive triangular pattern, but it requires that you manage tension more carefully while tying. It takes a little longer as it requires two tail pulls instead of one.

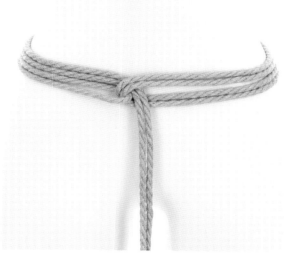

**1.** We want to make a band around the hips and have done the first part of the **Lark's Head Single Column** (p. 181). Now we need to lock it off.

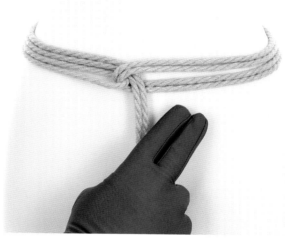

**2.** A forward-tension technique works in the direction that the tail is already naturally flowing. In this example, the tail is running through the secondary bight from left to right, so we will put the **Half Hitch** on the right.

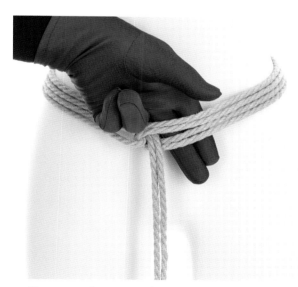

**3.** Place your fingers underneath the band on the forward-tension side.

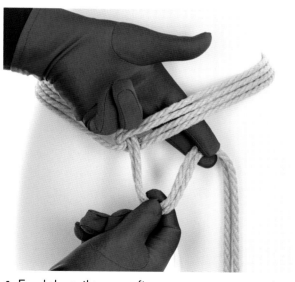

**4.** Feed the tail to your fingers. *continues...*

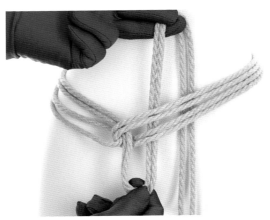

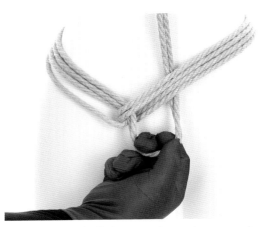

**5.** Protect a small loop of the tail so that it does not get pulled through while you use your finger as a hook to pull the tail underneath the band.

**6.** Pull the tail all the way through except for the small loop that you are protecting.

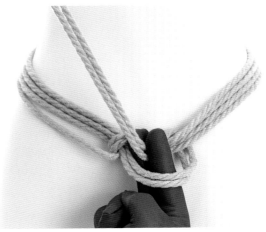

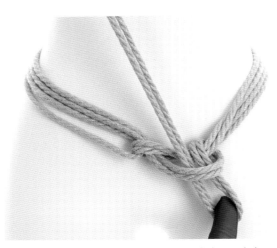

**7.** Reach through the loop you have been protecting and grab the tail.

**8.** Use your finger as a hook to pull the tail through. Note that I am pulling against the **Hitch**. This keeps the path open, allowing the tail to move through more easily.

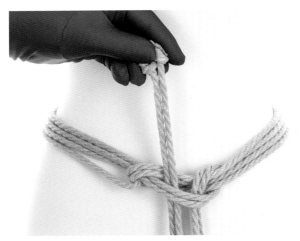

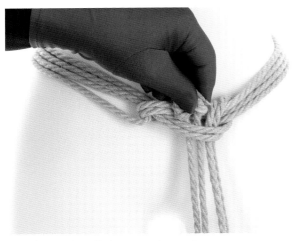

**9.** Keep hold of the other end and maintain tension on the rope as you are pulling it through. This way it does not flail around and hit things (like your partner's face).

**10.** Control it all the way through.

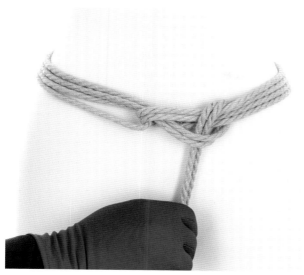

**11.** Here you can see the form of the **Half Hitch** around all the lines of the band. Now we need to set the tension and tighten the knot.

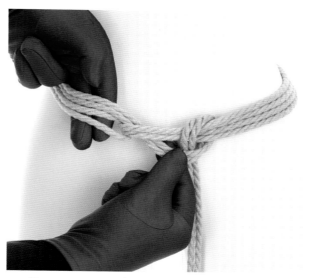

**12.** Place one hand (the left in this case) underneath the band on the opposite side of the bight so that you can feel all the lines making up the band. Adjust the lower node — the line running through the secondary bight — until all the lines of the band have the same tension and are lying flat.

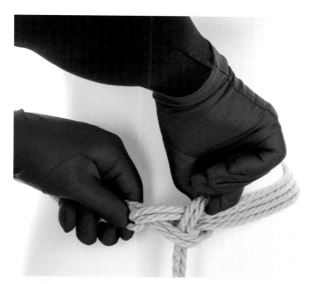

**13.** Change the grip of your left hand so that it holds all the lines in the band and secondary bight. This will keep things from moving around as you continue. Grab the upper node with your other hand.

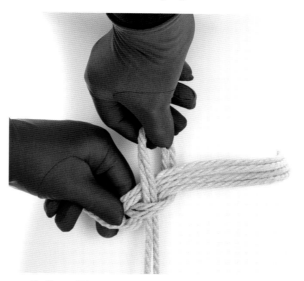

**14.** Pull up. This pulls the lower node tight around the tail, so that it will hold better when you tighten the tail. *continues...*

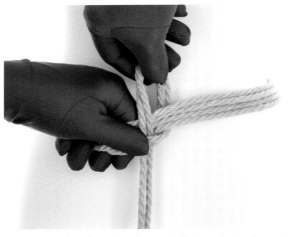

**15.** Move the thumb of your left hand a little to hold the lower node in place and keep it from loosening.

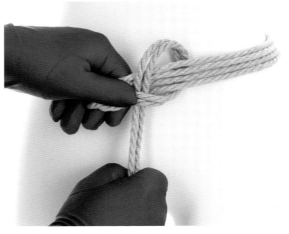

**16.** Keep the node steady while you pull the tail tight.

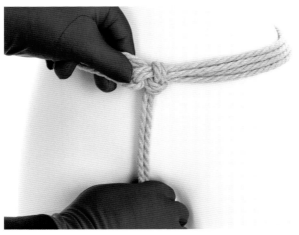

**17.** This completes a tight **Half Hitch** around the band.

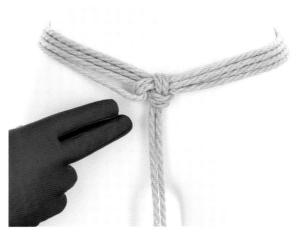

**18.** I personally prefer this version over the reverse-tension **Half Hitch** because I find this triangular pattern quite attractive.

## Locking Off a Band — Reverse-tension Style

This time we are going to reverse the direction of the rope one more time before locking it off. This version adds more friction, which makes it easier to maintain proper tension in the lines making up the band. Also, it is a bit faster! It only requires one tail pull as opposed to two for the forward-tension style. The downside is that it is a bit bulkier. It also has a different appearance.

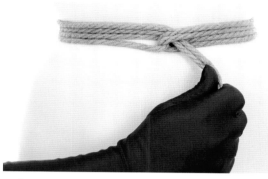

**1.** A reverse-tension technique works on the other side from that in which the tail is already naturally flowing. Just as with the previous example, the tail is running through the secondary bight from left to right, so we will put the **Half Hitch** on the *left*. The first thing we need to do is...

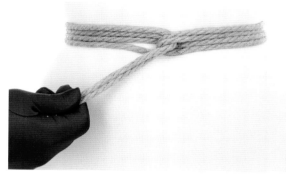

**2.** ...reverse the tension. In this case you want the tail of this rope to naturally flow downward when you are done, so position the tail on the downward side of the band before you start making your **Half Hitch**.

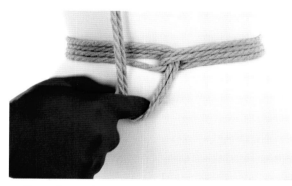

**3.** Put a finger between the tail and the band, then lay the tail over the band, making a sideways "4" shape.

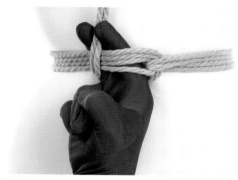

**4.** Reach through the loop you created, then under the band, and grab the tail.

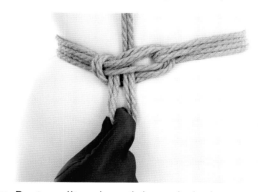

**5.** Begin pulling the tail through the loop...

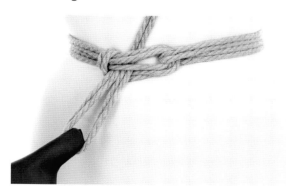

**6.** ...and immediately pull it against the **Half Hitch** like this.                    *continues...*

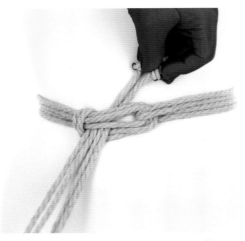

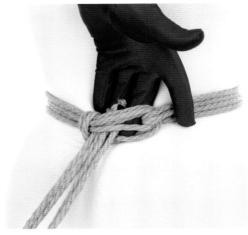

**7.** This keeps that passageway open, allowing the rope to move through with little resistance. Note that the rope remained straight as I have been moving it through. This is because I am holding the other end with my hands so that I can move the rope through this loop as if the rope was one solid straight line.

**8.** Once the end of the rope is about to be pulled through the loop, let go of the ends and just pull through. Moving rope like this reduces the overall friction on the rope and gives you greater control over how the rope is flowing. You will be less likely to accidentally hit your partner with flailing ends.

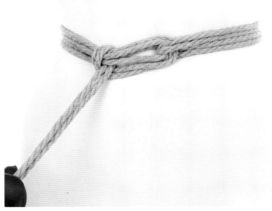

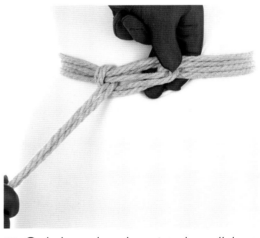

**9.** The form of the **Half Hitch** is now done. You now need to tighten it properly.

**10.** Grab the node — the point where all the strand come together — to keep all the strands in place as you...

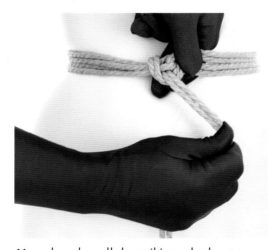

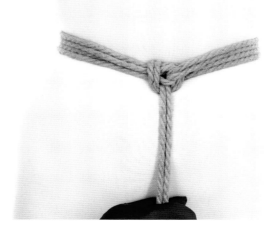

**11.** ...sharply pull the tail into the knot.

**12.** Then lock it off nicely!

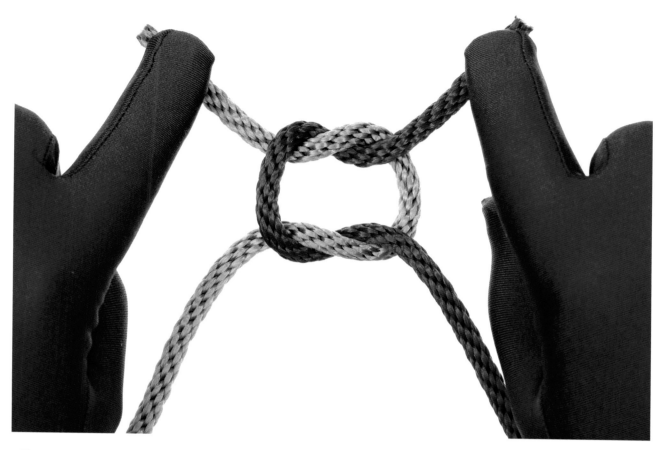

# Square Knot and Surgeon's Knot

This is the most common knot for holding two ends of rope together. It is also called a **Reef Knot**.

When you tie your shoes, you are using a "slipped" version of this knot. "Slipped" means you leave the last pull as loops instead of pulling them all the way through. This lets you untie the knot faster and more easily.

**Square Knots** are great for joining two ropes or for locking off two ends at the ending of a tie. However, it is important to avoid situations where they might capsize — when the tension in a knot changes and causes the knot to deform!

Also, if a **Square Knot** is subjected to strong tension, it has a tendency to jam and become difficult to untie, so it is best used in situations where it will not be under strong tension, such as those in this book. **The Surgeon's Knot** is better if there will be stronger tensions. One example of this is in applying the **Multi-loop Texas Handcuffs** (p. 260).

TheDuchy.com/square-knot/

# The Basic Square Knot Technique

This is the version taught around the world for all types of purposes: "Right-over-Left, Left-over-Right."

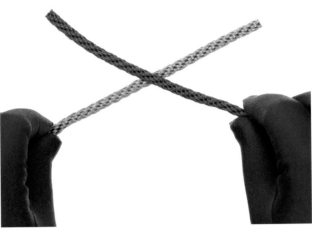

**1.** Cross the ends of the rope. Place the rope in your right hand on top of the one in your left. ("Right-over-Left.")

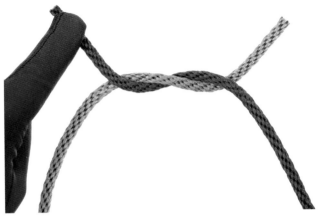

**2.** Make a twist. This is just an Overhand Knot. Note that the blue rope continues to move to the left and is on top of the grey on both ends of the knot.

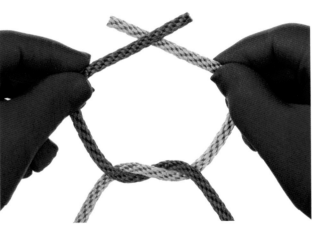

**3.** Now bend the ropes back the way they came. But this time, place the rope in your left hand (blue) on top of the one in your right (grey). ("Left-over-Right.")

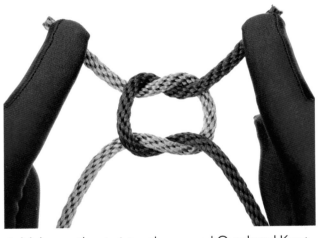

**4.** Make another twist — the second Overhand Knot. Again, the blue is on top of the grey on both ends.

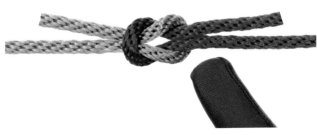

**5.** You know you have created it properly when both strands of one rope are on the same side, are parallel, and are contained inside a loop from the other rope.

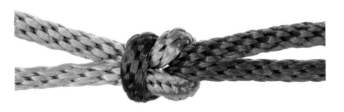

**6.** Tighten to complete the **Square Knot**.

## Capsizing a Square Knot

Caution: If you put tension on the same side of a Square Knot, it will "capsize" and come apart.

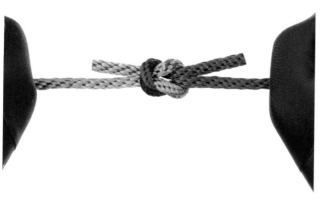

**1.** This knot is meant to hold two ropes on opposite sides.

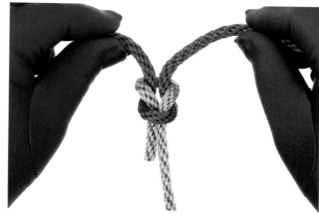

**2.** If you pull on both ends of the same cord...

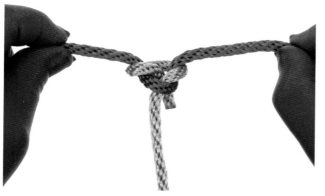

**3.** ...the tension will pull the knot apart...

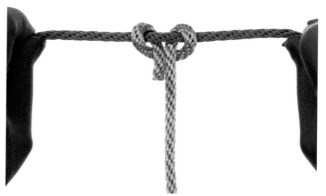

**4.** ...capsizing it...

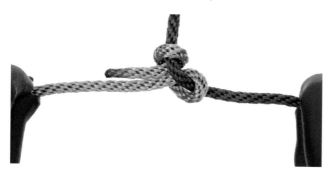

**5.** ...into a **Lark's Head Knot** around a straight rope.

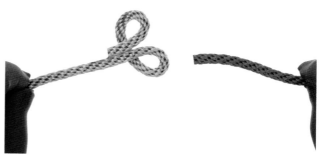

**6.** Once it has capsized, the ropes will just slip apart, making them useless for holding anything together.

# Granny Knot

If you ever accidentally do the same twist twice — "Right-over-Left, Right-over-Left" or "Left-over-Right, Left-over-Right" — you will end up with a **Granny Knot** instead. This knot will have the strands perpendicular to each other instead of parallel. It is not as strong as the **Square Knot**, but there are times when it is useful.

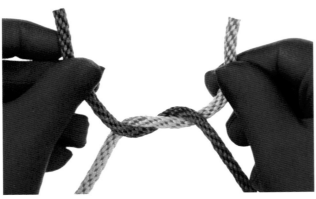

**1.** Start the same way: Right-over-Left...

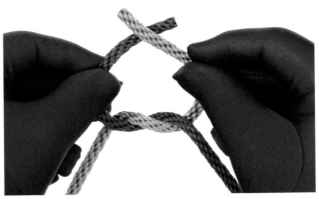

**2.** ...but do Right-over-Left again for the second twist.

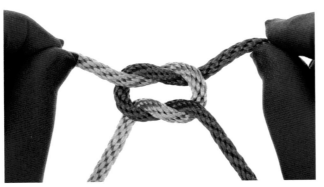

**3.** Like this.

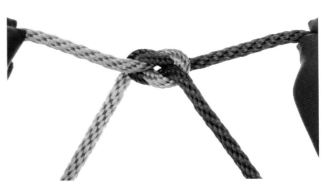

**4.** When you tighten this version...

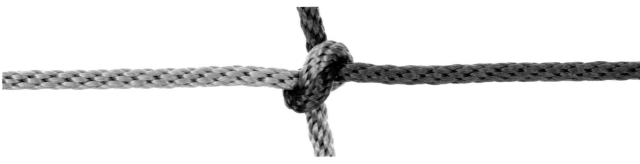

**5.** ...the lines will naturally leave the knot at right angles.

# Surgeon's Knot

A Surgeon's Knot is just a **Square Knot** with an extra twist on one side (or both). It does not jam as easily as the **Square Knot** can.

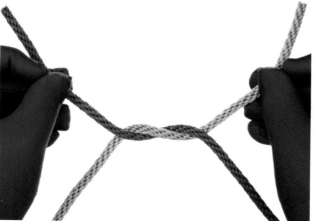

**1.** Start just as you would a **Square Knot**.

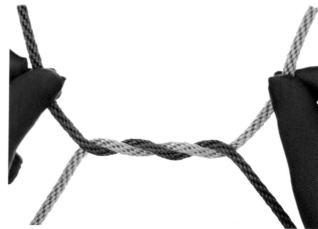

**2.** Add an extra twist to the first side...

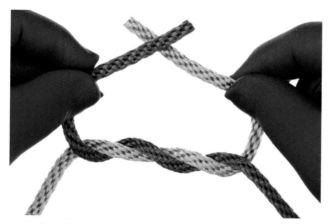

**3.** ...then finish normally.

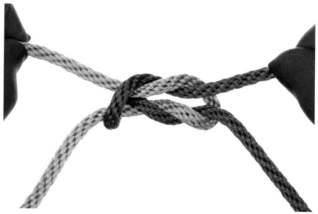

**4.** This second side can have the normal number of twists or an extra.

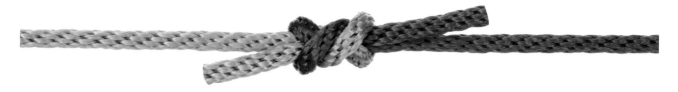

**5.** Tighten to finish.

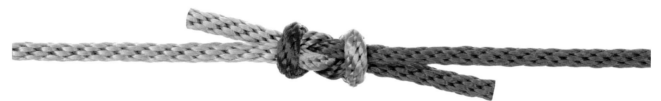

**6.** This is what it looks like from the other side.

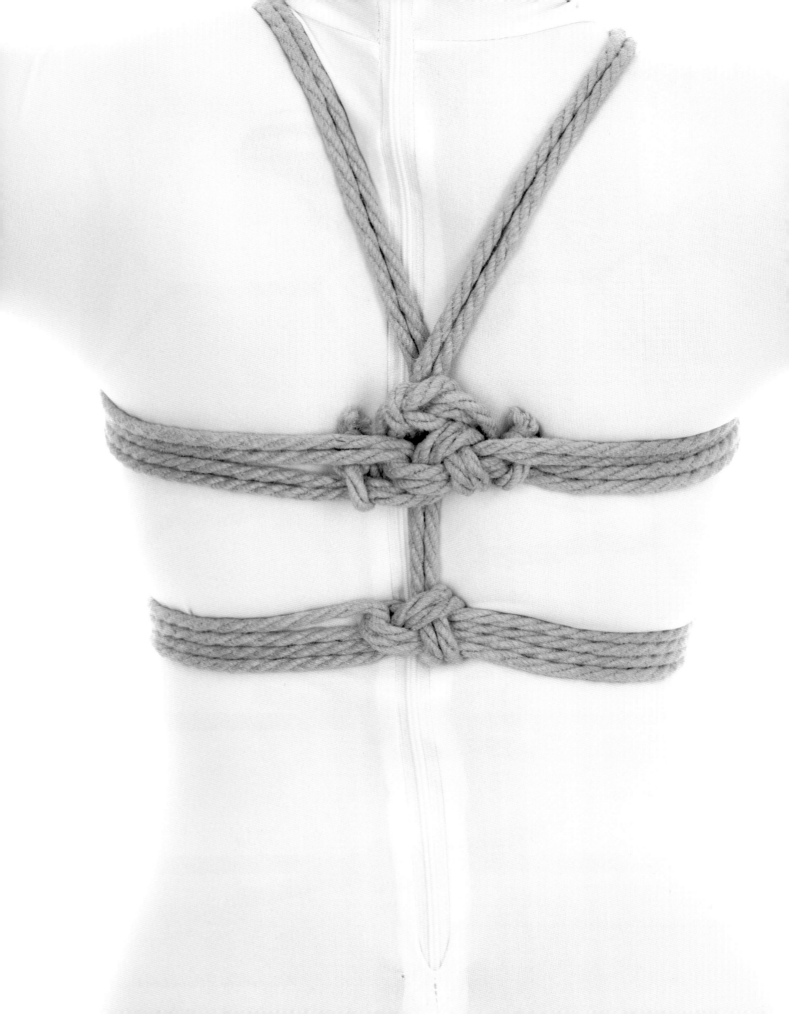

# 5
# Rope Handling Tips and Tricks

Rope bondage is an art. This can be true of not only the completed tie, but also the process itself. There are ways to handle rope, to move it and to manage its flow during the tying process, that make your tying look and feel like an art form.

These techniques are not difficult. They make the tying easier, reduce the risk of rope burn, and reduce the chances of having rope tails flailing around and possibly hitting your partner in unexpected ways and places.

The only way to get good at rope is to practice. You will need to practice these techniques over and over to build muscle memory. Speed will come with time and repetition but it is important to learn how to do these simple things the correct way.

You will see these specific techniques all throughout this book, but in this chapter, we will focus on the small details so that you can get a more comprehensive understanding.

## Handling Rope

Rope bottoms tend to enjoy a scene much more if they feel that the Top (the rigger) is knowledgeable and in control. One of the best ways to show that you are knowledgeable and in control is to move with precision and confidence. Mastering the tips in this section and practicing them until they become muscle memory will be beneficial and satisfying not only for you as the rigger, but also for your bottom.

How you handle the rope as you are doing the various ties — where you put your hands, how you hold and move the rope — is one of the most important elements of this. These techniques will allow you to move the rope more quickly, efficiently, and safely, helping you avoid rope burn and protecting your ropes from damage. If you like to perform or have an exhibitionist streak, moving with confidence, speed, and precision also makes watching a rope scene much more interesting and enjoyable.

These are fundamental skills that will help improve your rigging no matter what you tie:

- Pull rope, don't push it.
- Use the big hole, i.e. the path of least resistance.
- Control the rope during tail pulls.
- Protect your partner from rope burn.

**Pull Rope, Don't Push It**

When trying to move rope, do not push it; pull it instead.

There are a few rare cases where something is very tight, and it can be helpful to create a small bend in the rope and push it through the tight passage. In 99% of the cases, things will work much better if you reach through with your finger and hook the rope and then pull it through..

The following two techniques — The Hook and The Scissor — can be helpful.

# The Hook and The Scissor

Avoid using your fingers as pincers to grab the rope, especially with twisted-strand rope. You can accidentally grab just one of the strands and end up pulling that strand away from the other two, hyperthreading it. It is difficult to repair that damage and, if this happens, that piece of rope should never be trusted to be as strong as it once was. Use one of these techniques instead.

## The Hook Technique

This is the most common technique. It is very flexible and fast. It also works well in many tight areas.

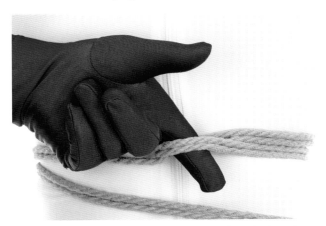 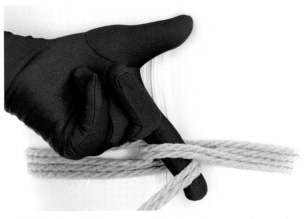

**1.** Put your finger through the desired path, but from the opposite direction.

**2.** Either hook the rope with that finger or loop the rope around that finger with your other hand.

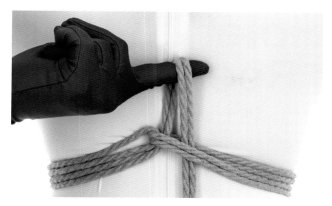

**3.** Then use that finger as a hook to draw the tail up through the intended path.

## The Scissor Technique

Alternatively, you can use two fingers in a scissor grip. This can sometimes be helpful in areas where using **The Hook** is difficult, and some people just prefer this style. This can also be a way to ensure that you are able to run two fingers under a band of rope, something that you should always be able to do for safety reasons (p. 60, 70). The technique is very similar to **The Hook**.

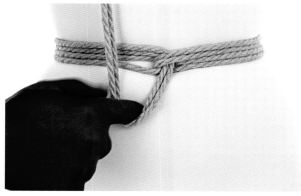

**1.** In this example, we want to run the tail behind the waist band and through the bend.

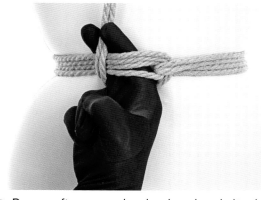

**2.** Put two fingers under that band and clip the rope between them.

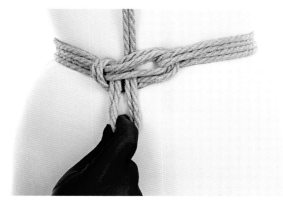

**3.** Flip your hand over and one of your fingers will automatically hook the rope. Pull it through.

# Use "The Big Hole" i.e. The Path of Least Resistance

If there is a path to run the rope so it will move through an area of lower resistance and friction, it is usually better to choose that path.

## Example 1 – Through a Bight

When you are running your rope through a bight or bend, do so in such a way that the rope passes through the path of least resistance. This can often be done with a simple twist of the wrist!

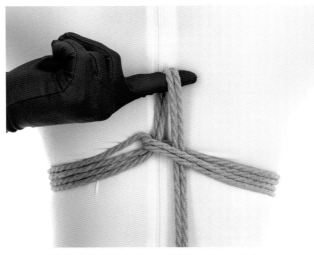

**1.** Use **The Hook** to begin pulling the tail through.

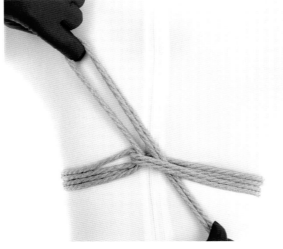

**2.** Once it is through, immediately reverse your tension a little to help keep the tension in the wraps.

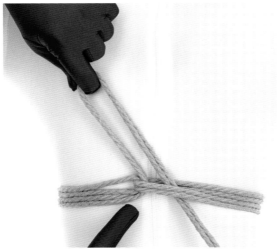

**3.** But twist your hand so that the part of the tail that will not be moving is against the bight...

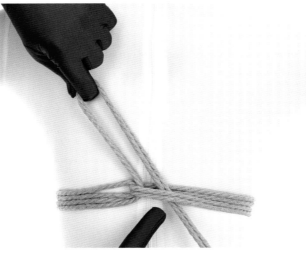

**4.** ...and the part of the tail that will be moving will move through this larger open area.

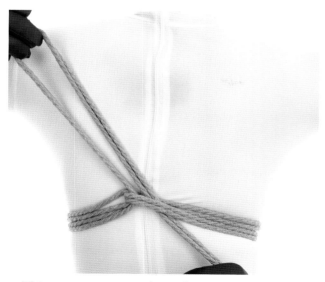

**5.** This way it moves easily, with much less friction!

Using this technique makes it easier to move and control the rope, while also increasing the life span of your rope because it reduces friction damage!

........................................................

## Example 2 – Through a Different Path, then Reposition

Run the rope though a location where you have more room, then reposition.

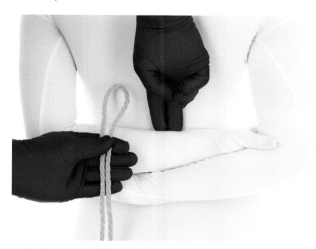

**1.** In this example, you want to run rope around the wrists to tie a **Somerville Bowline** (p. 188).

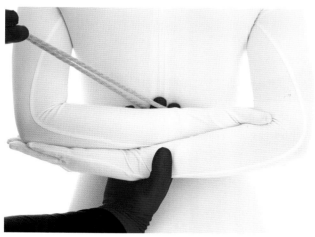

**2.** Yes, you *can* just reach behind the wrists, hook the bight and pull it through but, for most people, their wrists will be pressed quite tightly to their back in exactly the place we want to run the rope. Running a rope between the skin of their wrists and back at that point is harder to do and may result in rope burn. *continues...*

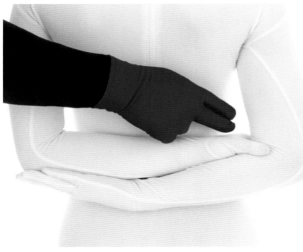

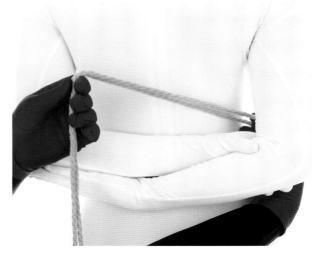

**3.** But if you instead run the rope around their arm through this open area ("the big hole") closer to the elbow, you can easily route the rope...

**4.** ...like this...

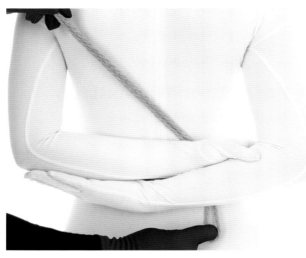

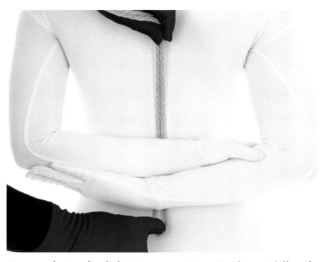

**5.** ...then, continuing to hold both top and bottom of the rope...

**6.** ...and simply slide it into position in the middle of the back.

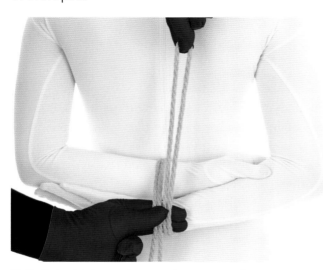

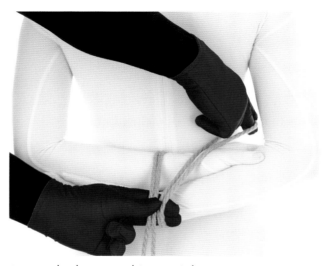

**7.** Pull the bight so that you have enough rope...

**8.** ...to do the same thing again!

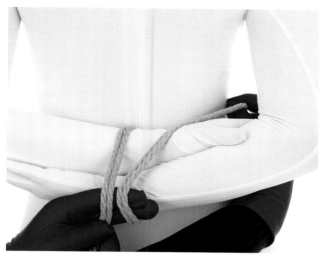

**9.** Run the bight through the big hole...

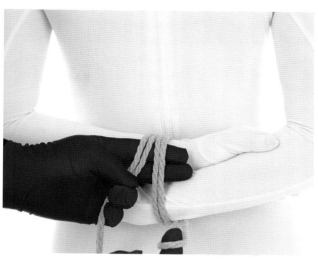

**10.** ...then reposition.

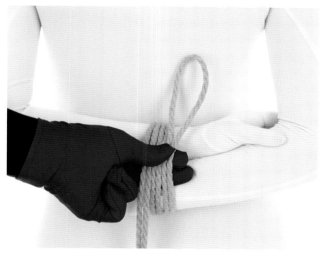

**11.** Repeat this for as many wraps as you like, then complete your tie.

In a case like this, which we will use in the **Box Tie** example (p. 397) we usually do three to four wraps for a total of six to eight strands.

# Control the Rope During Tail Pulls

One quality that marks experience in a rigger is how well they control the rope. How does the rope move around the area while being tied? Is it controlled, or do the ends fly all around, potentially hitting their partner or a bystander in unexpected ways? Are the rigger's movements swift and purposeful, or hesitant?

Big, rapid movements and long extensions of the arm when doing a tail pull are impressive. They are fun to watch and fun for both you and your partner to feel. But they need to be done with control. Without explicitly controlling how the rope moves, the ends will begin whipping around, perhaps hitting people. This will detract from the impression of how skilled you are.

For medium and short tail pulls, if you control both ends of the rope when moving it, you can control almost everything else you need. Let's walk through it and show how you can pull together all the tips in what to most people would look like a single move!

## Move the Rope like a Stick

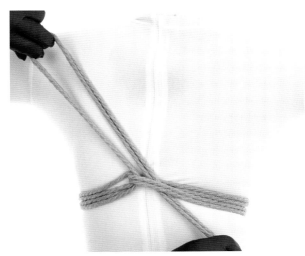 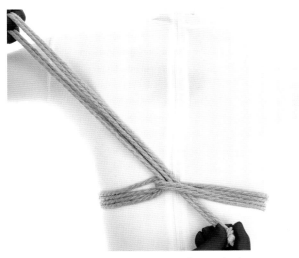

**1.** You have hooked the rope through the bight and flipped it so that the tail is traveling through the big hole.

**2.** As you are pulling the rope through, keep your other hand on the other end so that the whole rope is traveling in a straight line, like a stick.

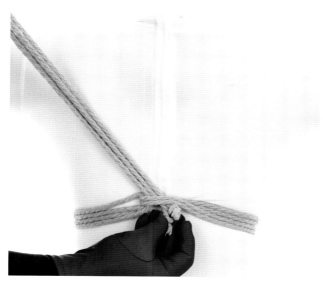

**3.** This will keep the ends from flying around. It can also be very helpful if you have knots in the end of your rope. Your hand is right there to help them through!

## Pull all the Strands, not Just the Free Ones

If you have a long tail pull, trying to move the rope like a stick doesn't work; your arms aren't long enough. But you can move the loose strands through by pulling them all. Only the tail strands that are free to move, will move.

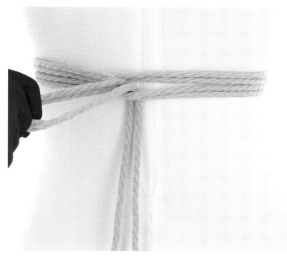

**1.** You have hooked the rope through the bight and flipped it so that the tail is traveling through the big hole.

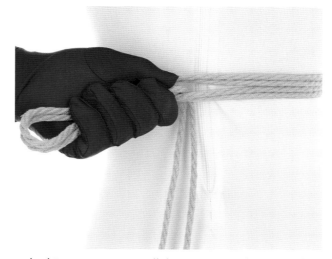

**2.** In this case you can pull the entire set of ropes with a medium-tight grip — sort of stroking the whole bundle.

*continues...*

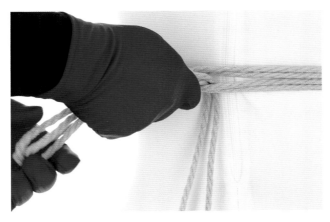

**3.** Only the loose strands will move. This saves lots of time compared to trying to keep track of which strands are free to move and which are anchored.

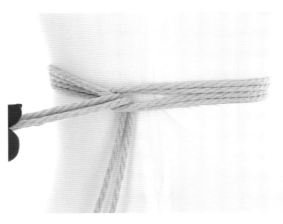

**4.** Also, you can do large movements with your arms, pulling more rope through with each movement and reducing the number of times you need to pull.

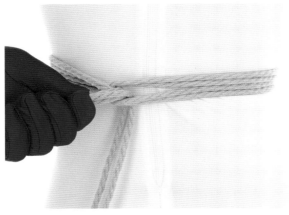

**5.** Just keep switching hands to keep tension on the bundle of ropes and continue to pull away in a stroking motion.

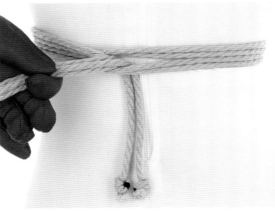

**6.** If you use this technique, change it up when you get close to the end.

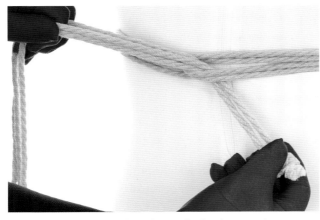

**7.** With one of your hands, grab the free ends as in "Move Rope Like a Stick."

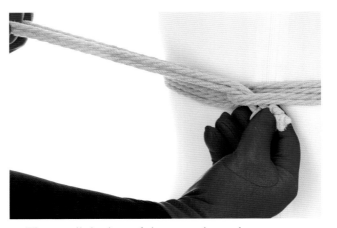

**8.** Then pull the last of the rope through.

By the way, this technique also helps protect your partner from rope burn. As you are pulling all the stands, you will naturally be pulling the moving rope away from your partner's skin.

# Protect Your Partner From Rope Burn

When doing a tail pull, moving rope may come into contact with your partner's skin. If it is moving too quickly or under too much friction, it can give your partner rope burn.

Some of the techniques we've covered already help with this. *Use the Big Hole* (p. 158) for example. Doing so helps the rope move more freely, with less contact and friction on the skin. But you can do more! *Use tension to pull the rope away from your partner's body during the tail pull.*

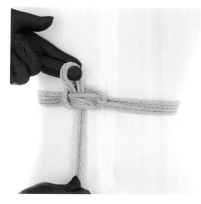

**1.** Here you are ready to do a tail pull, but this one will have the moving rope against your partner's skin.

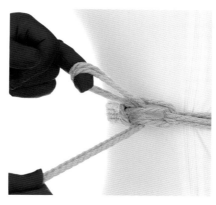

**2.** If you simply pull both sides of the tail away from the body a little bit, it will pull the moving rope away from the skin. (I am pulling at a sharper angle than is really needed so it is easier to see what I mean.)

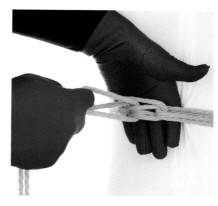

**3.** With just a little tension, there is plenty of space between the rope and the skin.

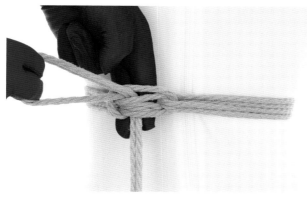

**4.** Another technique is for you to put *your* skin in the game! If you put your fingers between the moving rope and your partner...

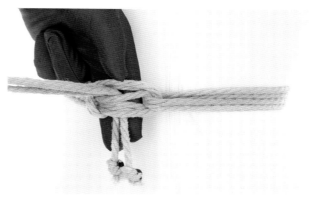

**5.** ...it will be your skin that feels the burn and you will naturally adjust your pull to a safe speed.

Another technique that helps keep moving rope off your partner's skin is to pull all the strands, not just the free ones (p. 163).

# Demonstration Time!

## Put All These Ideas Together as You Tie

We have covered a lot of tips, but they will become second nature as you practice them and you will naturally begin doing many of them at the same time with a few simple moves.

Let's do an example from the **Bikini Harness** (p. 332), looking at each action in terms of the tips we've discussed so far.

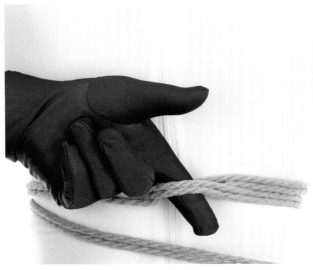

**1.** Place your finger under the lines.

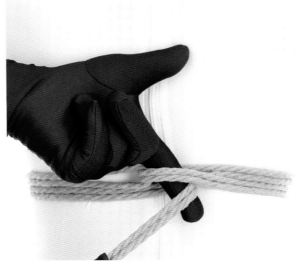

**2.** Loop the tail over your finger.

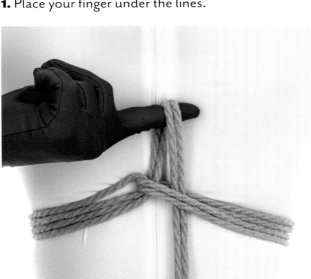

**3.** Twist your hand, bending your finger at the same time to form **The Hook**. Begin pulling the rope through.

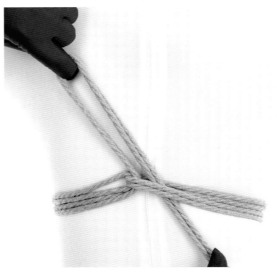

**4.** Be sure to position the tail so that it will move through **The Big Hole, The Path of Least Resistance**.

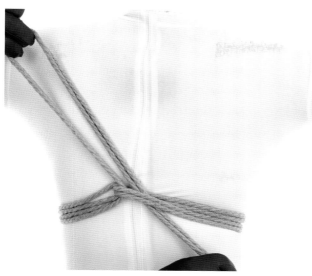

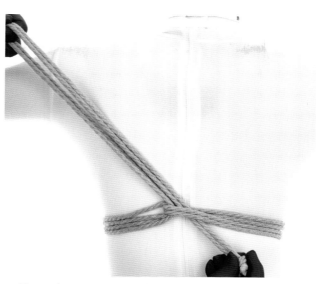

**5.** Hold both ends to keep the tail controlled. Pull the lines away from the body a little bit so that the moving rope is not touching the skin, **Reducing the Risk of Rope Burn**.

**6.** Keep that tension in place as you quickly **Move the Rope through Like a Stick**.

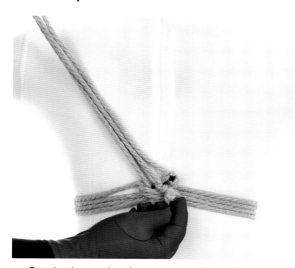

**7.** Guide the ends of your rope through.

### Use These Techniques for Both Tying *and* Untying

When *untying* your partner, continue to use **The Hook** and **Move the Rope Like a Stick** where you can. For example, when untying a single column, you will need to pull the tail under the band to release it.

Grab your rope not by using your fingers like a pincer, but just as you did while putting it on; by reaching under the band and hooking that tail. Doing it this way is generally faster and protects your rope.

To an observer that doesn't know much about rope, it looks like you just ran a rope through a node or under a band.

But in reality, you did so in a very efficient way that also protected your partner from rope burn and reduced the wear on your rope!

# How to "Lock Off"

When you hear the instruction: "lock off" or "lock it off", etc., it means that the tie itself is over and you just need to tie the end of the rope into the bondage so that the tie doesn't come undone. If you have rope left over, it also implies that you choose how you will use it up. See *Using Up Extra Rope* (p. 279) for more on this.

If the instructions do not specify a particular method to use to lock it off, it usually means that it doesn't really matter and you can use whatever seems appropriate in your particular situation. Here are a few common approaches:

## Use a Half Hitch
### Example 1 – Connecting to a Band
This example is from the **Crotch Rope** (p. 370).

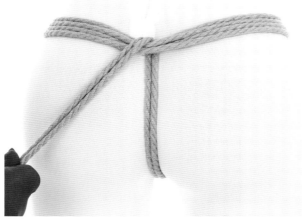

**1.** Run the tail under the thing you are anchoring to. Reverse tension on the tail, setting the tension on the incoming line.

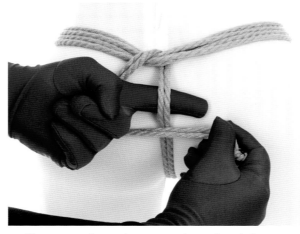

**2.** Place your finger between the tail and the incoming line and under the standing line. Make this "4" shape.

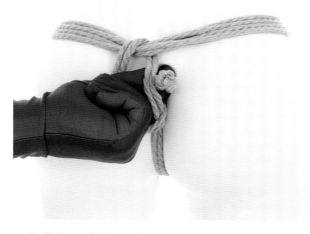

**3.** Pull the tail through.

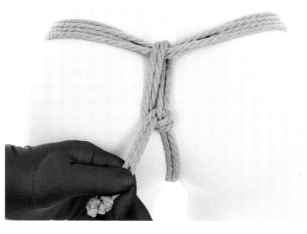

**4.** Like this.

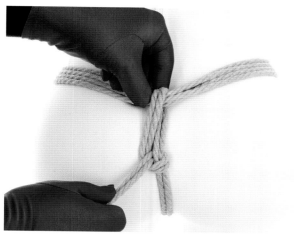

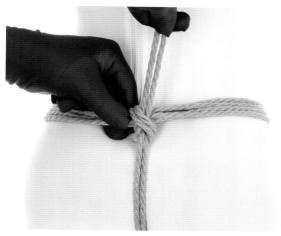

**5.** Hold the line in place.

**6.** Pull up to lock. Add a second **Half Hitch** to fully lock.

## Example 2 – Connecting to the Stem

This example is from the **Shinju** (p. 345).

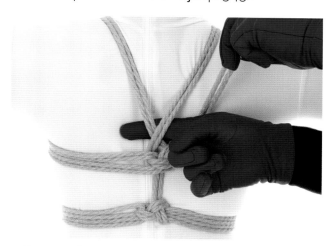

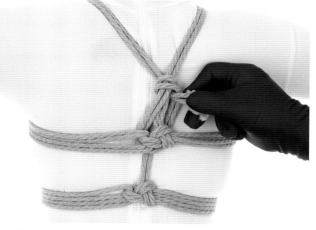

**1.** Put your finger on top of the tail and then under the lines of the shoulder bands.

**2.** Hook the tail over your finger and draw it through to complete the **Hitch**.

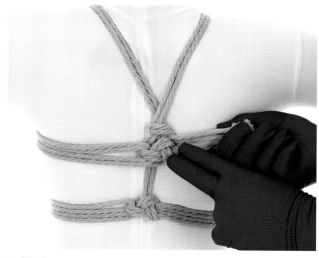

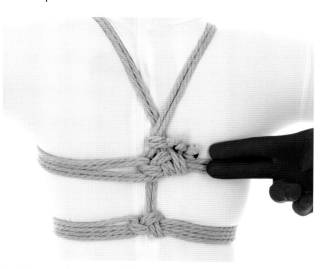

**3.** Tighten.

**4.** Use up the rest of the rope.

# Separate the Strands, Lock with a Square Knot

Separate the strands of the tail, run them around a band or stem,
and tie them together using a **Square Knot** (p. 149).

### Example 1 – Connecting to a Band

This example is from the **Crotch Rope** (p. 370).

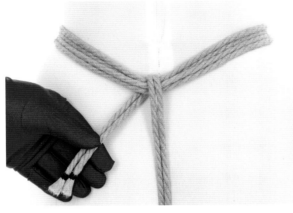

**1.** Reverse tension.

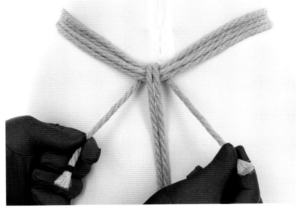

**2.** Separate the strands, place one on each side of some other line.

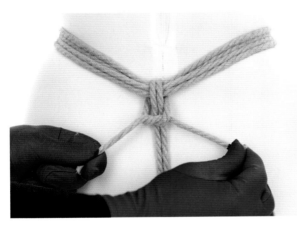

**3.** Add the first twist of the **Square Knot**.

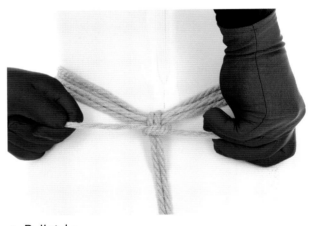

**4.** Pull tight.

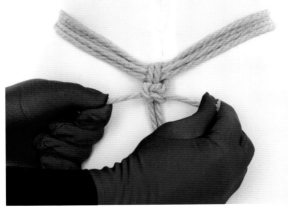

**5.** Add the second twist.

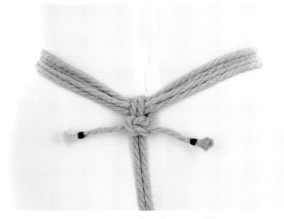

**6.** Tighten to complete the **Square Knot**.

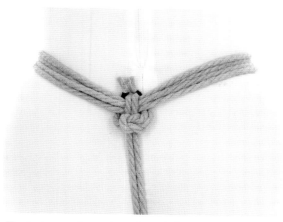

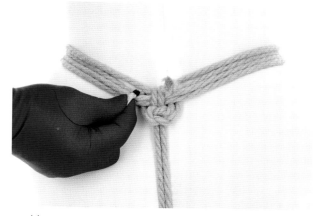

**7.** Tuck the ends under a band that is under tension.

**8.** Alternatively, you can tuck them between the strands. This is especially good if you have knots in the ends of your rope.

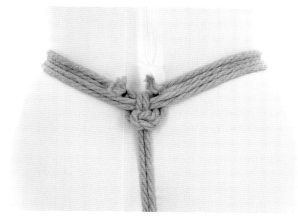

**9.** Done!

## Example 2 – Connecting to the Stem

This example is from the **Shinju** (p. 345).

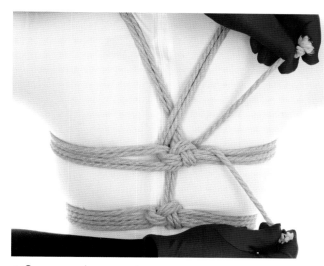

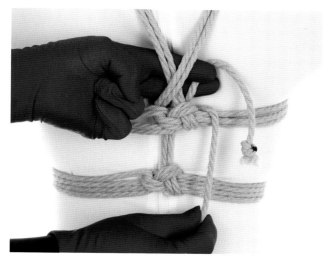

**1.** Separate the strands.

**2.** Reach under the shoulder bands to grab one of the tails. *continues...*

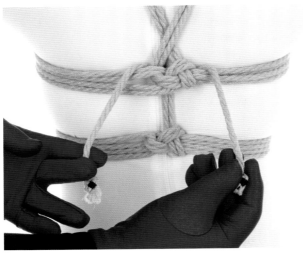

**3.** Pull it under so that one tail is on each side of the center line.

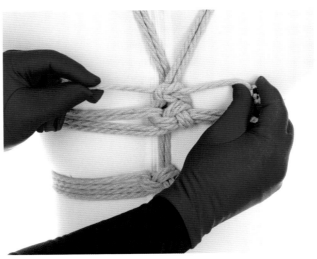

**4.** Tie a **Square Knot**. Pull tight.

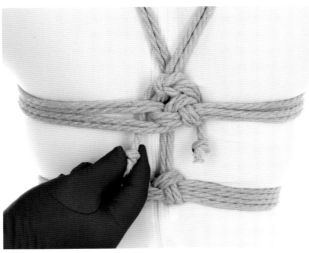

**5.** Tuck the ends under a band that is under tension.

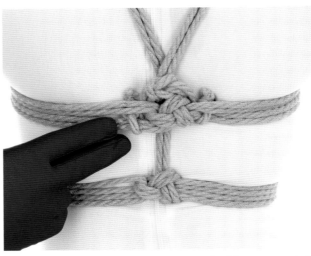

**6.** Or tuck them between the strands. This is good if you have knots in the ends of your rope.

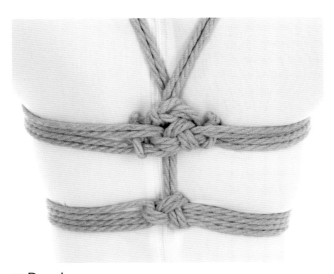

**7.** Done!

# Wrap and Tuck

Wrap the tail around a band that is under tension, then tuck the ends through some of those lines or make the last wrap a **Half Hitch**.

### Example 1 – Connecting to a Band (symmetrical)

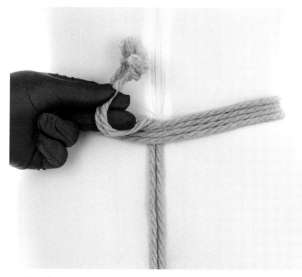

**1.** Set the tension.

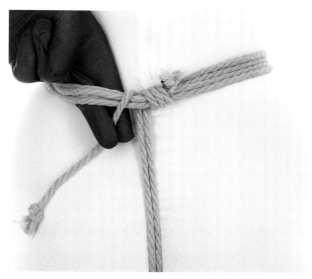

**2.** Wrap the tail around the band. (The other side is already done.)

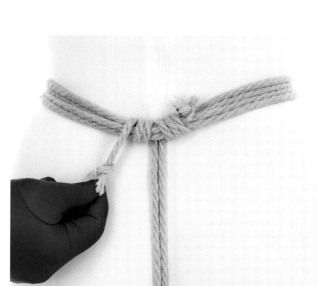

**3.** When you get to the end...

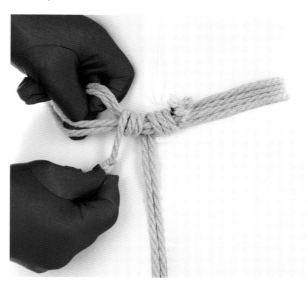

**4.** ...tuck the end between some of those lines.

*continues...*

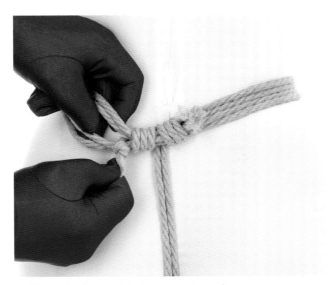

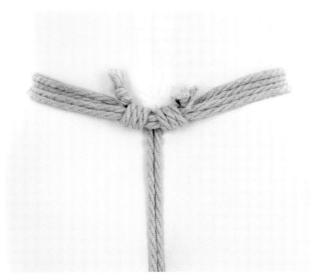

**5.** Push the knot tightly up against the wraps.

**6.** Done!

## Example 2 – Connecting to a Band (asymmetrical)

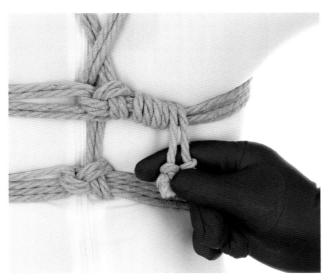

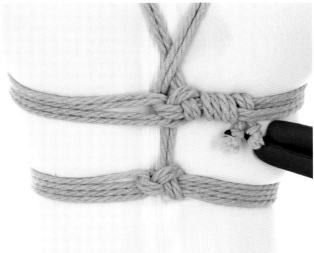

**1.** Wrap both strands around the band.

**2.** Tuck the knots between the lines.

# Style and Mood While Tying and Untying

Here are a few good style tips that will generally give you better presence. Doing these things will give your partner a stronger feeling that you are in control. You will demonstrate confidence and competence. Practice these things and you will both have a better time!

Practice and use all the tips in *Handling Rope* (p. 155). Most of this chapter is dedicated to those techniques. They are important!

Use those tips when you are untying, just as much as you do when tying!

Keep tension on the rope the entire time you are tying, don't drop it. Let your partner feel your strength and control throughout.

Even when using up rope at the end, keep tension so they can feel you moving the rope and pulling on them or holding it, and therefore them, still and in place.

Don't relinquish tension until the tie is completely finished.

The mood you set is just as important as your rope handling technique. The way you move and the way you interact with your partner can do more than almost anything else to set the mood of a scene. You can change up your style to meet your needs.

What do you and your partner(s) want your scene to be?

- Fast or slow?
- Light or dark?
- Playful or serious?
- Powerful or flowing?
- Sensual or demanding?
- Teasing or tormenting?
- Hands-off or hands-on?
- Passionate or peaceful?
- Intimate or objectifying?
- Worshipful or degrading?
- Exploratory or goal-oriented?
- Collaborative or domineering?

Be honest with yourself and your partner(s).

Make this part of your negotiation. Plan ahead. By making conscious choices about these things, you all have a much better chance of getting what you want.

Perhaps these questions will help:

*What is the purpose of the scene?*
Instructional? Demonstration? Exploratory? Professional (for photography, etc.)? Foreplay to sex?

*What mood?*
Playful? Serious? Sensual? Demanding? Dark?

*How proprietary do you want this scene to be?*
If you need them to be in a certain position or place, will you ask them to move? Order them? Physically force them to move where you want them to be?

*What is their role?*
Are they a stranger to you? Are they a play partner? A spouse?

*How do they want to be treated?*
As a respected partner? As a gift? As prey? As an object?

*What are the rules of contact?*
Will you be minimizing contact, touching their skin with yours only when absolutely necessary? Will it mostly be only the rope that touches them? Will you be casually and comfortably brushing their skin as you tie? Will you be all up in their business, teasing and tormenting them as you tie, i.e., the more touch the better?

*Is sex planned to be part of the scene?*
For some people, sex is an important aspect of a bondage scene, for others it is not part of it at all. IMPORTANT: If the answer to this is any type of "yes," make sure you know what that means! The spectrum of activities that can be called "sex" is huge. Be very clear and specific about what is allowed and what is not allowed. Your definition may not be the same as theirs!

Understanding what you both want can help you choose how you will behave in the scene. Here are a few examples:

You can set a dominating mood if you move quickly and with confidence. Use big movements when you are doing tail pulls, fast and sure tie-offs, etc. You can enhance this by physically moving them where you want them (spinning them, for example) without talking to them very much, demonstrating that you are in control. But it is important to understand that doing this to an extreme can make them feel extremely objectified. Feeling objectified can be very good or very bad depending on the person and how that person is feeling that day. Treating someone like an object without their consent is not likely to go well for you, but doing so when you have talked about it and are both into it can be hot as fuck.

You can set up a sensuous experience by moving slowly and gently, dragging the rope slowly across their skin as you tie. Letting it brush sensitive things like lips or nipples. Take your time, make the tying process itself a primary part of the experience. Even more, make untying just as much part of the experience. Untie just as slowly and sensuously and you will extend the scene and intimacy even longer.

If you are tying with someone that has never had rope on them or that you have never tied before, you can set an instructional and light mood by keeping your voice at a higher pitch (less intimate), explaining in detail what you will do before you do it, explaining again as you are doing it and checking in with them about how it feels each time you complete a phase. Keep skin contact to a minimum and let them feel just the rope. If you are clever or charming, use that to set them at ease. Do one short tie, let them feel it for a short time, and then untie them completely. Once they are completely out of the rope, take a step back, then smile and check in. Ask them how it felt and how they feel now. Let them process with you. Let them be heard.

There are as many moods and ways to set that mood as there are people. Your desires will change from day to day and encounter to encounter. Figure out what works for you. No matter what it is, I guarantee there are others that are just as into those things as you are. Once you understand yourself, find those other people that share your passions and pleasures. Those people are the path to amazing and fulfilling experiences.

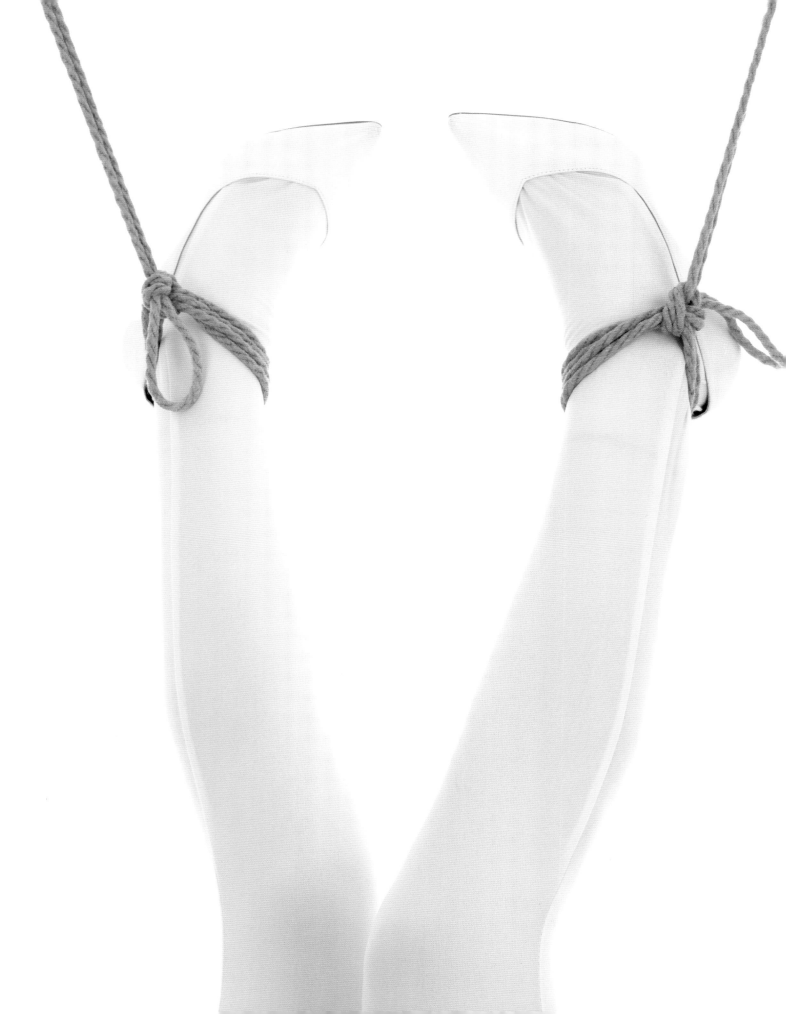

# 6
# Single Column Ties

**Single Column** ties create a non-collapsing cuff, belt, or band around any one of the following: Wrist, ankle, thighs, knee, arm, chest, waist, or hips.

The term "**Single Column**" refers to the fact that there is a single cuff or band. That often means there is only one wrist, ankle, waist, etc., in that cuff, but that is not always the case. If you put two wrists inside of just one cuff, as we commonly do for **Box Ties** (p. 397), it is still a **Single Column**; the act of putting two wrists into a single cuff does not make it a **Double Column**. To make it a **Double Column**, you add a cinch to the cuff so that each column — wrist, ankle, etc. — is inside its own cuff.

There are two general types of **Single Column** ties: Forward-tension and reverse-tension. Reverse-tension styles like the **Lark's Head Single Column** (p. 181) are slower to tie than forward-tension styles like the **Somerville Bowline** (p. 188), as they require tail pulls (the entire length of the rope must be pulled through some part of the knot while tying).

## Forward-tension

- Faster, no tail pulls.
- Can be untied from either end. This can be a useful safety feature, but sometimes it means the tie is less secure.

## Reverse-tension

- Slower, requires tail pulls.
- The tail must be released to fully untie the knot. This can be a security feature.
- Provides some control over your partner early in the tying process.

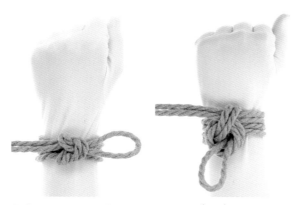

A **Square Knot Single Column** (left) and a **Somerville Bowline** (right).

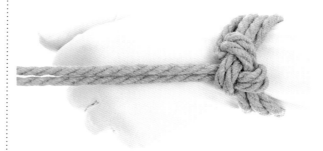

A **Lark's Head Single Column.**

# Important Safety Information!

Wrists are sensitive, they must be handled with care!

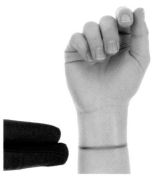

There are a lot of nerves and blood vessels near the skin on the inside of the wrists. Too much pressure there can impact blood flow or nerve conduction.

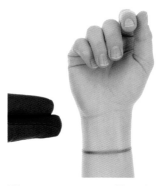

The wrist joint itself is also fragile. If you pull on wrists too hard, you could push some of those small wrist bones into the wrong position or damage that joint.

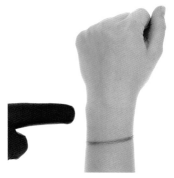

It is best to have cuffs positioned a little farther from the hand, on the other side of the ulnar styloid, that bump of bone on the wrist.

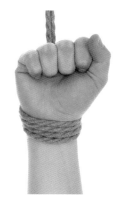

It is pretty common for cuffs to migrate up just below the hand like this. It can naturally happen in a wide variety of situations. If your partner is pulling strongly or jerking on the ropes and they are in this position, it can impact the wrist joint.

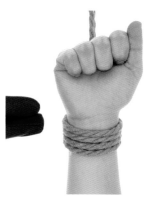

If you see the cuffs too close to the hand, slip your finger under the cuff and move it away a little.

## Always Remember:

- Cuffs should never be too tight; you should always be able to run two fingers under a cuff, more if you want the cuff to be able to easily rotate around the column.
- Never tie someone in a position where rope is applying heavy, continuous pressure on the wrists.
- NEVER suspend someone by the wrists alone.

### One Example of How this Could Happen:

You tie your partner's wrists to the bedposts then grab their feet and pull them sharply toward the foot of the bed. Their motion is brought to a jerking halt by the **Single Columns** on their wrists. In that scenario, you may end up applying too much pressure to the wrist joints. Tying your partner to a bed can be amazing fun, but make sure there is enough slack in the tie that they can move their arms and wrists enough to adjust the lay of the cuffs from time to time.

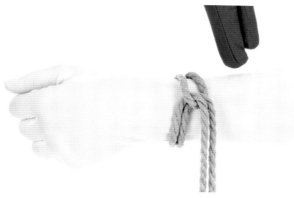

**7.** ...so do the wraps in the *opposite* direction.

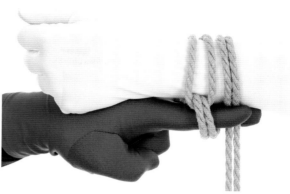

**8.** You can add one additional wrap (for a total of four strands) or two (for a total of six strands). You rarely want more than six strands in your cuff. More than that and the strands tend to start bunching up. This can be a safety issue, as the bunched-up cords can put too much pressure on the body in unpredictable ways.

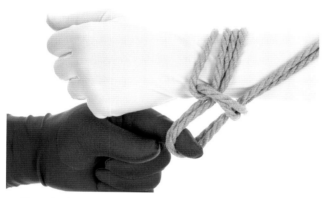

**9.** Reach through the secondary bight and hook the tail.

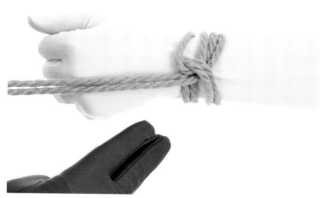

**10.** Note that the tail is naturally moving in the direction we want it to go when complete. Now we just lock it off with a **Half Hitch**.

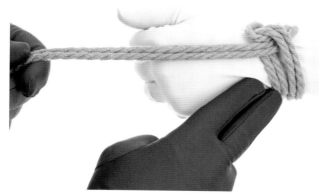

**11.** I will put the **Half Hitch** on the forward-tension side. I prefer it as I think it looks nicer. It is slimmer and less bulky. The reverse-tension approach (p. 147) is also perfectly fine. It is even a little faster as it requires only one tail pull.

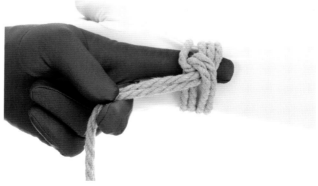

**12.** We need to run the rope through the cuffs in the direction my finger is going, so... *continues...*

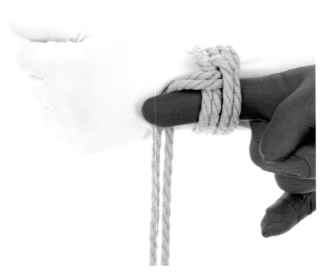

**13.** ...reach under the cuff from the opposite side and hook the tail.

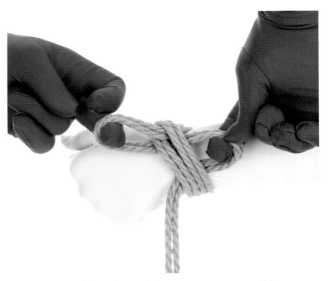

**14.** Begin pulling the tail, but protect a small loop from being pulled through.

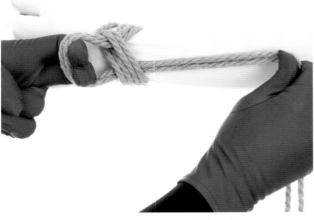

**15.** Pull the tail all the way through but keep your fingers in that protected loop.

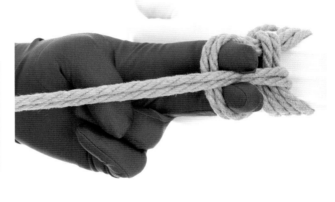

**16.** Feed the tail to those fingers.

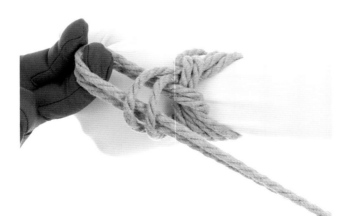

**17.** Pull the tail through that protected loop.

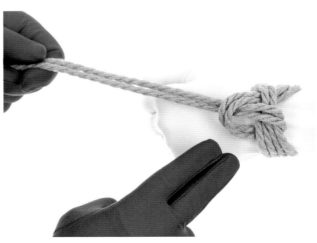

**18.** The shape of the **Half Hitch** is complete. Now we need to tighten it.

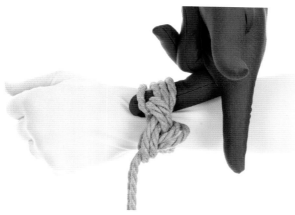

**19.** Place your finger under all the strands of the cuff on the opposite side of the knot from the **Half Hitch**.

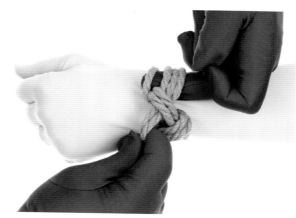

**20.** Grab the ropes at the point just after they have come through the secondary bight, the first lobe. Adjust them until all four (or six) strands of the cuff have the same tension. You will be able to feel this with the finger you have under the cuff.

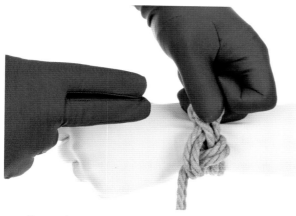

**21.** Once the strands all have the same tension, place your thumb on top of the secondary bight and squeeze. This will keep them in place as you continue.

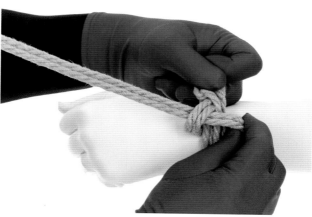

**22.** Pull the second lobe away from the knot.

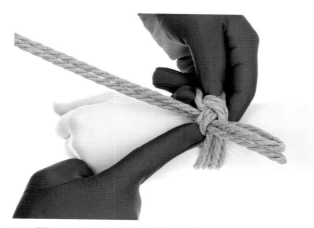

**23.** This makes the first lobe tighter, making it grip the tail firmly.

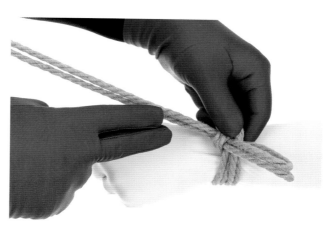

**24.** Move your grip slightly so that your fingers are behind the **Hitch**, holding the first lobe firmly in place.

*continues...*

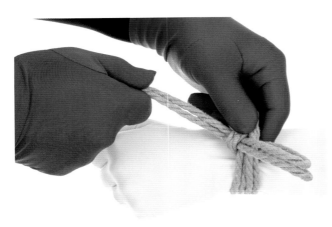

**25.** Grip the tail.

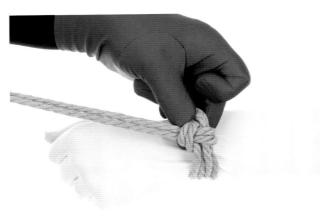

**26.** Pull it tight. This completes the **Half Hitch**. With practice, you can complete this tightening procedure in seconds. It will seem to others like you did almost nothing.

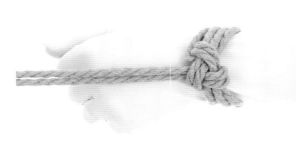

**27.** Done! Note that the cuff is not tight against the hand; it is just a little up the wrist. This is a better place for the cuff to be from a safety perspective — further from the wrist joint. The position of this cuff may change as your partner moves, so check it from time to time.

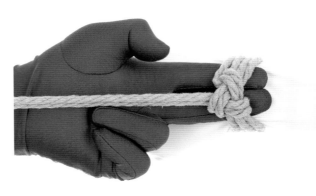

**28.** If you tightened the cuff as described, it should automatically be the right level of tightness, but it's good practice to double-check at the end. You should always be able to get two fingers under a cuff. If you cannot, it is too tight, and you risk injuring your partner.

**29.** It can be helpful to turn this cuff around so your partner can hold onto the rope.

# Leash

This can also be used to make a rope leash!

You may have heard of a general rule that goes "never put rope around the neck." That is the simple form of the rule that we tell people when they are new to rope bondage. The real rules are more complicated:

- Never put a collapsing loop or knot around the neck.
- Never allow sustained pressure across the front of the neck.
- Never jerk on a leash. That can cause whiplash or otherwise impact the cervical vertebrae.

But within these safety limits, many people love the sensation of a collar and leash made from rope.

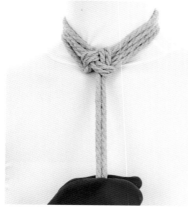

**1.** Tie a **Lark's Head Single Column** as usual, but...

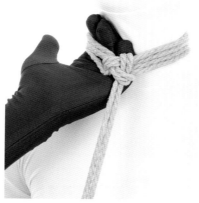

**2.** ...make sure to leave extra space inside the collar — you should be able to get at least three or four fingers under it.

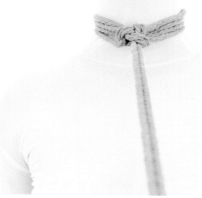

**3.** If you are going to use it to drag your partner around, pull only from the front so that any pressure comes across the back of the neck, not the front. Never jerk the leash.

# Stirrup Heel Tie

This can also be used to tie on a pair of heels. ("No, *I'll* decide when you can take them off!")

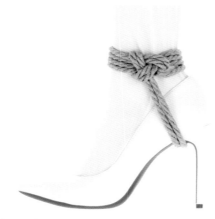

**1.** Use a short rope. Make the **Lark's Head Single Column**, then run the tail under the heel...

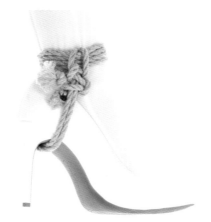

**2.** ...to the other side and lock off (p. 168) however you like.

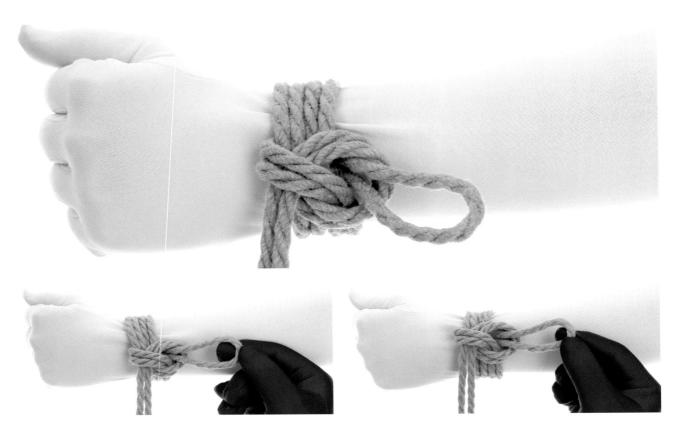

# Somerville Bowline

This is one of the most respected and widely-used forward-tension single column ties. It is my personal go-to forward-tension single column. Unlike reverse-tension single columns like the **Lark's Head Single Column** (p. 181), the **Somerville Bowline** requires no tail pulls and can therefore be used when the tail of the rope is already tied to something! Furthermore, it can be untied from either end. Once you have mastered the techniques, it can be tied very quickly.

This knot is very stable under tension. Some people use the term "bombproof." Properly tied, this knot will not deform and become self-tightening, a weakness of the **Classic Single Column** (p. 205). It is also possible to create a "slipped" version that lets you untie the knot in seconds — a great safety feature for any situation where untying quickly may be helpful. See **Box Ties** (p. 397) for a great example.

The **Somerville Bowline** is a little bulkier than some options, but that is a minor drawback given all of its advantages!

For a little historical context, this useful tie is a variation on the **Carrick Bend**. It was introduced to the BDSM community by Topologist in 2009 and further popularized by Wykd Dave and other riggers. It is one of the most widely taught ties not of Japanese origin.

TheDuchy.com/somerville-bowline/

# Core Technique

With practice, this can be tied in just a few seconds! This example shows the tie being done with two wraps (for a total of four strands), but you can do three wraps as well (for a total of six strands), which spreads the force over a larger area. This is particularly helpful when putting two wrists through one **Single Column** like you would in a **Box Tie** (p. 397).

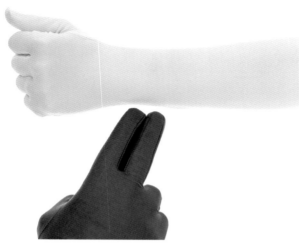

**1.** You can create a **Single Column** on anything. I'm choosing the wrist in this case. It is easier to learn this tie when you are perpendicular to the column you are tying.

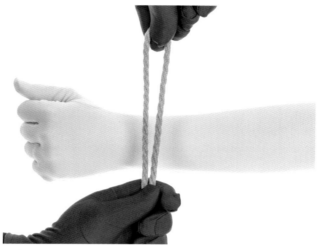

**2.** Begin with your rope folded in half. Grab the bight with your dominant hand. This will be your active hand. With your other hand — your guiding hand — grab the rope a few inches away from the bight. The guiding hand will remain mostly static while you are doing the wraps, simply helping to keep them in position and guide them as they slide. The other hand will be the active hand and do most of the moving of the rope.

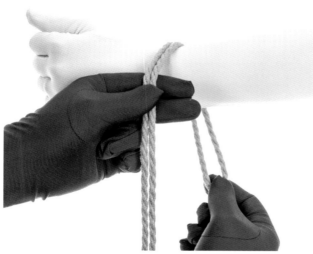

**3.** With the active hand, lay the rope on top of the column you are tying, positioning the bight going away from you. Then reach under the column and grab the bight.

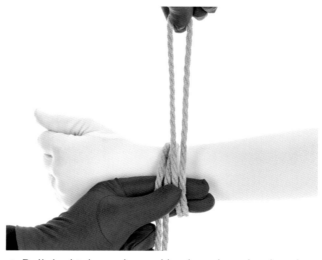

**4.** Pull the bight under and back to the other hand to make the first wrap. Pull out enough of the bight so there is sufficient rope to make a second wrap.

*continues...*

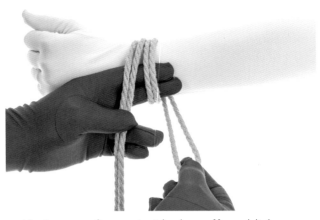

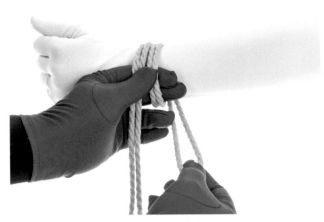

**5.** Having your fingers inside the cuff establishes a safe space between the skin and the ropes so you do not make the cuff too tight. It also helps keep the strands parallel and at the same tension while you are doing the wraps.

**6.** If you need more rope, hold the bight in place, then slide your other hand (the one under the cuff) back down, clip on to the cuff again, and....

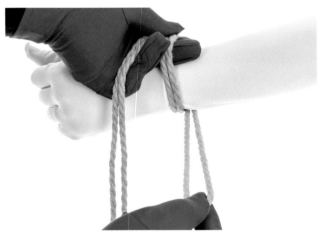

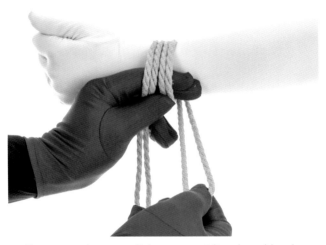

**7.** ...then grip the rope of the cuff and slide it back up and around again, "ratcheting" the rope around to build the cuff.

**8.** If you need more, slide your guiding hand back down...

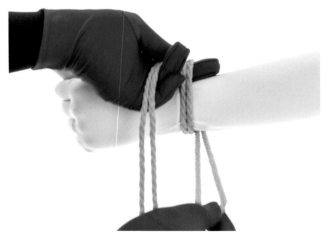

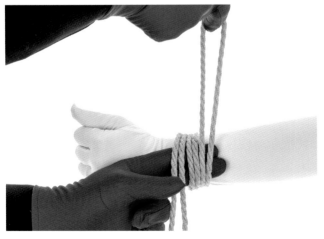

**9.** ...rotate some more. This way you can feed more rope around to get a better bight.

**10.** Do this until you have a completed cuff with 4-5 inches of bight.

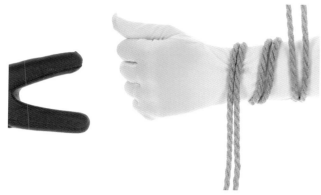 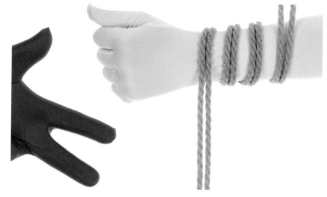

**11.** Normally you only go around twice, making a cuff of four total strands. This picture shows the individual wraps so you can see them more clearly. When actually tying this, you will keep all the strands close together as you wrap.

**12.** But in some cases, you may want to go around three times for six total strands. This will distribute force across a wider area and can be more comfortable. If you wrap more than this, take special care that you have even tension in each strand. They tend to bunch up, so it takes more attention to keep tension consistent with more wraps.

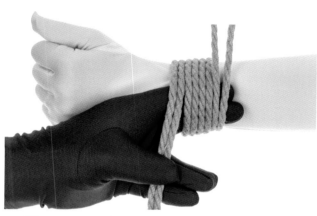 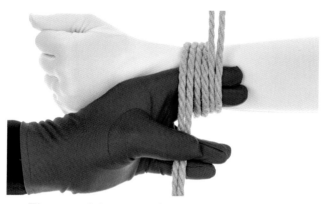

**13.** The pictures above were exaggerated so you could see the wraps. This is what you want it to look like for a three-wrap version.

**14.** The rest of this tutorial will be done using the more common two-wrap version. Make sure the strands are all close together, are parallel, have no twists, and are of even tension.

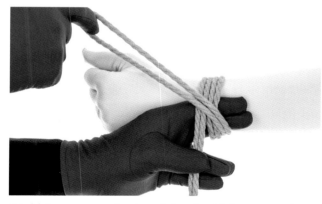 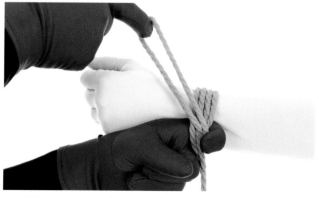

**15.** Using your active hand, lay the bight across the top of the wraps of the cuffs.

**16.** With your guiding hand, pinch the rope in the crook of your forefinger. You want to grip it with just your forefinger, so the thumb is free to help with the next steps.                        *continues...*

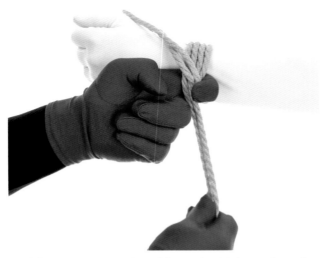

**17.** Move your active hand from the bight to the tail.

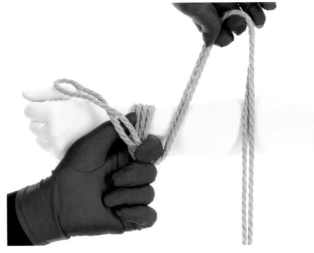

**18.** You are going to wrap the tail around the bight. To begin this, bring the tail around your forefinger. At the same time, slide your thumb under the bight.

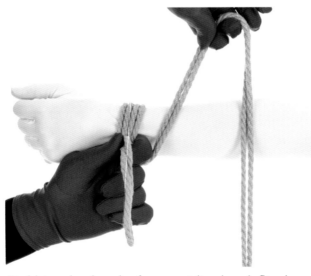

**19.** Using the thumb of your guiding hand, flip the bight down toward the tail.

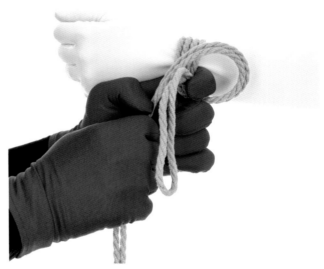

**20.** Continue bringing the tail around so that it is on the other side of the bight.

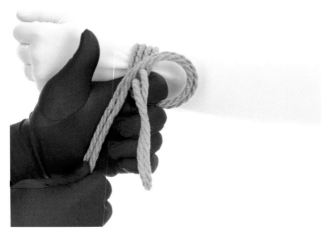

**21.** Pull your thumb out of the way...

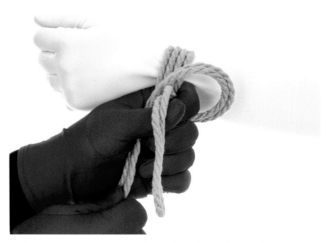

**22.** ...then move your thumb below the bight...

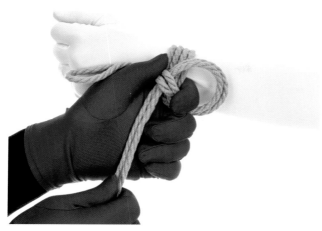

**23.** ...and flip it to the other side of the tail.

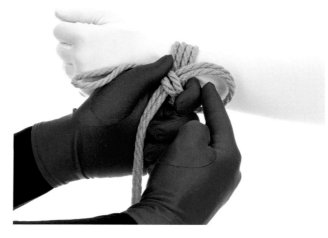

**24.** The next thing we need to do is run the bight underneath all the strands of the cuff...

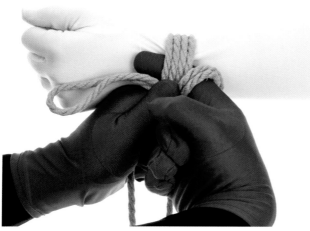

**25.** ...and up through this loop. You can do this in a single move by putting your finger through the loop and underneath the strands of the cuff, like this.

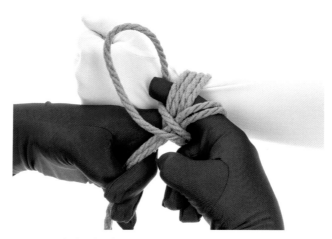

**26.** Hook the bight with that finger.

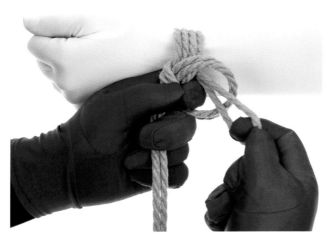

**27.** Draw the bight underneath the strands of the cuff and through that loop.

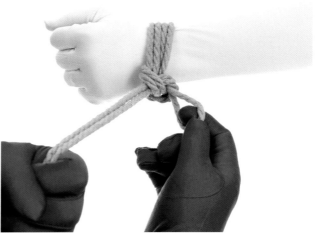

**28.** Keep tension on that bight, pulling it up and away from the cuff; it will hold the cuff together. You can then let go of all the strands of the rope and transfer the grip of your guiding hand to the tail.   *continues...*

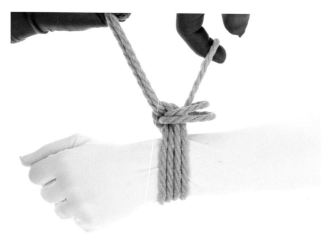

**29.** Here is what that looks like from another angle.

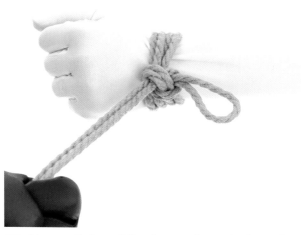

**30.** Now pull the tail firmly to tighten the loop (now a **Half Hitch**) around the bight.

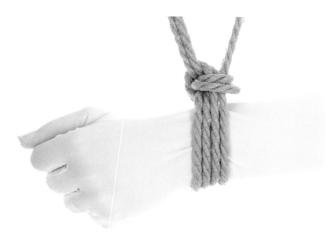

**31.** Here is another angle. The tail is in the process of being pulled tight.

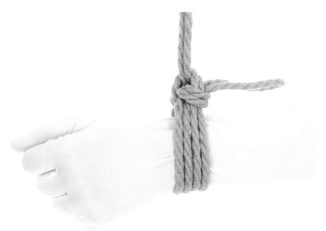

**32.** Here is the completed cuff, fully tightened. You now just need to go attach it to something!

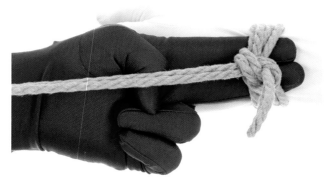

**33.** If you have been following this procedure step-by-step, the cuff should automatically be the correct level of tightness but double-check to make sure!

# Untying the Somerville Bowline

There is a cool trick for untying a **Somerville Bowline** quickly!

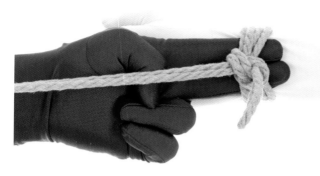

**1.** Put your finger inside the cuff below the knot to give it some stability. Optionally, you can also grip all the lines of the cuff with your thumb (not shown).

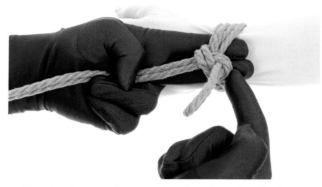

**2.** Put the finger of your other hand under the loop that encircles the bight.

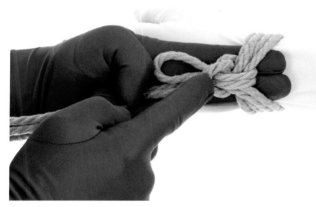

**3.** Pull that loop across the cuff. This breaks the hold of the knot.

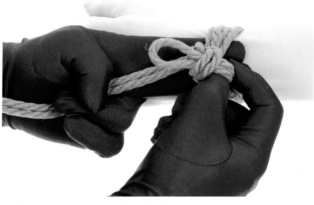

**4.** Now you can easily pull the bight free of that loop.

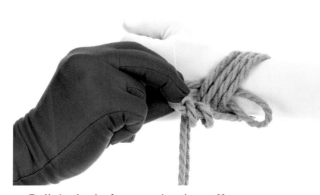

**5.** Pull the bight from under the cuff...

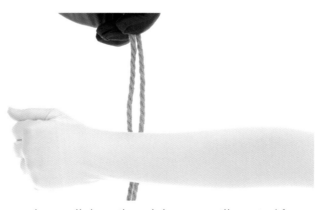

**6.** ...then pull the tail, and the rope will unwind from the cuff.

# The Slipped Somerville Bowline

Sometimes it is helpful to tie a **Single Column** so that it can be untied very quickly in cases of discomfort or numbness. Here is where the slipped version of the **Somerville Bowline** can be very helpful, especially for **Box Ties**.

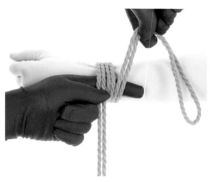

**1.** To tie the slipped version, you need a longer bight.

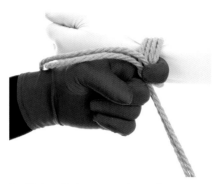

**2.** Grip all the strands with your forefinger.

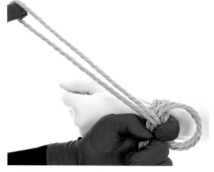

**3.** Then create the loop around the bight with your tail.

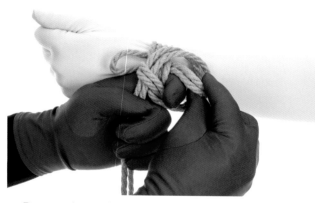

**4.** Begin to bring the bight under the cuff and up through the loop, but do not pull it all the way through.

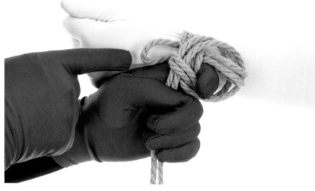

**5.** Leave the bight on the other side like this.

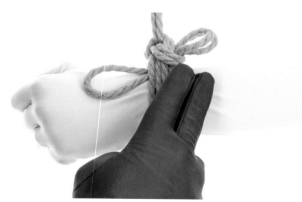

**6.** Tighten the knot as usual. You will have the folded-over rope on this side...

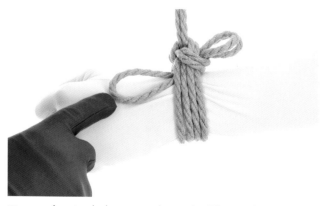

**7.** ...and a single loop on this side. This is the emergency release. This example was shown with two wraps so you can more easily compare it to the core technique. If you use this for a **Box Tie** (p. 397), I recommend three wraps (six strands).

## Using the Quick-Release

The Slipped Somerville Bowline can be released in seconds!

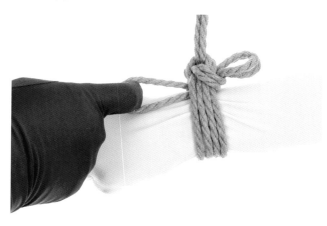

**1.** Grip the release loop firmly.

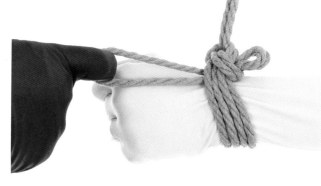

**2.** Give it a sharp pull.

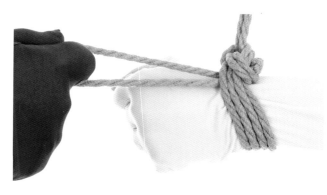

**3.** This pulls the bight out of the loop.

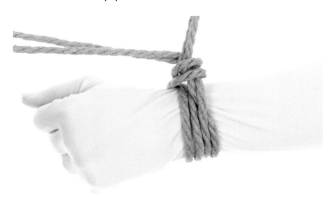

**4.** Now let go of the bight.

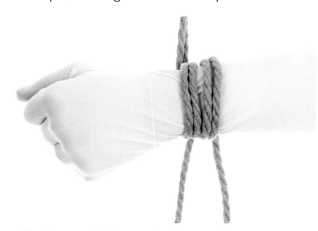

**5.** The loop will fall away, leaving just the wraps...

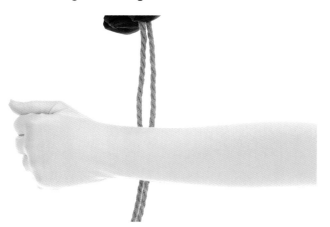

**6.** ...which can simply be pulled off your partner.

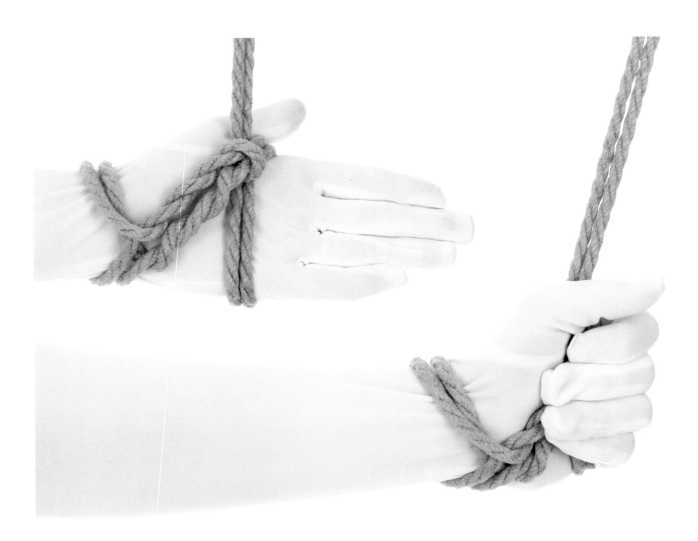

# Cat's Paw Single Column and Flogging Cuff

This **Single Column** is very fast to create and apply and is reasonably attractive. It is not intended to be secure; it is entirely escapable. It is more intended to help your partner maintain position. As far as I am aware, the **Flogging Cuff** variant of this tie was developed by the inimitable Two Knotty Boys!

**Warning:** Improperly applied, this can become a collapsing knot and can cinch down over time. It will also do so if the person likes to fight or struggle. This is good for the person that just wants to feel the sensation of being held in position by rope, but this is *not* for eels. The general rule "never leave a person unattended when bound" is particularly important with this knot.

TheDuchy.com/flogging-cuff/

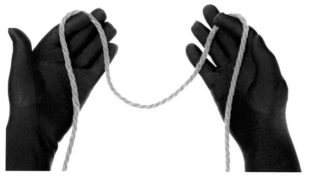

**1.** Make an "M" where you want the cuff. The middle of my rope is at the bottom/middle of the "M."

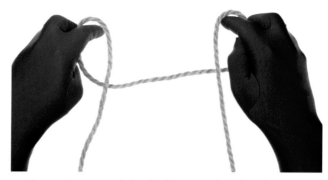

**2.** Twist the tops of the "M" toward each other...

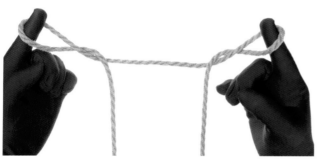

**3.** ...and back making one full twist on each side.

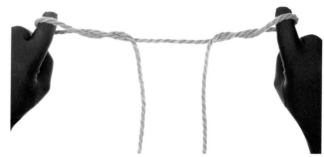

**4.** Keep twisting...

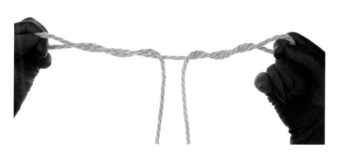

**5.** ...and twisting...

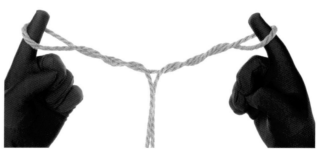

**6.** ...until you have three full twists.

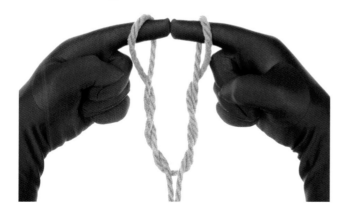

**7.** Touch your fingers together.

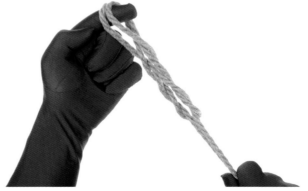

**8.** Slide both loops onto one finger. This is the **Cat's Paw Knot**...

*continues...*

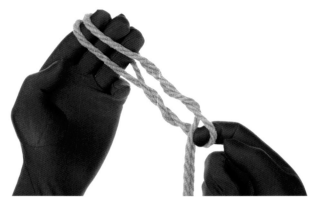

**9.** …but the loop is too small to fit a wrist into, so we need to make it bigger. To do so, hook the bight…

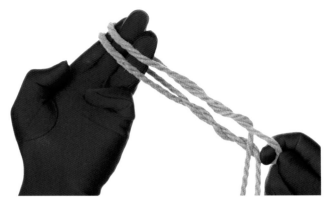

**10.** …and pull it away from the cuff.

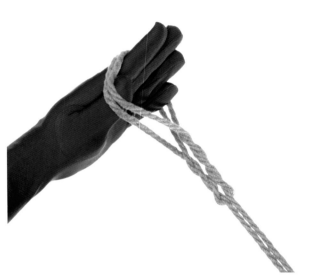

**11.** Now it is big enough to be usable!

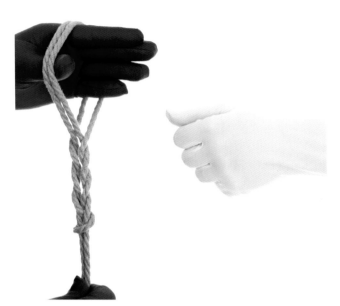

**12.** Place the knot over the wrist.

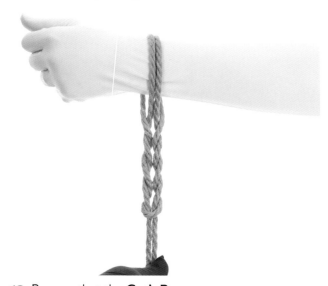

**13.** Be sure that the **Cat's Paw** stays even, symmetrical, and elongated like this.

# Do Not do this. This Form is Not Safe to Use

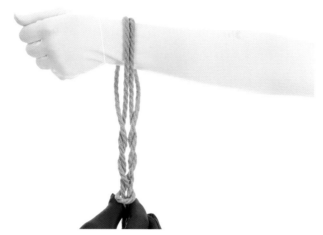

**1.** DO NOT push the knot from the bottom! If you do...

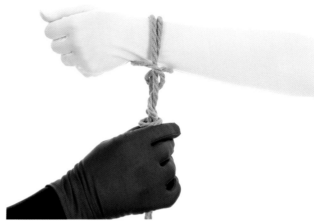

**2.** ...you deform the **Cat's Paw** and end with just a bunch of loops around the standing line.

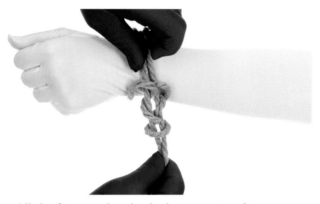

**3.** All the friction they had when entwined is gone and this is now a dangerous collapsing knot.

# Do this!

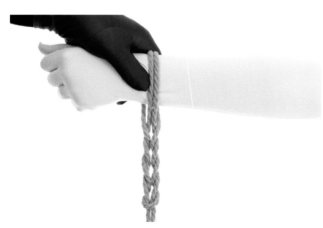

**1.** Instead, hold the cuff at the top and "ratchet" the knot tighter.

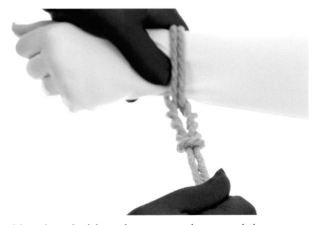

**2.** Here I am holding the rope at the top while my hand on the tail moves toward the camera. As I do this, the knot will tighten. *continues...*

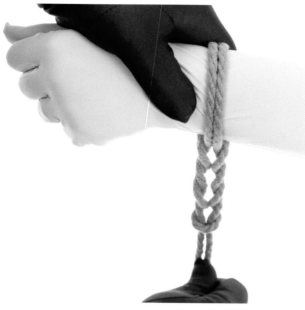

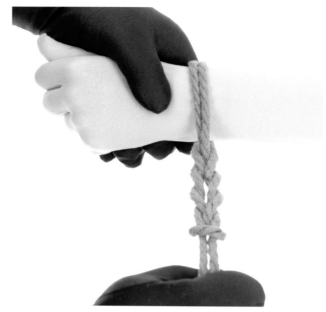

**3.** Now my lower hand moves away from the camera.

**4.** Toward.

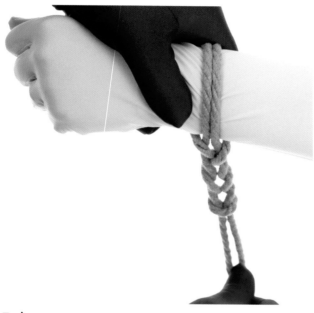

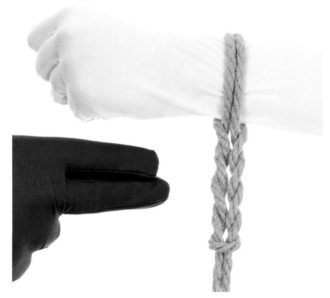

**5.** Away.

**6.** The **Cat's Paw** crawls tighter each time.

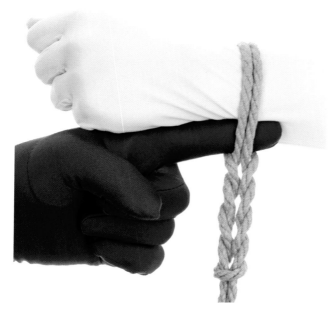

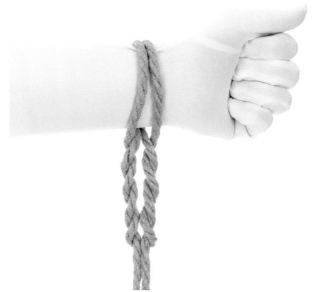

**7.** Remember to check for tightness. DO NOT release tension on the tail when testing the tightness. If you do, the **Cat's Paw** will lose its integrity and will not work properly.

**8.** Note that the **Cat's Paw Knot** is still elongated and symmetrical. This is important. When properly constructed, there is enough friction in the **Cat's Paw** to prevent this loop from collapsing.

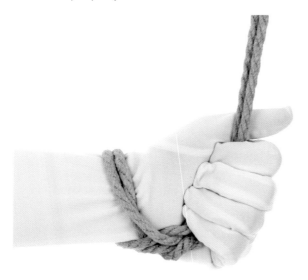

**9.** Lay the knot across your partner's palm to give them something to grab onto.

You can use it just like this, but there is a fun variation that many prefer on the following page.

# The Flogging Cuff

To make this a **Flogging Cuff**, simply add a loop around the hand for added stability.

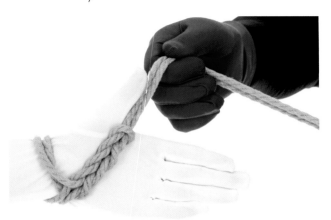

**1.** To do this, place the **Cat's Paw Knot** in your partner's palm, then...

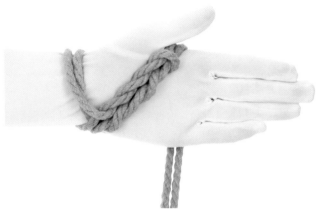

**2.** ...run the tail around the back of your partner's hand...

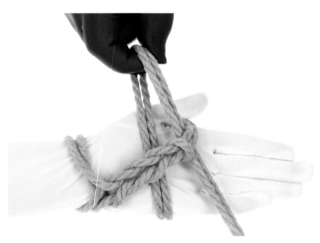

**3.** ...across the palm, and under the **Cat's Paw Knot**.

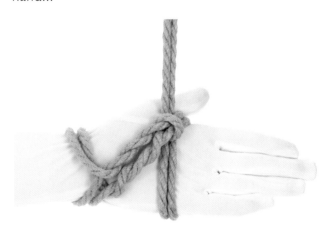

**4.** Done. That is it!

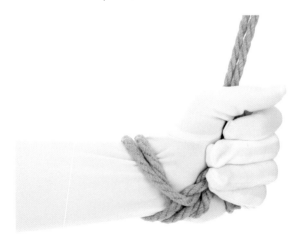

**5.** When your partner grasps the knot, there is enough bulk there for a handhold that feels good.

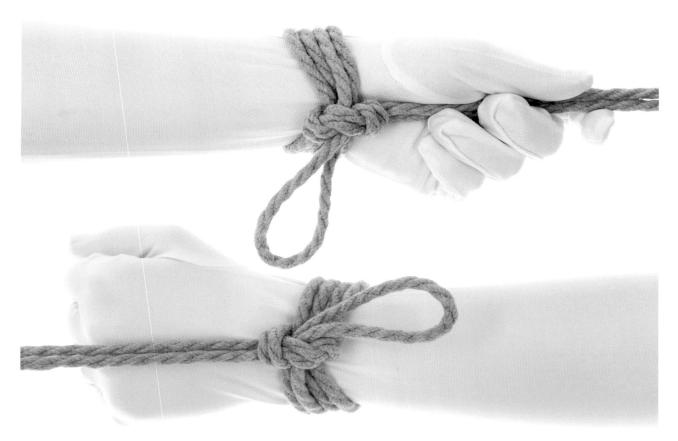

# Classic Single Column

When a rigger says "**Single Column**" without further specification, such as "**Lark's Head Single Column**," this tie is probably what they are talking about (or they are saying that you can use any **Single Column** you like).

This is a forward-tension **Single Column**, using a variation on a simple **Square Knot** or **Granny Knot**. As such, these ties are sometimes called by the names "**Square Knot Single Column**" or "**Granny Knot Single Column**" depending on which variant is specifically meant, but this is not common.

This technique is common in classical shibari because it is intuitive, fast to tie, and easy to untie. By choosing the **Square Knot** or **Granny Knot** approach, you can also choose which direction you want the tail to be naturally flowing as it leaves the cuff, thereby making your finished bondage more attractive.

There are four phases, five if it will be under strong tension:
- Create the cuff wraps.
- Create the first twist and adjust the tightness of the cuff.
- Add a second twist to create a **Square Knot** or **Granny Knot**.
- Tighten the knot to lock the cuff.
- If strong tension is anticipated, reinforce the knot.

TheDuchy.com/square-knot-single-column/

**Personal Note:**

I personally do not often use this type of **Single Column**. I include it because it is very well known and widely used, so you need to recognize it and know how to tie it. When I need a forward-tension **Single Column**, I prefer the **Somerville Bowline** as it is far easier to get right, more stable, and very fast to tie.

# Phase 1 – Create the Cuff Wraps

Phase 1 utlizes a procedure covered earlier in this chapter. The steps below are a brief recap. For full instructions on creating the cuff wraps, refer to Steps 1-15 of the **Somerville Bowline** (p. 189).

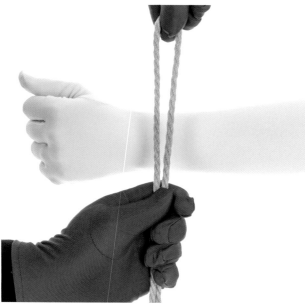

**1.** Begin with your rope folded in half. Grab the bight with your dominant hand.

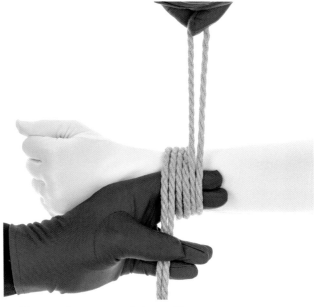

**2.** Create the wraps of the cuff.

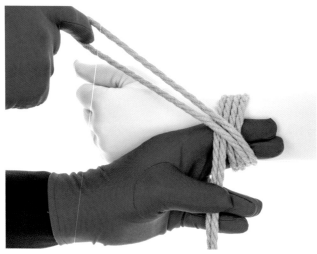

**3.** Using your active hand, lay the bight across the top of the wraps of the cuffs.

# Phase 2 – Create the First Twist

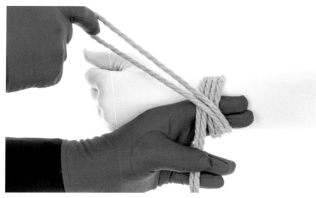

**1.** To make the cuff non-collapsing, you need to use a knot that catches all the lines of the cuff. To do this, keep a grip on all the strands with your guiding hand and use your active hand to lay the bight end over all of them.

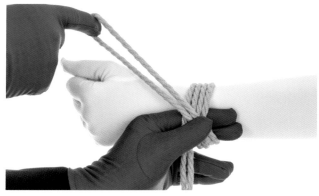

**2.** Use the thumb of your guiding hand to clip the bight in place on top of the lines of the cuff.

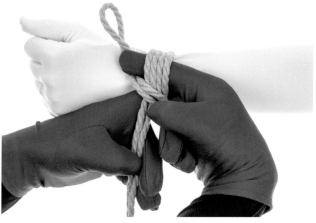

**3.** Then run the forefinger of your active hand underneath the cuff and hook the bight.

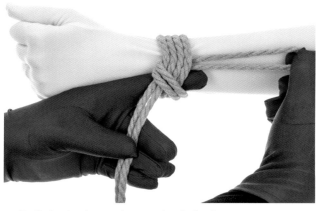

**4.** Pull the bight underneath all the lines.

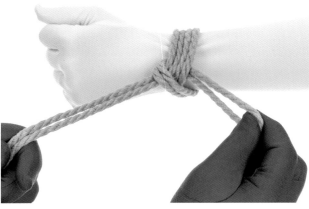

**5.** Keep tension on both the bight and the tail while you slide your guiding hand away from under the cuff, up the tail a little.

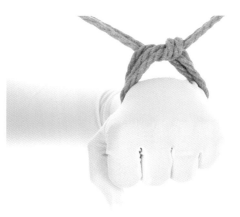

**6.** Here is what that looks like from the front.

*continues...*

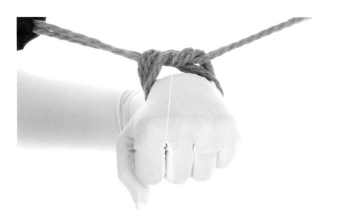
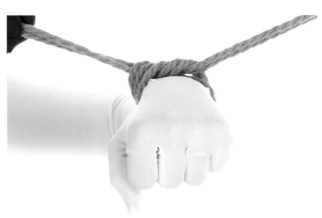

**7.** Now you can tighten the cuff to your desired level. To do this, pull the tail and bight *away* from the wrist (up in this picture) at the same time you are pulling them away from *each other* (right and left in this picture) to tighten the knot.

**8.** This technique helps ensure that you maintain the same tension in all the strands. It also helps you see what you are doing so that you do not over tighten.

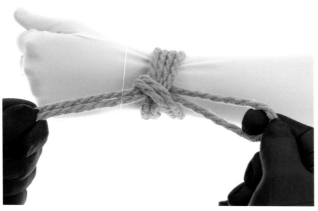

**9.** Be sure to keep tension on both the bight and the tail as you move on to Phase 3.

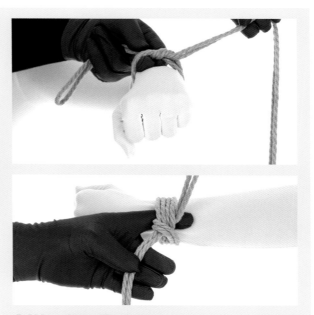

### A Word on Tightness

With practice, you will not need to release your grip to do this test; you should be able to see that it is not too tight. I took my hand off to demonstrate this point. You should always be able to easily slip a finger or two under the cuff. If it is any tighter than that, it is too tight, and you risk causing compression injuries (p. 60, 70). When tying onto a wrist or ankle, etc., where you might want the **Single Column** to be able to move freely and easily around the limb, you may want it even looser — three to four fingers.

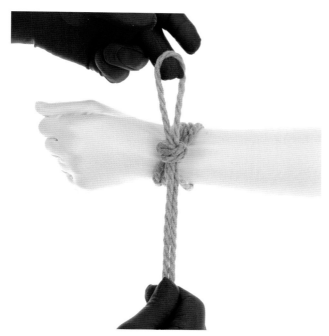

**11.** Now pull the tail again very firmly.

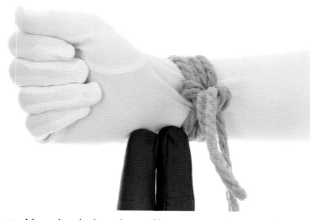

**12.** Also check that the cuff is not too close to the hand and thus not putting too much pressure on the bones of the wrist.

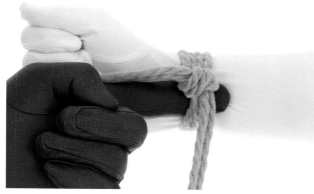

**13.** Ensure that the cuff is not too tight against the skin of the wrist and thus potentially impacting blood vessels or nerves.

## Direction of Tail

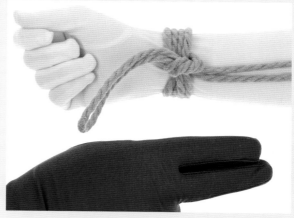

Note that the tail is naturally flowing toward this direction. This is because when we did our first wraps, the bight was on that side.

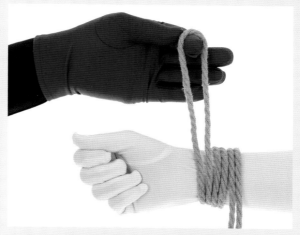

With the **Granny Knot**, the tail is going to naturally flow out the same side of the cuff as the bight in the original wrap.

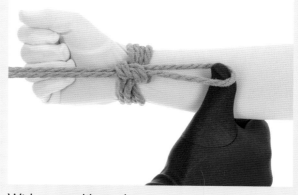

With a wrap like in the previous picture, the tail will end up flowing in the direction of the fingers like this.

## Alternative 2 — Reverse the Tail to Create a Square Knot

This version creates a **Square Knot Single Column** and tends to result in a more compact, tighter knot. Some people find this version more attractive and sometimes choose it for the aesthetics. With a **Square Knot** approach, the tail and bight will be parallel to the strands of the cuff. This can be useful, for example, if tying an ankle cuff when you plan to then tie that ankle to the thigh; the natural flow of the rope will be going in the direction needed.

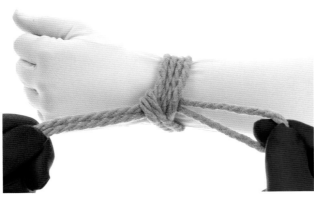

**1.** Finish the first twist (Phase 2). Remember to keep tension on the bight as you proceed.

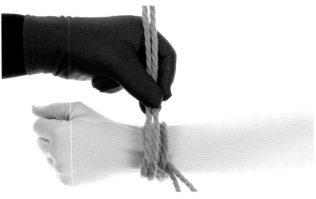

**2.** Reverse the direction of the tail, laying it on top of the cuff to form a U shape — a secondary bight.

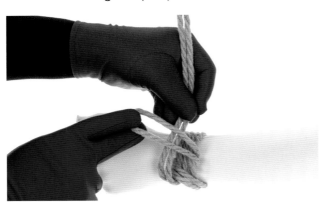

**3.** Lay the primary bight on top of the tail.

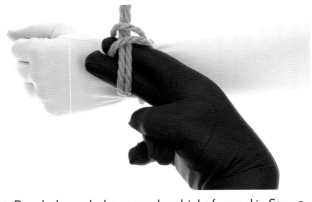

**4.** Reach through the secondary bight formed in Step 2.

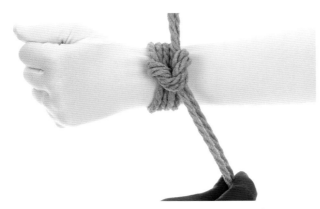

**5.** Hook the primary bight and pull it through.

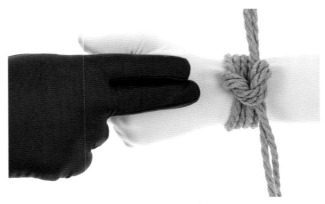

**6.** (Do not tighten too much yet.) You will know that you have achieved the correct general shape when there are three lobes with double lines like this.

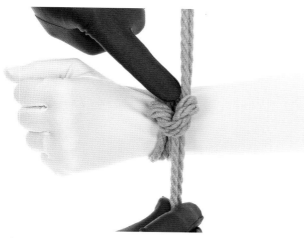

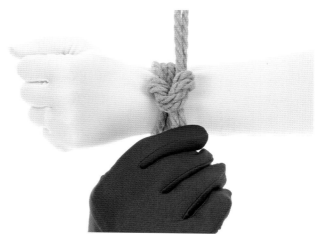

**7.** Not everyone does this, but I like to do one more thing before tightening this knot. When you hook the bight through, it will normally fold itself over like this. The knot can be made more stable if you make one quick adjustment to flatten it before tightening.

**8.** To do this, I just firmly grab the strands of the bight end like this...

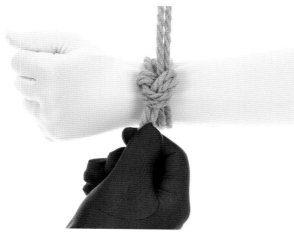

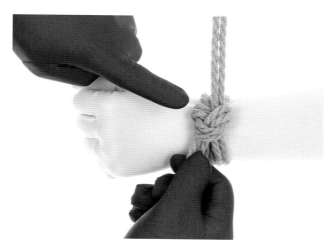

**9.** ...and then flip my hand over as I would when tightening a screw.

**10.** The strands are now lying flat on top of themselves instead of being folded over. This adds a little more friction, making it a little more stable.

This version of the knot is great for any application where the tail will be leading away from the column in the direction shown.

If you want the rope to flow toward the opposite direction, put on the whole cuff the opposite way. If you try to just reverse tension on the tail and pull, you will capsize the **Square Knot** into a **Lark's Head** and the whole cuff will become a collapsing knot.

If you want the tail to naturally flow out of the knot parallel to the column, choose the **Granny Knot** technique on the next page.

## Alternative 3 – Reverse the Bight to Create a Granny Knot

You can also make the second twist the other way. Like Alternative 1, this will make a **Granny Knot**, as opposed to a **Square Knot**, but it does so in a different way. The tail and bight will naturally flow away from the knot perpendicular to the lines of the cuff instead of parallel. This can be useful when tying a wrist or ankle to a bedpost because the tail will naturally be flowing out the end of the wrist or ankle toward the post. If tension is expected on this knot, it is very important to reinforce (p. 218) it first.

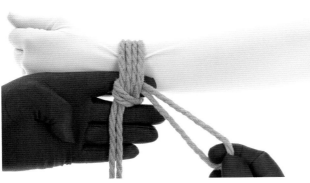

**1.** For this version, I like to slip my finger into the cuff, where the bight crosses under the strands of the cuff. This keeps it in place for the next few steps. Then bring the bight…

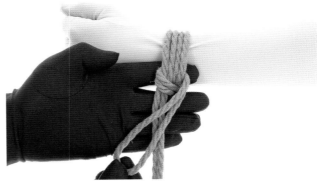

**2.** …across the tail.

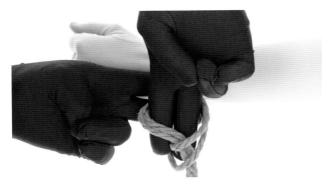

**3.** Reach between the two lines and hook the end of the bight.

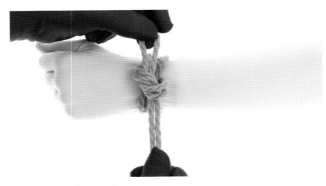

**4.** Draw it through.

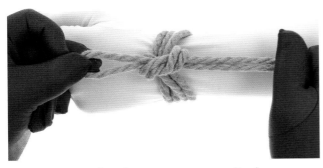

**5.** Rotate it so that this twist is perpendicular to the lines of the cuff. **Important:** The bight is on the opposite side from where it began. Check that the bight and the tail are nicely twisted into each other.

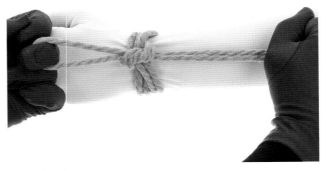

**6.** Pull tight.

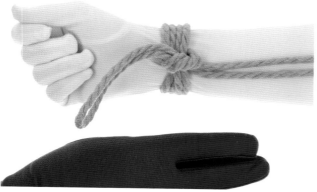

**7.** Note that the tail is naturally flowing this direction. This is because when we did our first wraps, the bight was on this side.

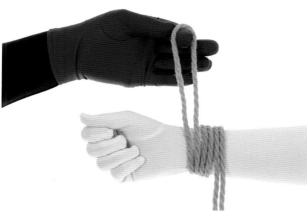

**8.** With the **Granny Knot**, the tail is going to naturally flow out the same side of the cuff as the bight in the original wrap.

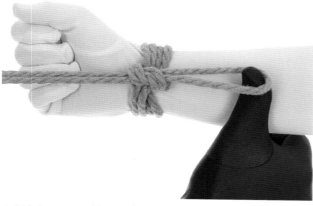

**9.** With a wrap like in the previous picture, the tail will end up like this.

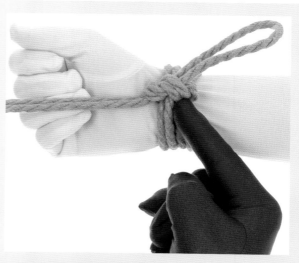

## This Version Can be Less Stable

Note that with the **Granny Knot** version, the tail is not fully reversed into a "U" shape as it is with the **Square Knot**; it is more at a right angle. This is one of the reasons why this version can collapse more easily.

If the tension remains parallel to the column — for example, when this is tied to a wrist, and the ropes run past the hand as shown in this picture — the knot will usually hold up well. But if tension is put on it in a different direction, this knot can pop open, capsizing and turning the cuff into a collapsing loop (sometimes also called a noose).

This is why if tension is expected on this knot — especially if that tension is in some other direction than the natural flow of the tail — it is very important to reinforce (p. 218) it first.

# Phase 4 – Tighten the Knot to Lock the Cuff

Regardless of how you create the second twist, it is important that you tighten this knot very firmly. If you do not, it can loosen easily and may even result in the cuff becoming self-tightening, i.e., turning into a collapsing loop, which presents an unsafe situation. It helps to tighten this knot in three stages. This can be done very quickly with practice.

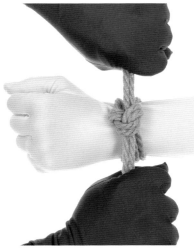

**1.** Pull the tail and bight very firmly away from each other.

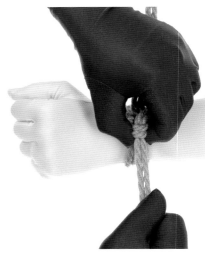

**2.** Hold the knot itself in one hand, then grab the bight and pull it away from the knot.

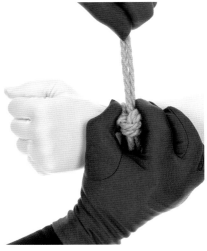

**3.** Switch hands and pull just the tail while keeping a firm hold on the knot.

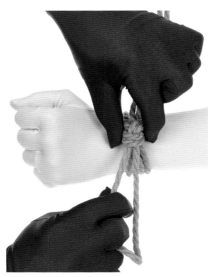

**4.** Keep holding the knot itself, then pull each individual strand tight. You will be surprised how much more space you can pull out of that knot.

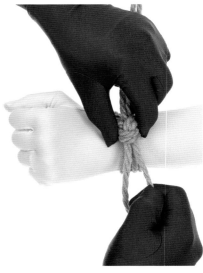

**5.** Make sure to do this for both strands of the bight.

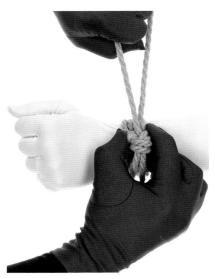

**6.** Then for one strand of the tail...

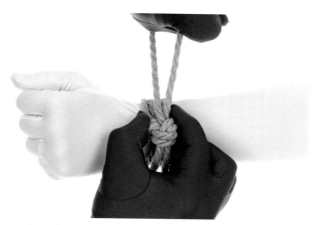

**7.** ...then the other.

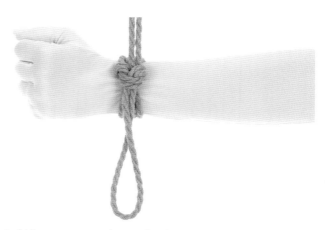

**8.** When you are done, this knot should feel very hard to the touch.

This is the completed **Square Knot Single Column.**

## A Word of Caution

IMPORTANT! If you plan to use this tie in such a way that the tail is going to be under strong tension — particularly if that is in a direction other than the natural flow of the tail (in a suspension, for example) — you are not done yet! In this simple form, the knot can deform and become a collapsing loop which can cinch down. That is not good!

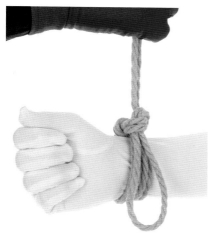

Here I am pulling straight up on the tail, adding strong tension perpendicular to the cuffs.

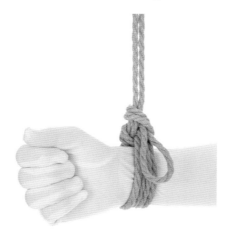

As I do, this knot deforms — the **Square Knot** capsizes into a **Lark's Head**.

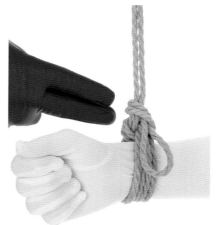

The **Lark's Head** is still around the tail, but the tail can just slide through it, turning this tie into a collapsing loop (or noose).

To demonstrate this to yourself, tie this on your own leg up to Phase 4, using Alternative 2 or 3 to complete Phase 3. Then pull on the tail upward strongly. Your knot will probably capsize, and you will notice that one set of strands in your **Single Column** begins getting tighter.

If you want to use this technique in a situation where it will be under strong tension, you must take additional steps to make it more stable.

# Phase 5 – Reinforce the Knot

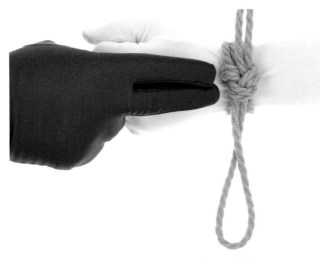

**1.** To reinforce this knot, you need to add just one more twist.

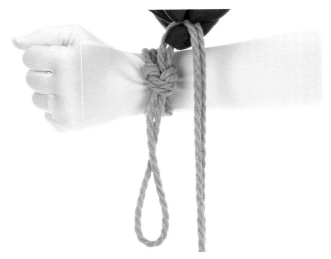

**2.** Use whichever approach you prefer. Here I am using Alternative 2 of the Second Twist options (p. 212): Reverse the direction of the tail.

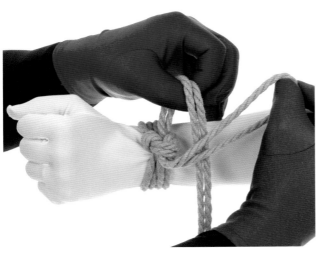

**3.** Lay the bight on top of the tail.

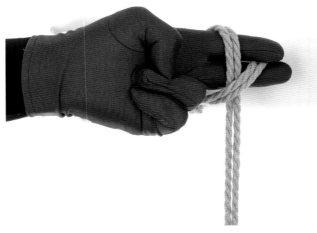

**4.** Reach through the loop and grab the bight.

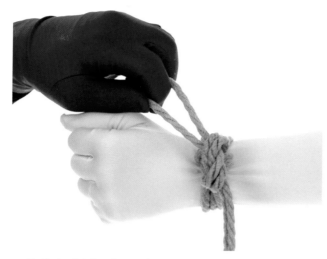

**5.** Pull the bight through.

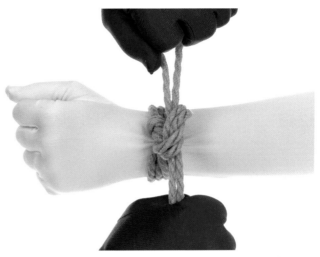

**6.** Tighten in phases again. Both cords together, then...

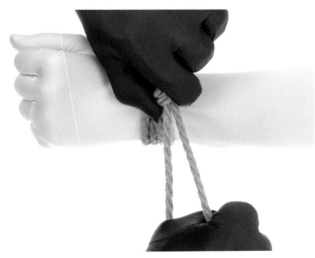

**7.** ...each cord individually.

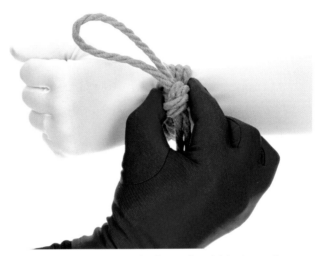

**8.** If properly tightened, the knot should feel very firm to the touch.

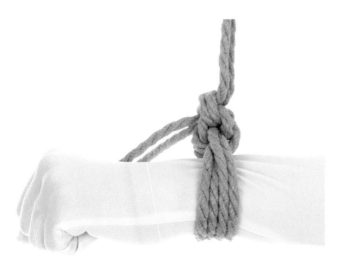

**9.** Now if tension is added to the tail, the top twist might deform somewhat, but it should protect the two twists below it from being deformed.

## Rapidly Untying this Single Column

You can use the fact that this knot can capsize to your advantage:
To rapidly untie it!

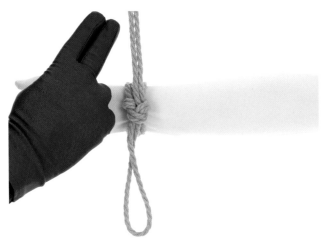

**1.** See how the tail of the knot is naturally flowing in this direction?

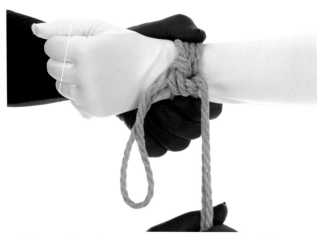

**2.** To quickly release or "pop" this knot, pull the rope in the opposite direction...

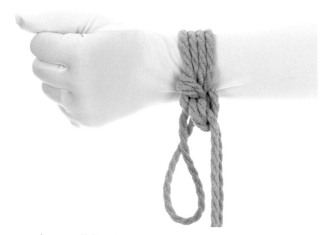

**3.** ...then pull firmly.

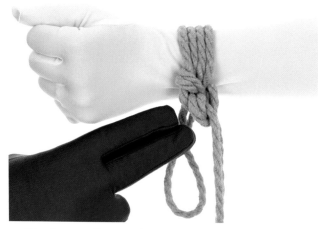

**4.** The knot will come loose.

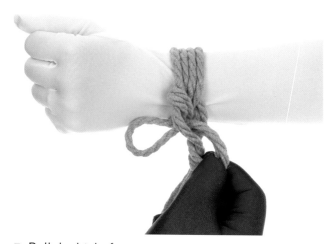

**5.** Pull the bight free.

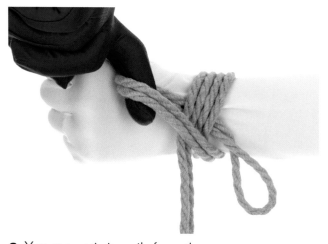

**6.** You can untie it easily from there.

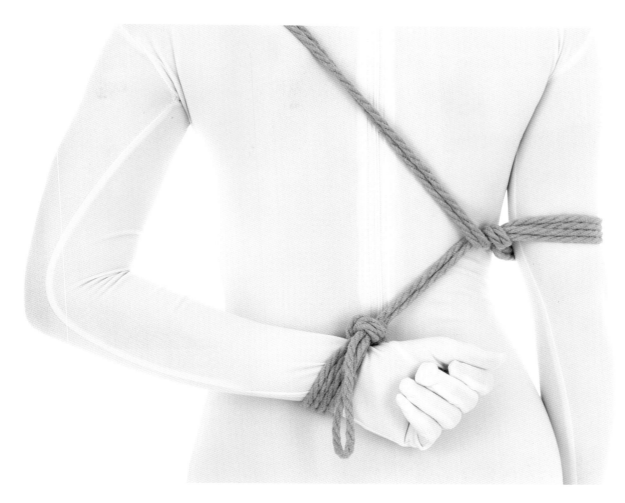

# Hojo Cuff

A quick, useful way to add a cuff in the middle of your rope!

This is a forward-tension **Single Column** that starts the same way as the **Classic Single Column** (p. 205). It is intuitive, fast, and easy to tie and untie.

**Warning:** This technique should only be used in situations where the tensions on both sets of ropes — the ones leading into the cuff and the ones coming out — are either the same, or perhaps there is slightly more tension on the outgoing side.

In cases where the tension on the incoming line is greater than the outgoing line, it is possible for this cuff to tighten down on your partner. You DO NOT want this to happen; it can lead to nerve damage or blood flow issues. Always keep safety in mind.

**Another note:** This knot is best reserved for rope with greater inherent friction, like natural fiber rope. If this is done with more slippery rope, it can collapse more easily, so if you do use it with such rope, keep a special watch on it and adjust as needed.

TheDuchy.com/hojo-cuff/

# The Hojo Cuff — Core Technique

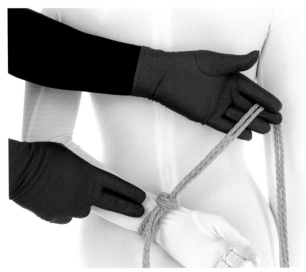

**1.** In this example, one end of the rope is anchored...

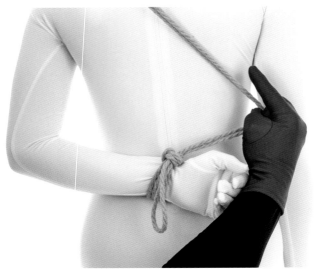

**2.** ...and you want to add a cuff around the upper arm using the same rope. Here is where the **Hojo Cuff** can be helpful! In this case, we want the tail to continue on upward after the tie.

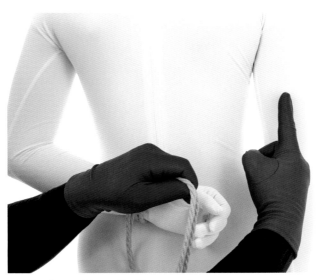

**3.** The basic **Hojo Cuff** is just the first half of the **Classic Single Column**, but you need to make sure you do your wraps the same direction as you want the tail to travel at the end: In this case, up. If the tail is going to come straight out of the **Hojo Cuff**, perpendicular to the column you are tying, it does not matter which way you wrap it.

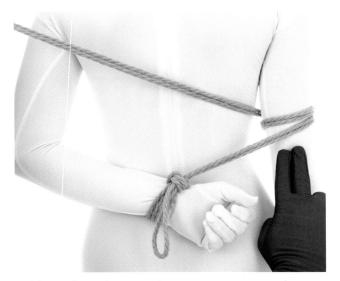

**4.** Using this rule, wrap the rope going upward.

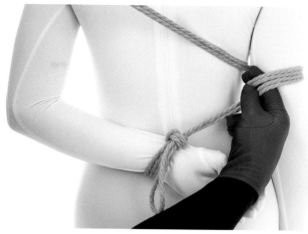

**5.** Place two fingers under the wraps from the incoming side.

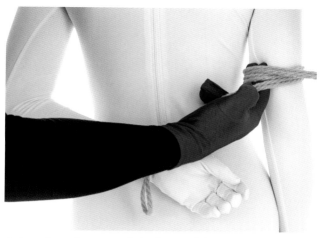

**6.** Lay the tail across all the lines of the cuff.

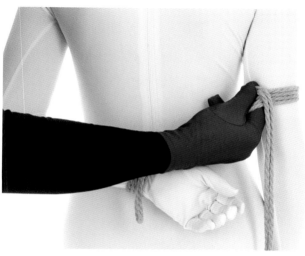

**7.** Clip the tail in place.

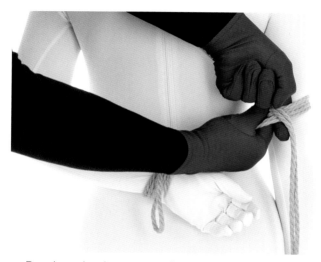

**8.** Reach under those wraps from the tail side.

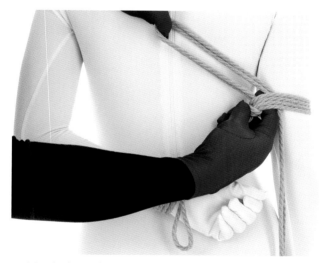

**9.** Hook the tail with your finger. Pull the tail under the lines of the cuff.

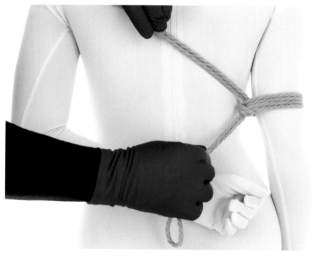

**10.** This is the completed **Hojo Cuff**. As long as the tension is the same on both sides or is a little stronger on the outgoing side, this cuff will not collapse.

*continues...*

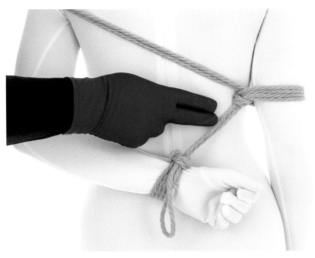

**11.** I personally like to add a little extra friction to the cuff by adding one more wrap around the incoming line. This is not foolproof, but it helps.

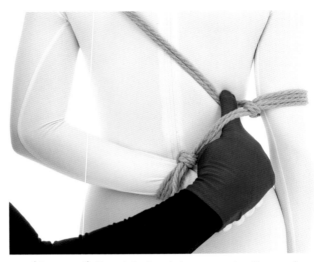

**12.** (Optional) Reach behind the incoming line and hook the tail.

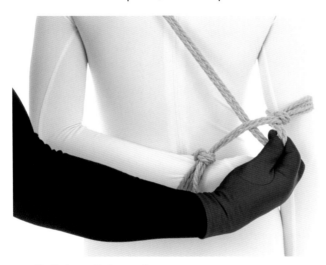

**13.** Pull the tail through.

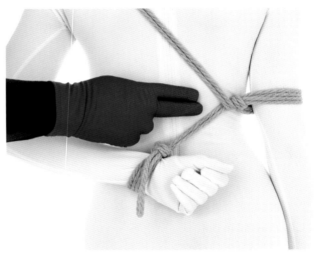

**14.** Wrap it around the incoming line.

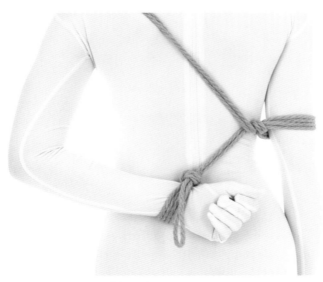

**15.** This also adds a decorative twist.

## Untying the Hojo Cuff

If you release tension on the outgoing line, the cuff will collapse, making it difficult to untie. Untying it like this stops that from being an issue.

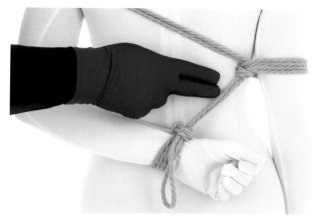

**1.** Untie the **Hojo Cuff** to this point; the tail is no longer around the incoming line, but **keep tension on the tail**.

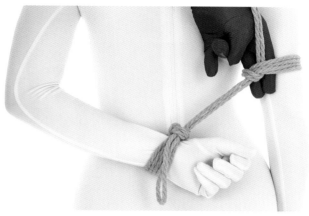

**2.** Before you release that tension, insert your fingers inside the cuff. This will prevent it from collapsing.

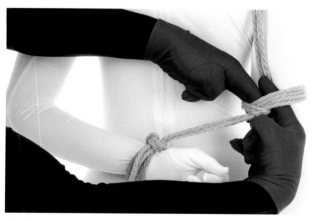

**3.** Now you can release the tail, run your finger under the cuff, hook the tail, and...

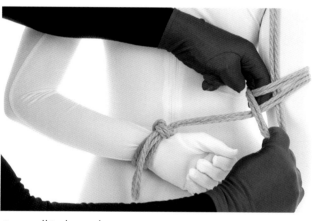

**4.** ...pull it through.

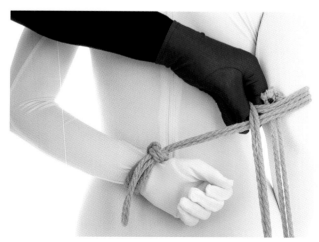

**5.** It is also helpful to have your fingers there to help guide the knotted ends through.

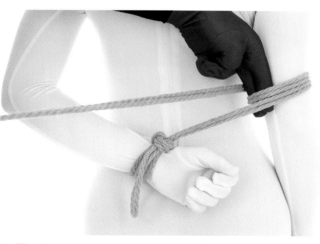

**6.** The knot has now been removed and the rope can be unwrapped.

## The Quick-Release Hojo Cuff

This technique gives you the ability to release the tension on a **Hojo Cuff** very quickly without untying either end! It does not allow the rope to be removed entirely, but it gives back a lot of slack, which can be useful in an emergency.

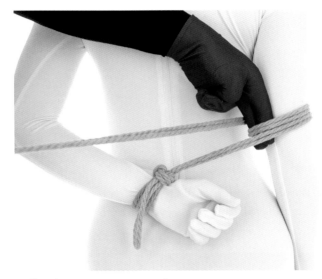

**1.** Do the wraps as normal.

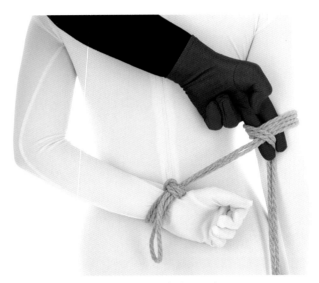

**2.** Reach through and hook the tail...

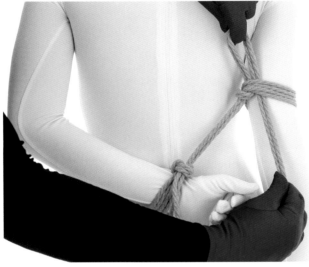

**3.** ...but only pull a small loop through. Hold that loop in place, while you...

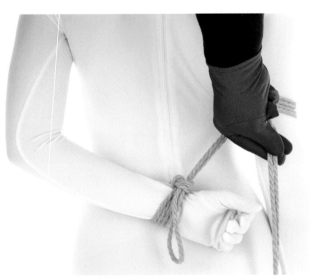

**4.** ...flip your other hand over and grab the tail.

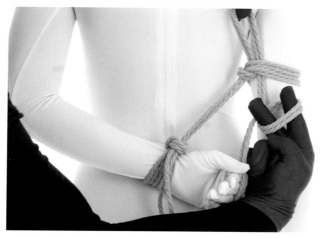

**5.** Flip that hand over again and bring the tail up into a **Hitch**.

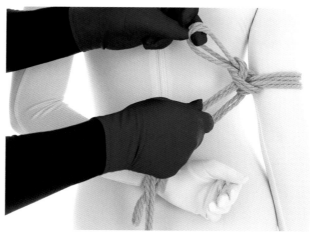

**6.** Drop that **Hitch** on top of the loop you made in Step 3.

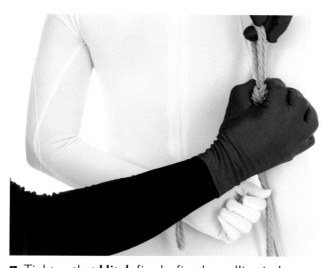

**7.** Tighten that **Hitch** firmly, first by pulling it down into the knot, then pulling the tail firmly.

Now let's see how to utilize the quick-release!

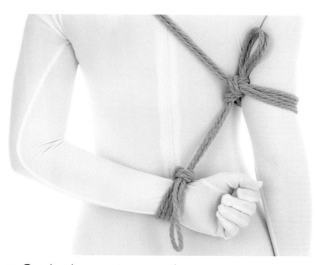

**8.** Quick-release variant complete.

## Releasing the Quick-Release Hojo Cuff

If you need to release the tension in this cuff, you can quickly do so.

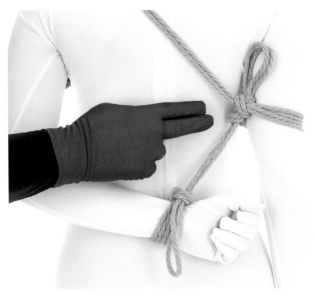

**1.** When ready to release it...

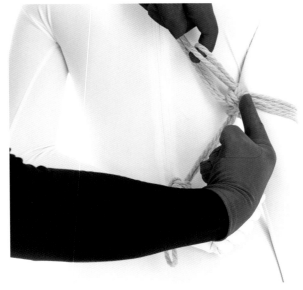

**2.** ...find the **Hitch** that you dropped onto the loop.

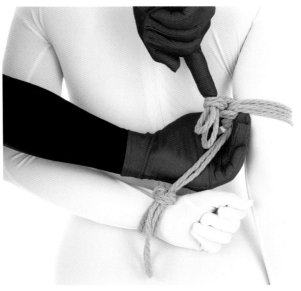

**3.** Pull that **Hitch** away from the knot, up the length of the loop.

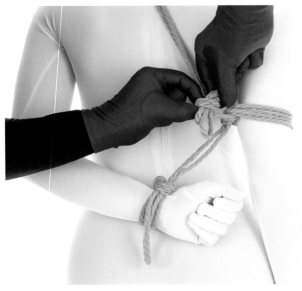

**4.** When it has been loosened, grab the loop and...

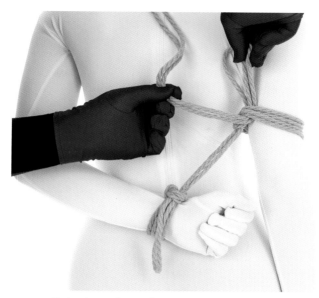

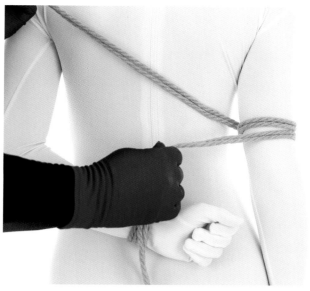

**5.** ...pull the loop free of the **Hitch**.

**6.** You will immediately have released the tension on the cuff. If you want to fully remove it, you will have to free one end of the rope or work the loops over the end of the limb, if possible.

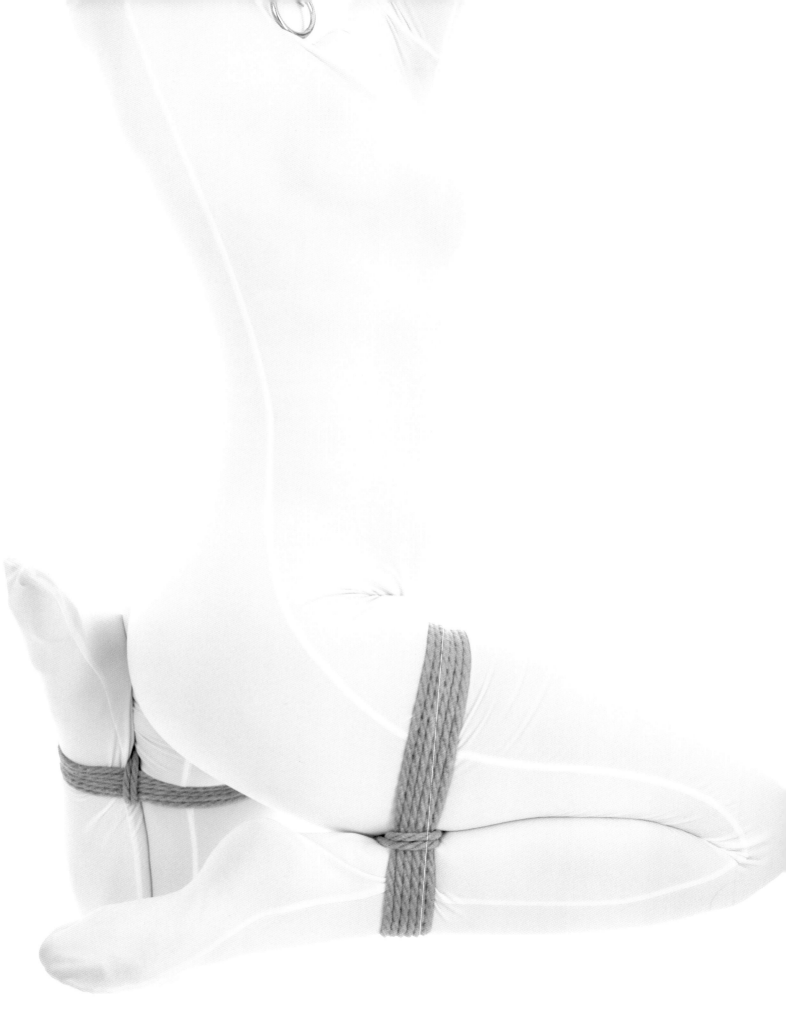

# 7
# Double Column Ties

A **Double Column** tie is often just a **Single Column** tie separated into two parts with a cinch. You may also hear the word *kannuki*, which is the Japanese term for this same idea of a cinch. This chapter will cover the **Classic, Wrap & Cinch**, and **Lark's Head Double Columns**.

*Double Columns* are great for tying any two things together. Wrists, ankles, and much more! See *Building Great Scenes Using Multiple Ties* section (p. 383) for lots of fun ideas!

How to convert any **Double Column** into a load-bearing version.

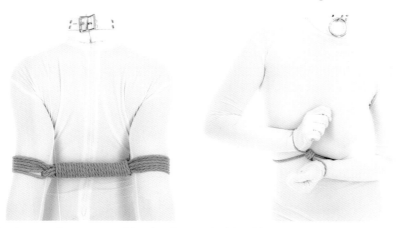

And special variations like the **Extended Lark's Head Double Column** and **Multi-loop Texas Handcuffs**.

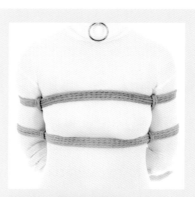

## More Than Two Columns

The idea of separating a **Single Column** into parts using a cinch is sometimes extended beyond just two. Example: In the **Takate Kote**, this idea is used to create a **Triple Column**: The chest and each arm. The **TK** is a well-known form of **Gote Shibari** (roughly translated: "hands tied behind the back").

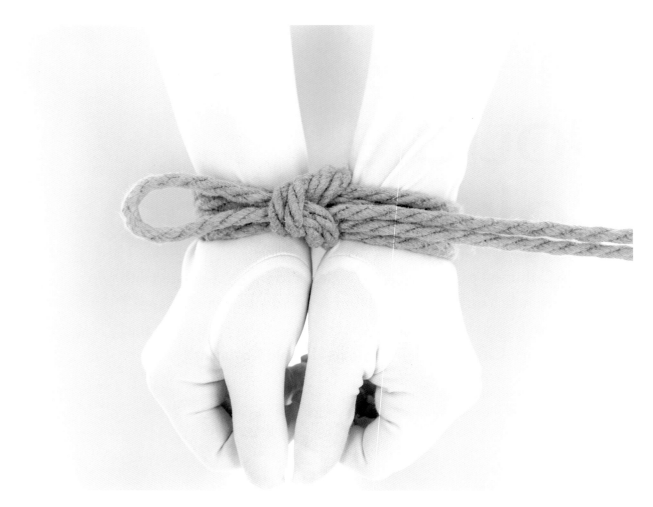

# Classic Double Column

When a rigger says "**Double Column**" without further specification, such as "**Lark's Head Double Column**," this is probably what they are talking about (or they are saying that you can use any **Double Column** you like).

This is a very quick and intuitive method of tying a forward-tension **Double Column**, using a variation on a **Square Knot** or **Granny Knot**. This version is commonly used in classical shibari.

On the downside, it is not as stable as the other options in this chapter and can collapse if not properly formed or if too much tension is put on the knot without reinforcing it.

**Important:** See the *Reducing Risk* chapter (p. 49) for important safety information about tying the wrists.

TheDuchy.com/square-knot-double-column/

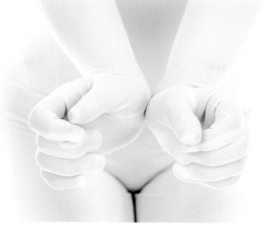

**1.** For this example, we will tie the wrists.

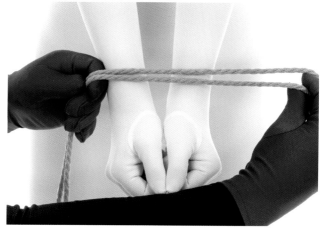

**2.** Begin with your rope folded in half. Hold the rope in your guiding hand while your active hand lays the bight on top of what you are tying.

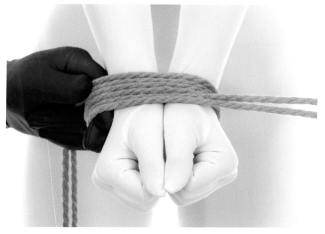

**3.** Make two to three wraps for a total of four to six strands in the cuff. You will need a longer bight than you had for the **Classic Single Column**, roughly 10 to 14 inches, to have enough to finish the tie.

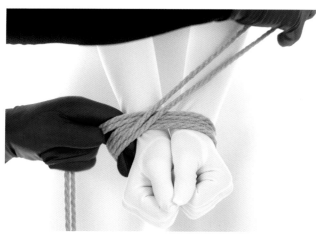

**4.** Keep a grip on all the strands with your guiding hand and use your active hand to lay the bight end over top of all of them...

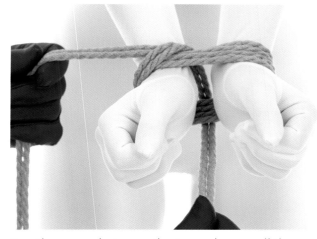

**5.** ...then wrap between the two columns, all the way to the other side.

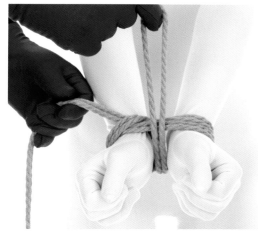

**6.** Bring the bight around all the lines and back up to where you started. *continues...*

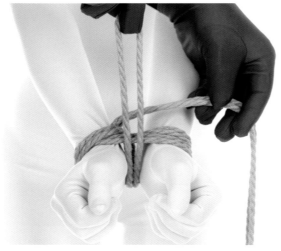

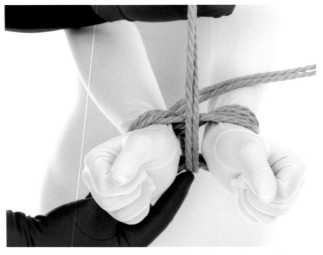

**7.** Now we need to lock the cuff. First, reverse the direction of the tail to make a bend in the rope. (This, along with the crossing in Steps 4-5, creates the first twist of the **Square Knot**.)

**8.** Pull the bight straight up to begin cinching the lines of the cuff. This will tighten all the strands at the same time and to the same level.

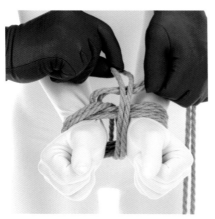

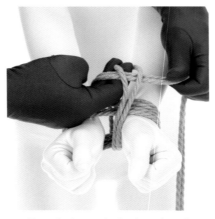

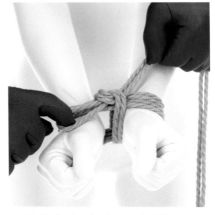

**9.** Lay the bight on top of the bend in the tail.

**10.** Reach through the bend and hook the bight.

**11.** Pull the bight through. This is the second twist of the **Square Knot**.

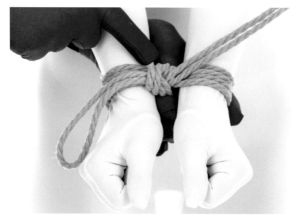

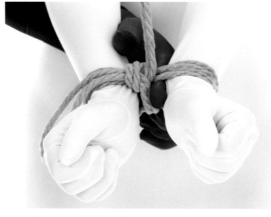

**12.** If you have tied it correctly, you will have this distinctive shape with three lobes.

**13.** Confirm the cuffs are at the desired level of tightness. You need to be able to get two fingers under the cuffs. If not, it is too tight, and you risk impacting blood flow or causing nerve damage.

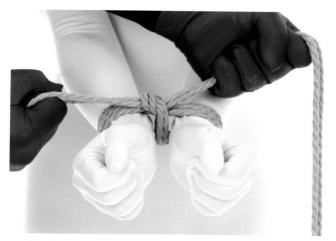

**14.** Tighten the knot very tightly as shown in the **Single Column** tutorial (p. 216).

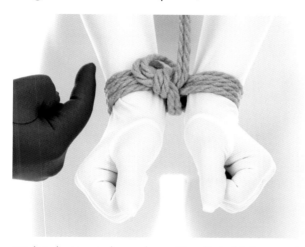

**15.** It is better to have the cuffs a little higher on the wrists so they do not impact the small bones of the wrists. The rope may have naturally migrated tight up to the hand while tying. If so, place your fingers inside the cuff and move them away slightly.

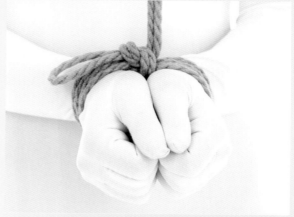

If strong tension is added perpendicular to the cuffs (I am pulling straight up on the tail)...

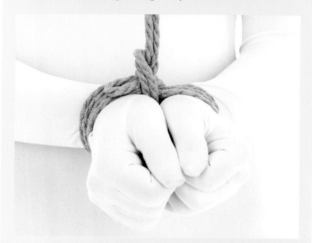

...this knot will deform and can either untie or result in this becoming a collapsing tie.

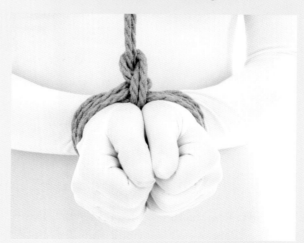

If you plan to have the tail in this configuration, reinforce the knot as shown on the next page or use the load-bearing technique (p. 248).

# Reinforcing the Knot

Add an additional twist so that you have a full Square Knot above the cuffs.

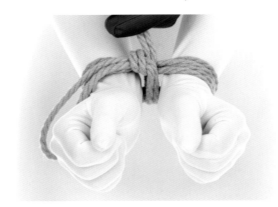

**1.** Grab the tail.

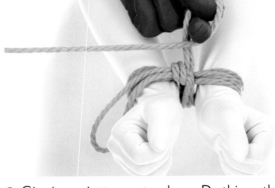

**2.** Give it a twist to create a loop. Do this so that the lines of the tail lay parallel to the lines of the cuffs.

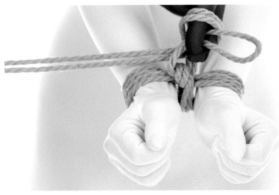

**3.** Reach through that loop and grab the bight.

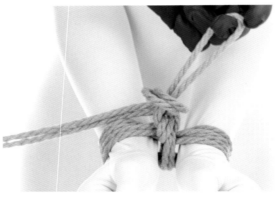

**4.** Pull the bight all the way through. Now that that loop is around something, it is a **Hitch**. That is why this technique is often called "dropping a Hitch."

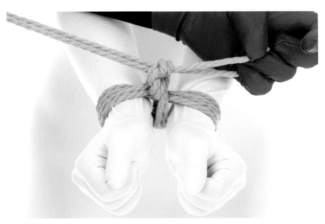

**5.** Pull the tail and bight away from each other very firmly. Then tighten each individual strand as shown in the **Single Column** tutorial (p.216, tightening part).

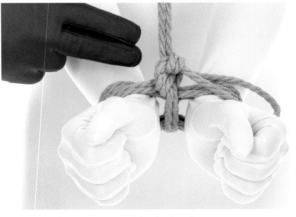

**6.** Now, if tension is added, the first twist may deform somewhat, but it protects the second and third twists from deforming.

This technique can also be used to create the second twist when doing the original tie in steps 7-12.

# Rapidly Untying this Double Column

The lack of stability in this tie can be a feature! This allows it to be rapidly untied.

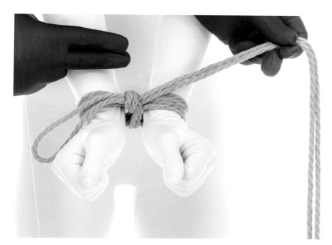

**1.** See how the tail of the knot is naturally flowing in this direction?

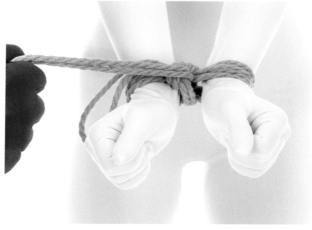

**2.** To quickly release or "pop" this knot, pull the rope in the opposite direction...

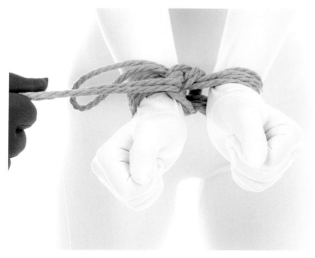

**3.** ...then pull firmly.

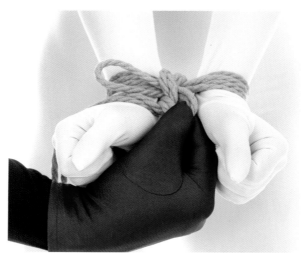

**4.** The knot will pop loose.

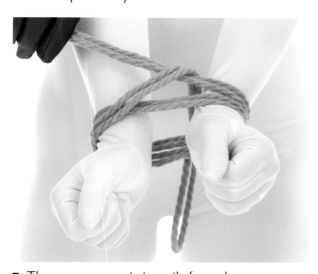

**5.** Then you can untie it easily from there.

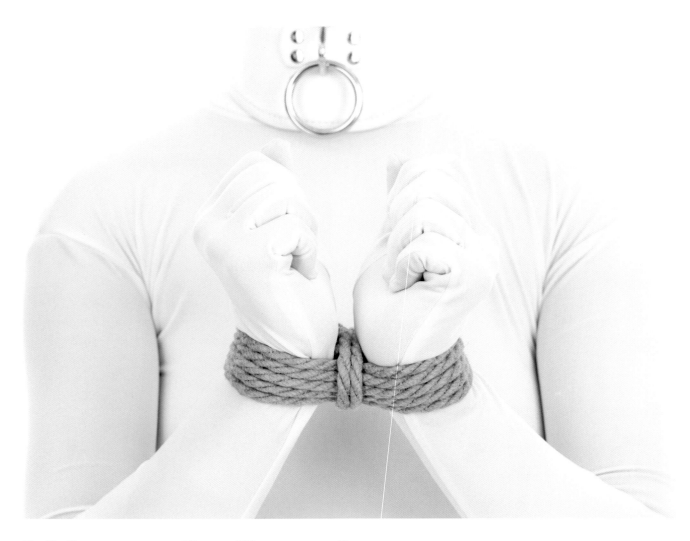

# Wrap & Cinch Double Column

This is a forward-tension **Double Column**. It is very fast and efficient; you can do this with as little as 5 feet of rope.

It is great for a just-tie-them-up-quick scenario. If you plan to tie these cuffs to some hard point — perhaps to a bedpost or some overhead point — and anticipate that your bottom might want to struggle or pull on their cuffs — put the tie under tension — convert this tie to a load-bearing version (p. 248) first, so that the cuffs do not get tighter as the bottom pulls on them.

    **Important:** See the *Reducing Risk* chapter (p. 49) for important safety information about tying the wrists.

    This is the only Western-style tie in this book. That is, it starts from the end of the rope instead of the middle.

TheDuchy.com/wrap-cinch-double-column/

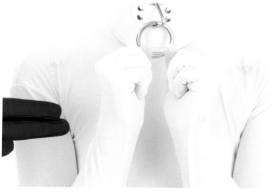

**1.** Find someone with two things you (and they) want tied together. We have chosen the wrists for this example.

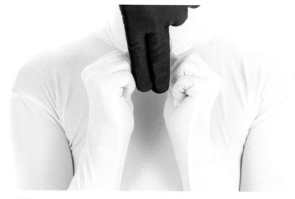

**2.** When tying wrists, it can be helpful to have your partner try to hold their wrists a little apart like this and to provide a little resistance. This helps you hold the tension in your ropes while making it easier to not make the cuffs too tight later in the tie. Plus, it helps give you both the feeling of struggling, which can make a scene really hot.

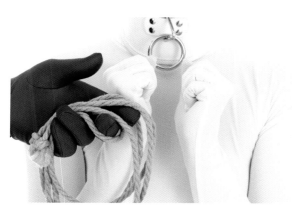

**3.** Start with a short length of rope. Some riggers keep very short lengths — only 5 feet or so — for tying wrists or ankles.

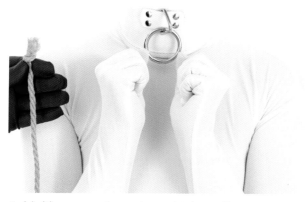

**4.** Unlike most of our ties, which are Eastern-style and start with the rope folded in half, this is a Western-style tie and begins with the end of the rope, tying with only one strand at a time.

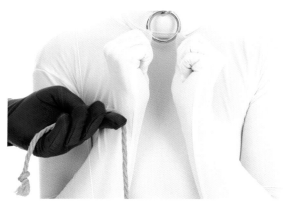

**5.** Start about 8-10 inches in.

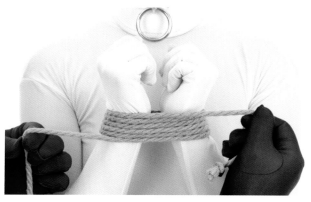

**6.** Wrap it around the wrists four to six times. This distributes the pressure across the wrists. Be sure to keep the lines in order, parallel to each other and with the same tension. *continues...*

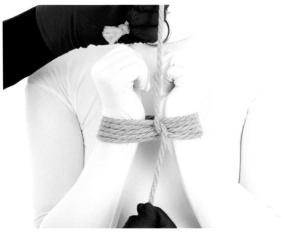

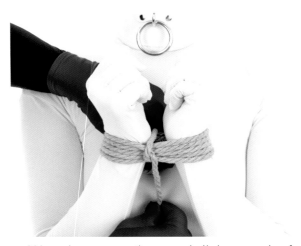

**7.** Bring the two tail ends together and twist them around each other once as shown so that they are now traveling perpendicularly to the strands of the cuffs.

**8.** Wrap these two tails around all the strands of the cuffs...

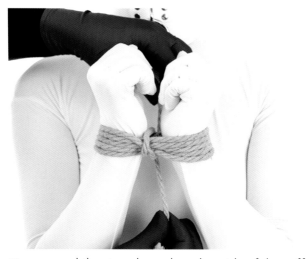

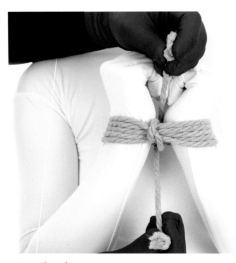

**9.** ...around the strands on the other side of the cuff...

**10.** ...back to your starting point.

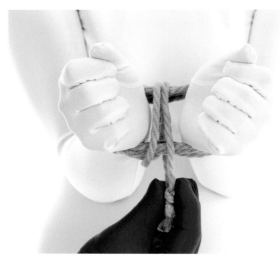

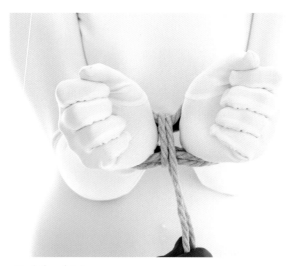

**11.** Now if you pull on the two tail ends, it will cinch all the cords of the cuffs together at the same time and at the same level of tension.

**12.** Like this!

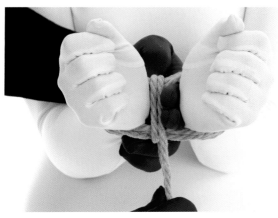

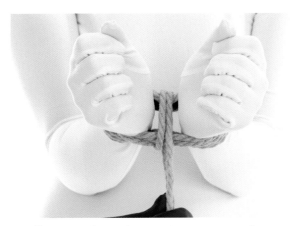

**13.** Important safety tip! There are lots of blood vessels and nerves very close to the skin on the inside of the wrist. You should be able to get two fingers into each cuff. If you cannot, they are too tight.

**14.** Once you have the tension set properly...

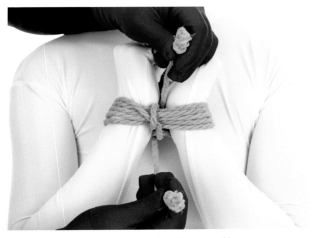

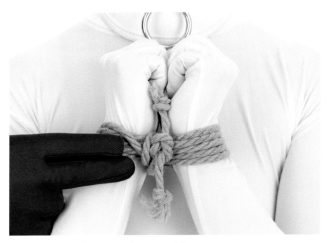

**15.** ...come back to the side of the cuffs you were working on, and...

**16.** ...lock off with a **Square Knot**.

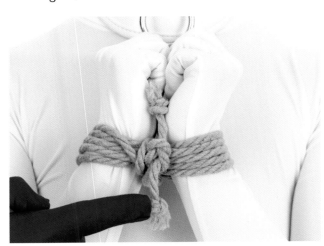

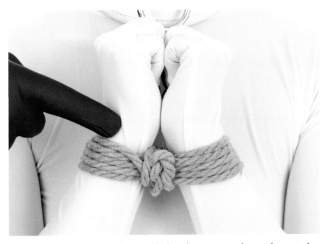

**17.** Tuck the ends inside or deal with them in some other way.

**18.** Done! Note: I showed this being tied on the pinky side of the hand for a reason. If you put the knot on the thumb side, it can be easy for your partner to untie it with hand or mouth. *continues...*

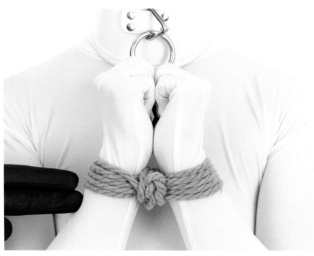

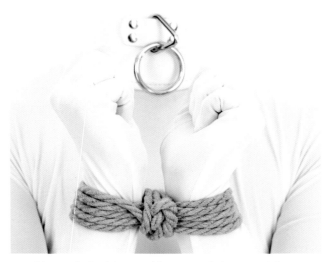

**19.** Note that it is generally better to have the cuffs a little further away from the hands, so they do not impact the small bones of the wrists. The rope may have naturally migrated tight up to the hand while tying. If so, place you fingers inside the cuff and move them away slightly.

**20.** Not only is this good because it lowers risk a little, but it also tends to be a bit more comfortable.

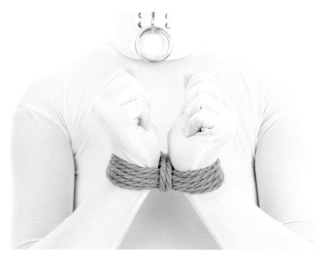

**21.** The knot side of this tie is not especially attractive. If you are doing this tie for photography, you may want to have the knot facing away from the camera because the other side looks much nicer.

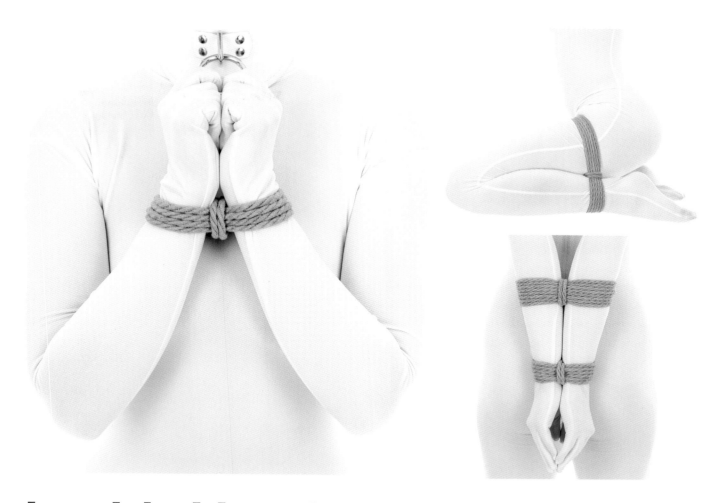

# Lark's Head Double Column

This is a popular reverse-tension **Double Column**. It is simple to apply and results in a snug and secure tie.

As this is a reverse-tension technique, it has an advantage over forward-tension techniques like the **Wrap & Cinch**: You can gain some control over your partner early in the tie. If they want to play struggle games, you can quickly cinch it tight for a moment to get them under control, and then loosen it to the appropriate level to continue the tie.

 **Important:** See the *Reducing Risk* chapter (p. 49) for important safety information about wrists.

 If you plan to tie these cuffs to some hard point — perhaps to a bedpost or some overhead point — and anticipate that your partner might want to struggle or pull on their cuffs, convert this tie to a load-bearing version (p. 248) first, so that the cuffs do not get tighter under tension.

TheDuchy.com/larks-head-double-column/

## Lark's Head Double Column

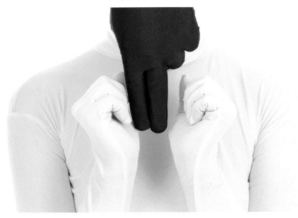

**1.** In this example, we will tie together two wrists. It can be useful to have your partner hold them a little bit apart like this so that you have some resistance to work against as you tie without having the cinches become too tight at the end.

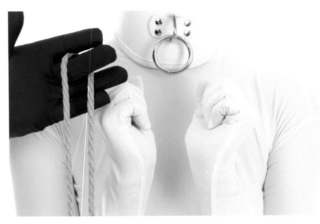

**2.** Fold the rope in half.

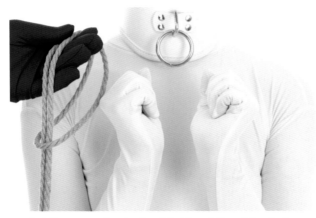

**3.** Oddly enough, the **Lark's Head Double Column** begins with a **Lark's Head**. There are two ways to get the initial **Lark's Head** around your partner's wrists. One way is to create your **Lark's Head** first...

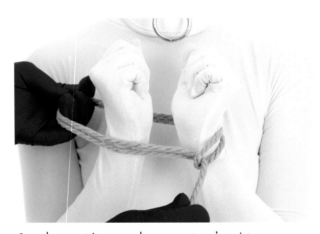

**4.** ...then put it around your partner's wrists.

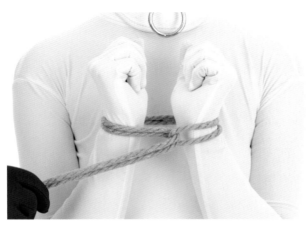

**5.** Like this.

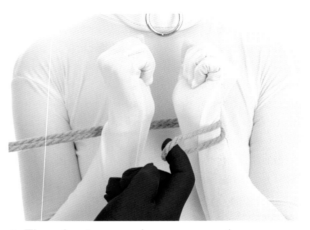

**6.** The other is to put the rope around your partner's wrists.

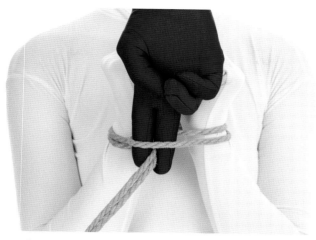

**7.** Reach through the bight to grab the tail...

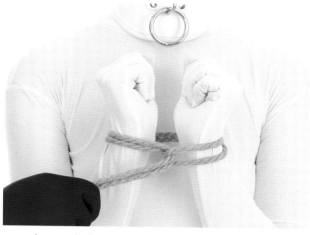

**8.** ...then pull the tail through and reverse the tension.

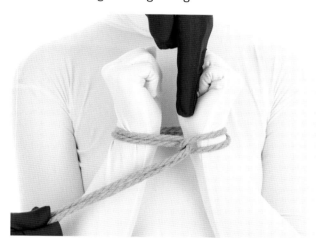

**9.** Place the bight just a little off center.

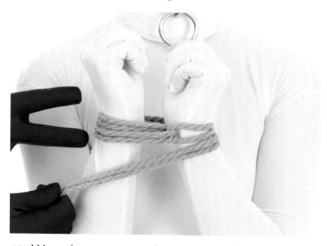

**10.** Wrap the rope around your partner's wrists at least once more (for a total of two wraps or four strands).

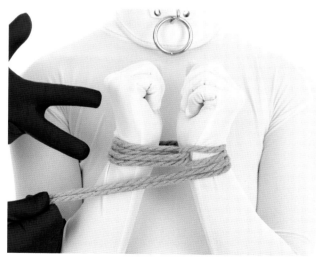

**11.** You can wrap it around an additional time if you wish (for a total of three wraps or six strands). You typically do not want more wraps than this, or you will start getting uneven tension in the strands when you cinch them tight.

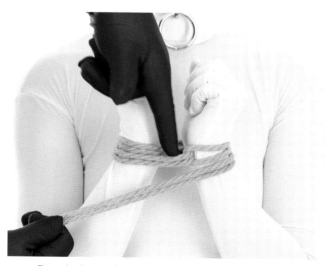

**12.** Reach through the secondary bight. *continues...*

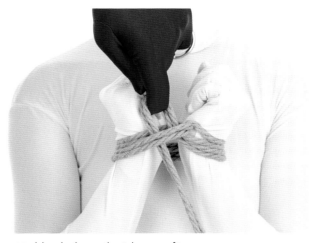

**13.** Hook the tail with your finger.

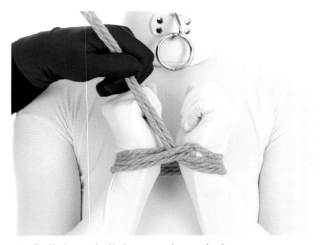

**14.** Pull the tail all the way through the secondary bight.

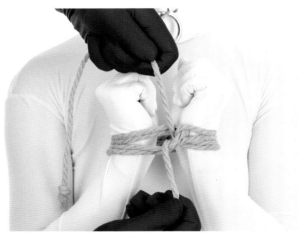

**15.** Separate the tails. (Sometimes called "splitting" the tails.)

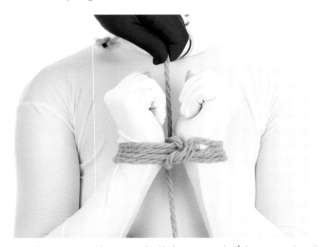

**16.** Run one tail around all the strands (those on both sides of the wrists) in one direction and the other tail around all the strands in the other direction.

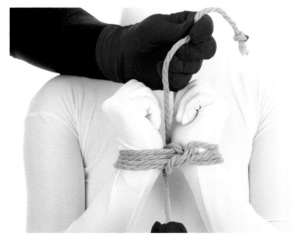

**17.** Come back to your starting point.

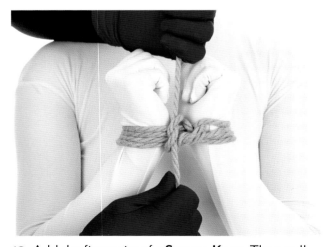

**18.** Add the first twist of a **Square Knot**. Then pull the ends apart a little. This will cinch the rope around all strands of the cuffs at the same time, tightening them all evenly!

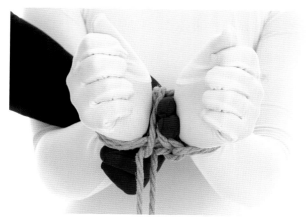

**19.** It is important that these cuffs not be too tight. You should always be able to slip two fingers inside of each cuff. If you cannot, they are too tight. Safety first!

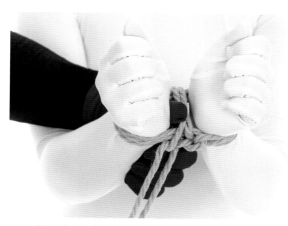

**20.** Check both sides.

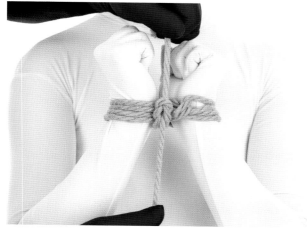

**21.** Once you have the correct level of tension set, add the second twist of the **Square Knot** to lock everything off.

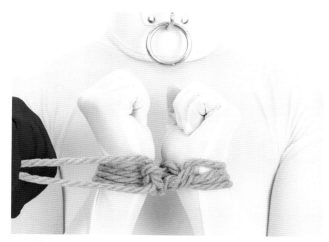

**22.** Done.

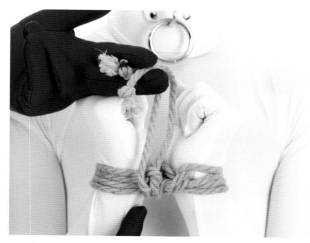

**23.** Use up the tails. Sometimes people add more wraps around the cinch (Steps 16-17) before tying them off.

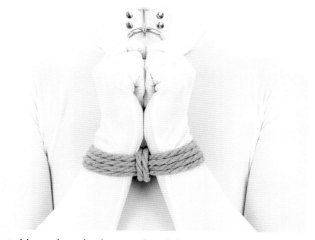

**24.** Note that the knot side of this tie is not especially attractive. If you are doing this tie for photography, you may want to have the knot facing away from the camera because the other side looks much nicer.

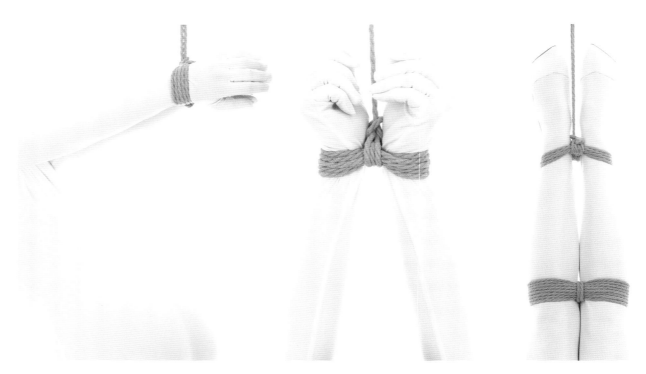

# Load–bearing Double Column

If you plan to have any tension or load on your **Double Column** — for example, if you plan to tie your partner to a bed so they can struggle or tie them to an overhead hard point — it is extremely important do so in such a way that the cords of the cuffs do not cinch down more tightly. Here is one good way to do so.

**Warning!** Wrists are sensitive; they must be handled with care. "Load-bearing" means *reasonable* amounts of load. Hands *attached* overhead is fine, as long as your partner's feet are still touching the ground. NEVER suspend someone by the wrists alone; you *will* cause injury.

   The wrist joint itself is also fragile. If you pull on the wrist too hard, you can damage that joint or even push some of those small wrist bones into the wrong position. Never tie someone in a position where rope is applying heavy continual stress on the wrists.

**For Example**

You put **Double Columns** on your partner's wrists and ankles and then tie them diagonally across the bed to opposite bedposts. In the scene you have planned, they may want to fight and thrash around. Using this technique would help reduce risk. They could pull on their wrist and ankle bindings like in the pictures above without those bindings tightening down.

TheDuchy.com/load-bearing-double-column/

# The Problem

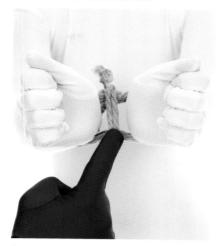

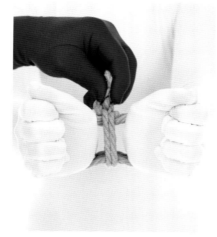

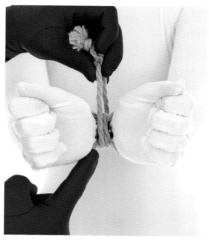

Remember that it is these cinch lines that cause the cords of the cuff to get tighter. (The wrists are wider apart than usual, to better demonstrate this point.)

If the tails coming out of the cuff itself — those that create the cinch — get pulled on...

...the cuffs will get tighter. Having rope clamped around a wrist like this is **bad**. It can impact the nerves and blood flow through the wrist, which can quickly cause injury.

## One Good Solution

If you want to do something where your partner might put tension on the **Double Column**, you need to convert it to a load-bearing version first. You do this by adding a **Lark's Head Knot** around just the cords of the cinch; this way, the tension pulls only on the cinch cords and not the cords of the cuffs themselves.

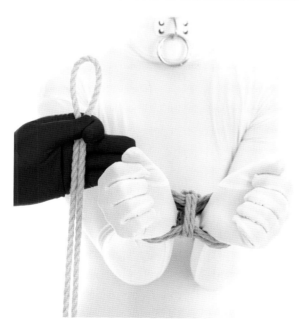

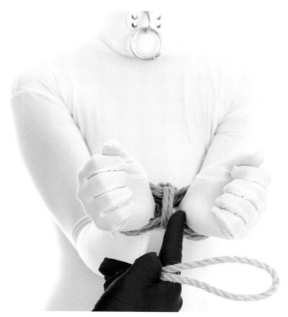

**1.** To do this, grab a new rope.

**2.** We are going to create a **Lark's Head Knot** around the **Cinch Cords** themselves. If your cuffs are properly tight (i.e., not too tight), you should have gaps like these next to the wrists. *continues...*

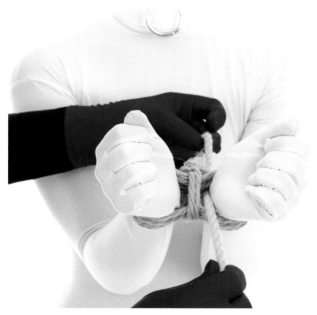

**3.** Run the bight of the new rope through the inside of the cuff on one wrist from the hand side toward the elbow...

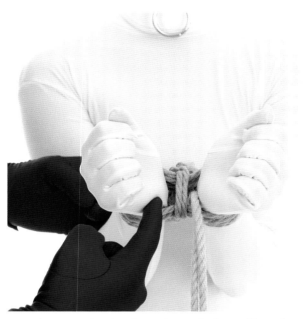

**4.** ...then coming back up through the cuff on the other side of the cinch...

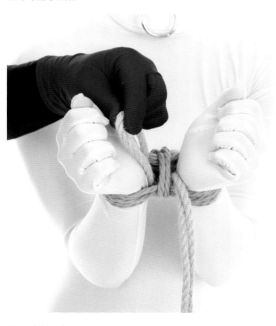

**5.** ...like this.

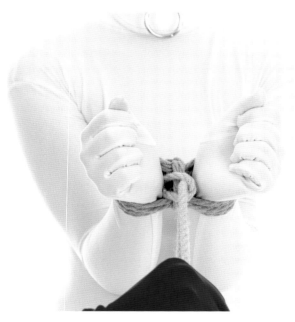

**6.** Now run your tail through the bight and tighten. You now have a **Lark's Head** around just the cinch lines. Now any tension you add to the new rope will tighten around the cords of the cinch. This way the cords of the cuffs themselves do not clamp down on the wrists. You can also lock off using **Two Half Hitches** instead of a **Lark's Head**. Doing so takes a little more time but makes it easier to untie.

You have earned a break. Use that lead you just tied to drag your partner off for a bit of fun... as long as they are also into it!

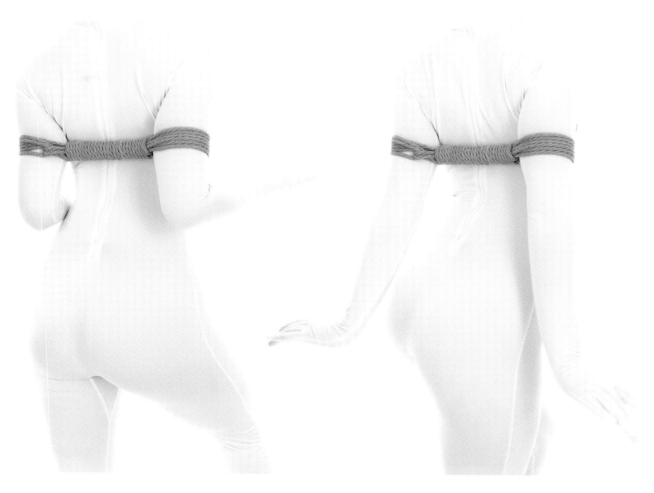

# Extended Lark's Head Double Column

This is a great technique for binding two things that either cannot be brought fully together or that you purposely want to leave slightly apart. For example:

- An elbow tie (since most people cannot touch their elbows together behind their backs).
- A hobble on the ankles so they can walk, but not run.

This is basically just a **Lark's Head Double Column**, but with an extra twist or two (bad pun very much intended). You will soon see what I mean.

There are nerves that run on the outside of the arms above the elbows. The radial and median nerves run through this area (p. 70-75). Putting too much pressure on these nerves can cause a person's fingers to go numb or otherwise feel strange. Be sure to *instruct your partner to inform you if they feel anything unusual:* Numb, cold, tingling, anything out of the ordinary.

TheDuchy.com/extended-larks-head-double-column/

If they report an issue, first try to move the cuff up or down on their arm an inch or two. If the sensation goes away in 15 seconds, you can continue with the tie. If the sensation remains, untie them quickly. Perhaps the tie is too tight, or their nerves run close to the skin and/or are easy to compress. Or perhaps the issue is not the rope, but the position itself. Never leave bottoms in a condition where their fingers are tingling; that can very quickly lead to nerve damage.

Nerves in the *shoulder* can be impacted by elbow ties too.

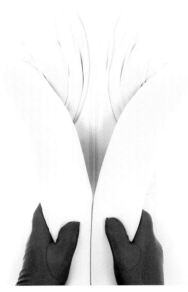

Despite what you may have seen in pictures or videos, most people cannot touch their elbows together behind their back. The ability to do this is quite rare and being able to *maintain* this position for more than a few minutes is *even* rarer.

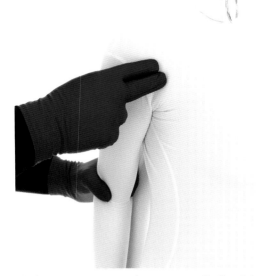

Unless your partner has unusually flexible shoulders, staying in this position can put pressure across the nerves in the front of the shoulder (the brachial plexus, p. 70) and cause potential nerve damage in a very short time.

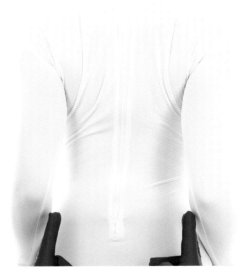

It is a much more common for a person to only be able to put their elbows a little behind them, like this. **But you CAN still tie their elbows together!**

## Extended Lark's Head Double Column – Core Technique

For this tutorial, I used one 30 foot piece of ¼-inch rope.

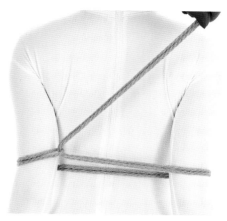

**1.** Begin just as you would with a **Lark's Head Double Column**. Place the bight near, but not touching, one of the elbows.

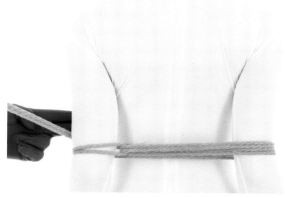

**2.** Wrap the tails around the arms. You can wrap up or down. I personally prefer wrapping up because of where the lock knot ends up after the tie is complete, but it makes little difference.

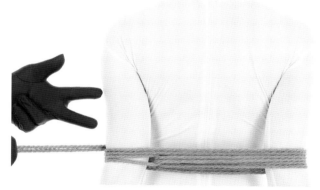

**3.** You need to have at least two wraps total, but I personally like to do three wraps (six total strands of rope) because it makes a wider cuff that distributes pressure over a larger area. See the aforementioned nerve warning for more.

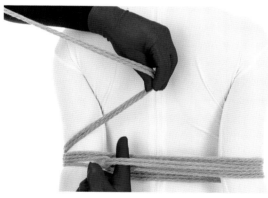

**4.** Reach through the secondary bight.

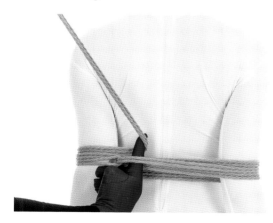

**5.** Hook the tail.

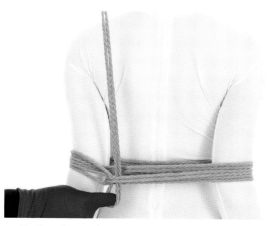

**6.** Pull it through.

*continues...*

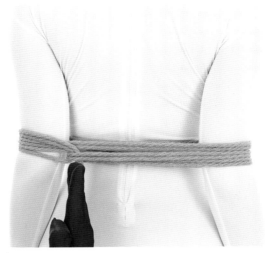

**7.** Confirm that the bight is near the arm.

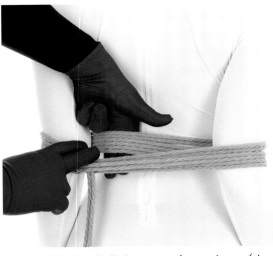

**8.** Reach behind all the ropes from above (the back of your fingers should be touching your partner's body)...

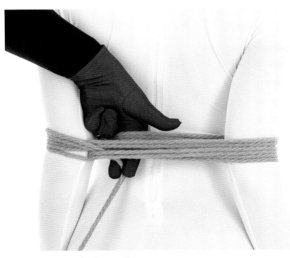

**9.** ...and hook the tail.

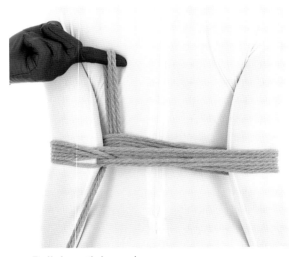

**10.** Pull the tail through.

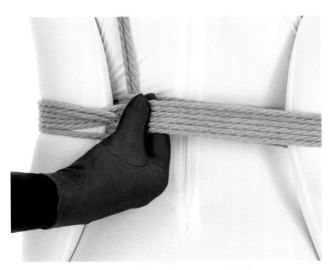

**11.** Hold the horizontal cords in an orderly fashion, and...

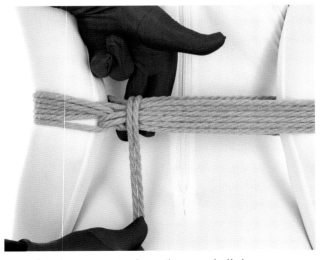

**12.** ...begin wrapping the tail around all the ropes.

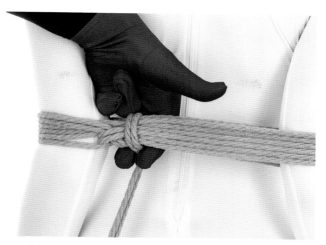

**13.** Complete two to three wraps.

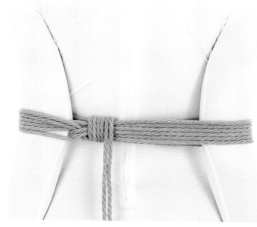

**14.** Before you continue, you can adjust the tightness of the first cuff.

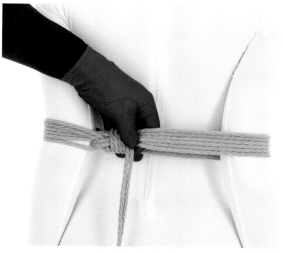

**15.** To do this, grip the knot and the cords on the outside with one hand.

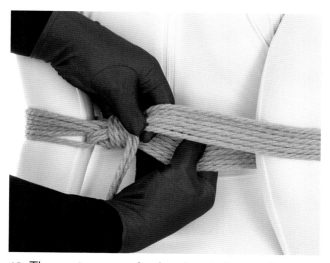

**16.** Then, using your other hand, grab the set of horizontal cords that are closer to the body.

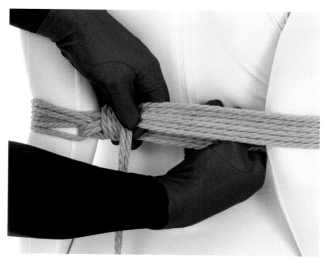

**17.** Now you can pull the wraps you just made (Step 13) towards the elbow to tighten the cuff.

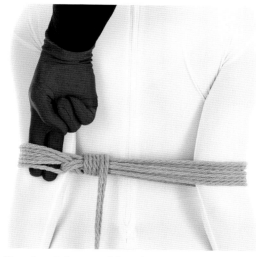

**18.** Test for tightness. You should be able to comfortably get two to three fingers between the ropes and their arm. *continues...*

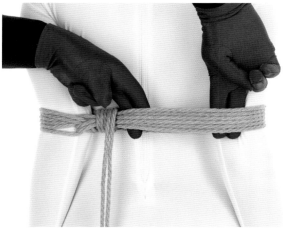

**19.** Dress the cords. Confirm they are parallel and have the same tension.

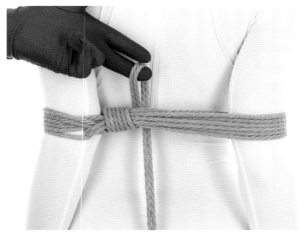

**20.** Continue wrapping the tail around the cuff cords.

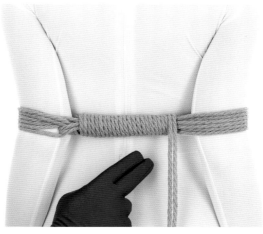

**21.** When you get close to the other elbow, separate the ends to tie them off.

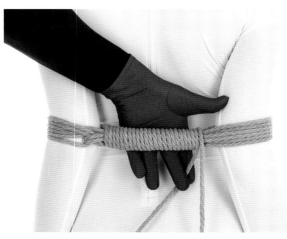

**22.** Take the cord farther from the elbow and run it up behind the wraps as you have been doing. (After doing so, I will temporarily drape it over the shoulder so you can see the next step more clearly.)

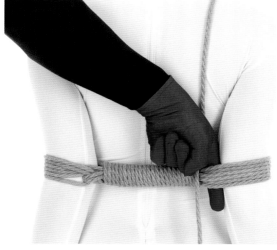

**23.** Run the other line up through the cuff itself. To do this, put your finger inside the cuff

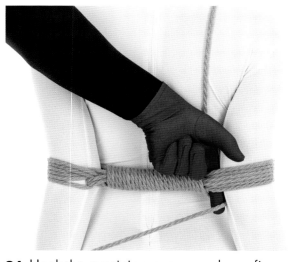

**24.** Hook the remaining rope around your finger...

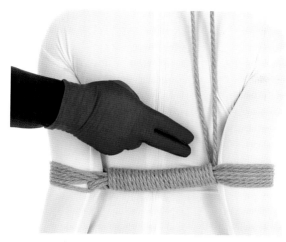

**25.** ...and run it up through the cuff.

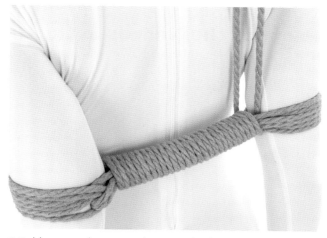

**26.** Now you have one line inside the cuff and one outside.

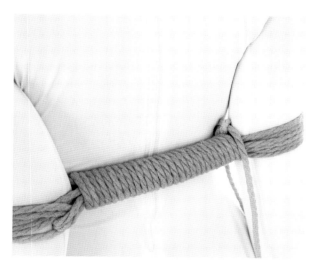

**27.** Tie it off with a **Square Knot**, then...

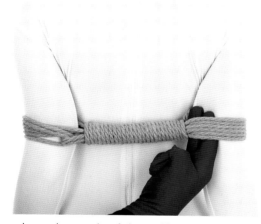

**28.** ...dress the cords of the cuff. That means: Run your fingers under the ropes in the cuffs to ensure that they are not too tight, and that the cords are lying flat and parallel.

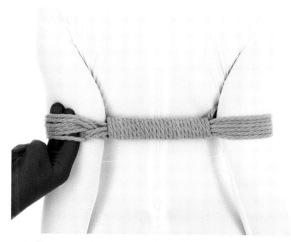

**29.** Double-check the other side, too.

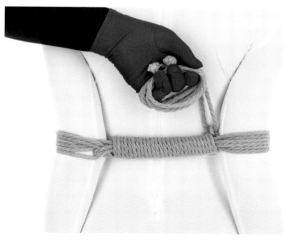

**30.** Use up any remaining rope however you wish.

# Protect the Nerves in the Upper Arm

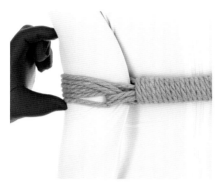
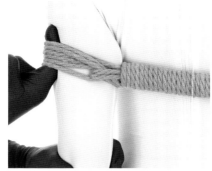
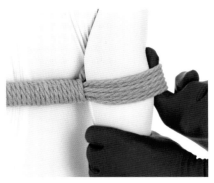

There are nerves that run on the outside of the arm in this range. This tie can put pressure on those nerves, resulting in numbness, tingling, a hot or cold feeling, or other weird sensations. Make sure your partner knows that it is important to tell you immediately if anything like this happens. Instruct — or even command — them to tell you. This gives them the permission they may need.

Everybody is different, so the exact location and depth of those nerves will be different, but if your partner reports anything weird, the first thing to do is to just move the cuff up or down an inch or two. Do this by holding their arm, running your finger under the cuff and sliding your finger back and forth under the strands of the cuff while pushing it up or down.

Adjust the other side as well, just in case. If the weird sensation goes away in 10-15 seconds, the pressure on the nerves has been alleviated and you can continue to use the cuffs, but if it does not go away, remove this tie immediately. It may be that the issue is in the shoulder and not the arm. You will need to decide for yourself if you want to stop the entire scene, but definitely remove this rope.

# Ankle Example

This tie can be used for other things too, such as tying the ankles together. This gives your bottom more stability than tying the ankles directly together because they can shift their feet to maintain their balance. When in a hobble, they can walk slowly, but not run.

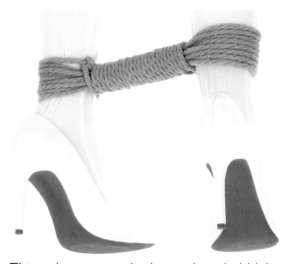

This technique can also be used as a hobble!

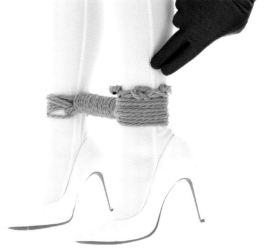

If you have a little rope left over, one option is to run it around the ankle and tie it off with a **Square Knot**.

# Use Up Extra Rope

Create a sash that also helps keep the cuffs from migrating downward. This is just one of many options. For other ideas, see *Using Up Rope* (p. 279).

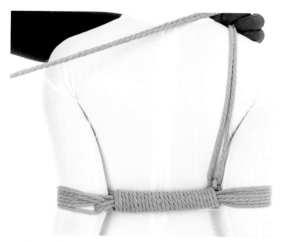

**1.** Bring the remaining tail over the shoulder...

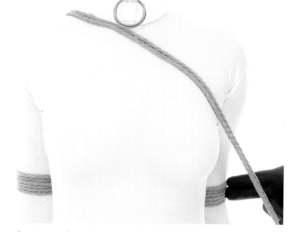

**2.** ...and across the chest to the cuff on the other side.

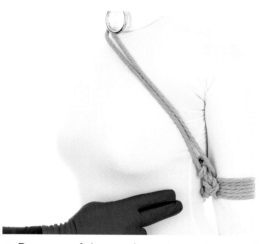

**3.** Run one of the two lines through the cuff. Lock the two ends together with a **Square Knot**.

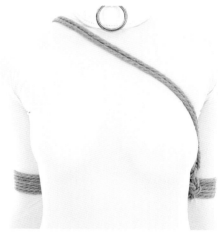

**4.** Done from the front.

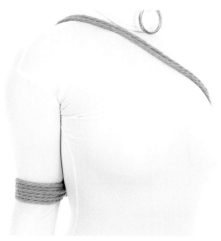

**5.** Done from the side.

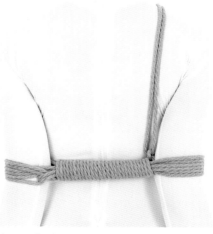

**6.** Done from the back.

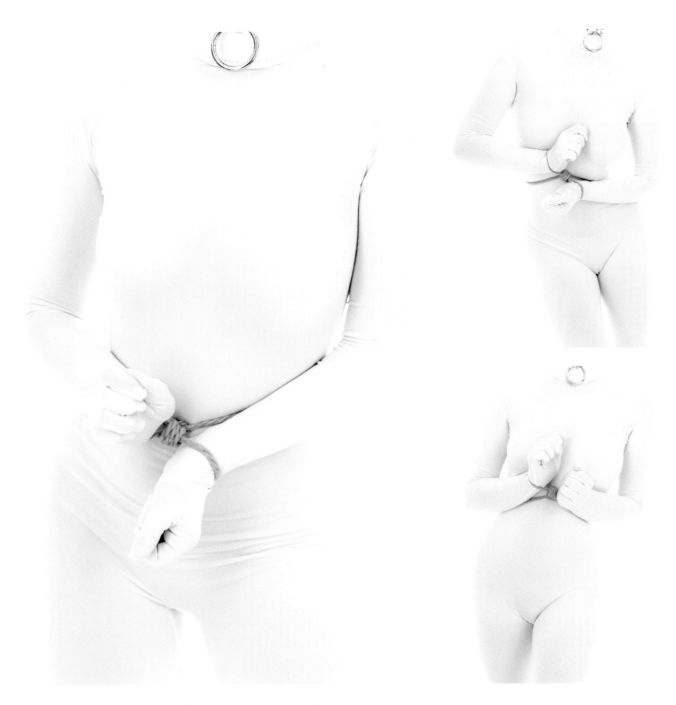

# Multi-loop Texas Handcuffs

This is one of several types of rope handcuffs. It is quick to tie and is very difficult to escape when properly applied. It can be a fun option if your partner is an eel — someone that likes to try to escape.

TheDuchy.com/multi-loop-handcuffs/

Pro Tip: Most rope bottoms find it disappointing if they can escape. If your partner is a "brat" or an "eel" they *will* try to escape. They will become much more turned on if they find themselves helpless.

But this technique has a few risks you need to understand and manage.

This is a collapsing knot, so make sure you read through the instructions on how to properly apply it in order to not endanger your partner.

Also, it has a single strand around the wrist instead of four or more. This increases the risk of rope burn. It also increases the risk of injury to the bones in the wrist if your partner struggles too hard. Keep an eye on them. Keep good communication. Do not let them get so competitive with the knot that they hurt themselves.

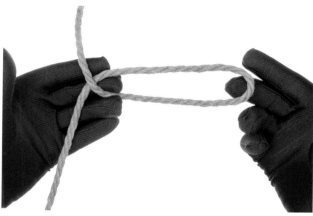

**1.** Create a loop like this. The line leading upward is the working line; it should lie on top.

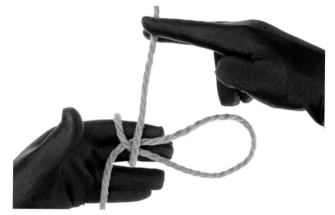

**2.** Grab the working line and wrap it around the loop and your fingers...

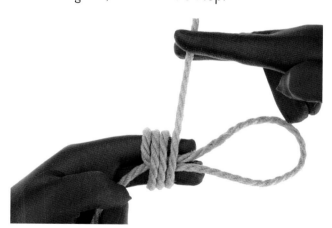

**3.** ...three to four times.

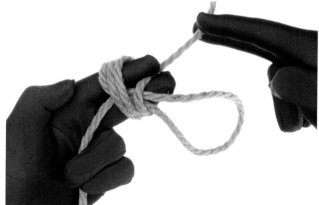

**4.** Place the working line between the two fingers you have been wrapping around. *continues...*

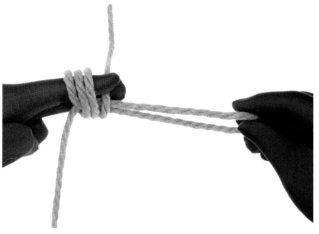

**5.** Pull the working line through the coil of rope...

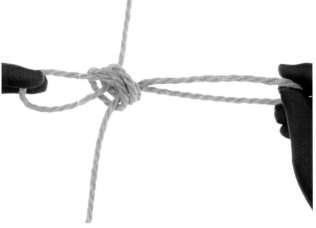

**6.** ...pull slowly and smoothly...

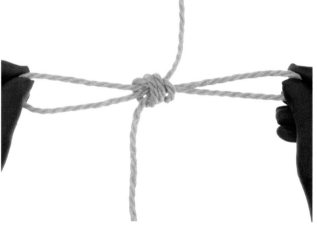

**7.** ...and the coil will naturally tighten down. You may have to adjust your grip as you are pulling.

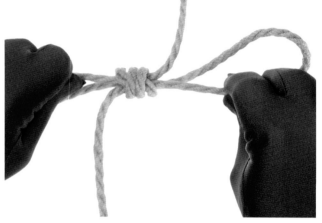

**8.** Pull it somewhat tight, but not too much. Dress the knot, making sure the cords lie evenly and have even tension.

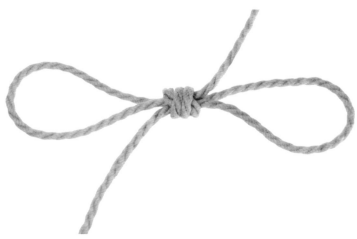

**9.** You want the knot to have a grip on the sliding lines, so you feel some resistance when you move them, but they are not cinched down too tightly.

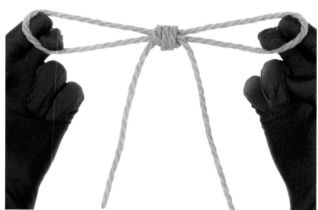

**10.** It is now ready to use!

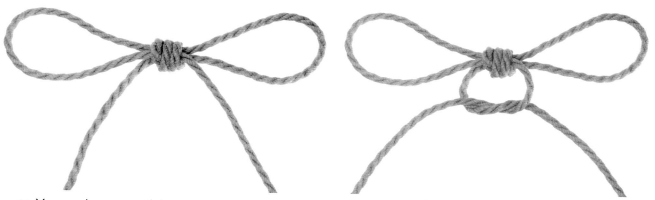

**11.** You can have one of these pre-created in your rope bag and be ready in a moment's notice!

**12.** To lock it (once on your partner's wrists), use an **Overhand Knot** like this.

## Applying a Handcuff Knot

This is one great way to apply a handcuff knot: As a belly chain! Properly applied, this configuration keeps the wrists away from the mouth so they cannot use their teeth to pull the knot apart. That and other features make it very difficult for someone to escape when this is properly applied!

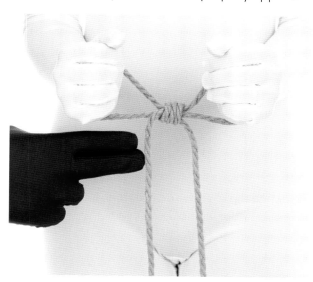

**1.** Place the loops over the hands with the knot and tail ends on the pinky side. This keeps the knot a way from the thumbs and makes it more difficult to away.

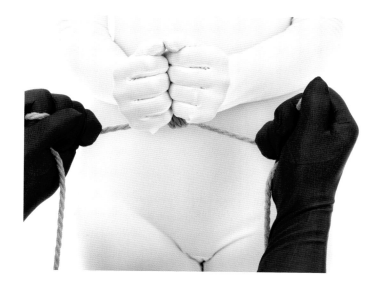

**2.** Tighten the loops.

*continues...*

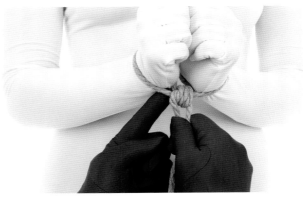

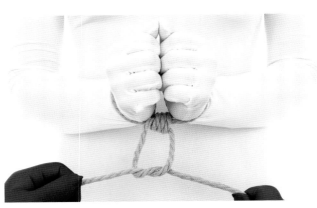

**3.** Tighten more than you normally would, to the point that your smallest finger can just barely be forced under the rope. The bottom will pull some slack out of the knot when they pull, and the cuffs will settle into a better size. That said, as always, remember to check in with your partner and remind them to routinely do their safety checks (p. 72).

**4.** Lock the cuffs by doing a single **Overhand Knot** like this.

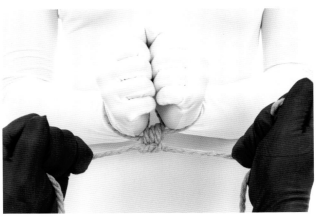

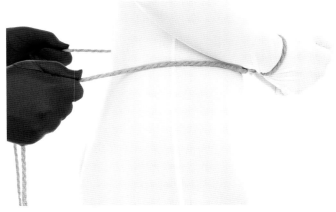

**5.** Tighten this **Overhand Knot** very firmly. Do not turn this into a **Square Knot**. As the person struggles, the knot will get much tighter and a **Square Knot** might become difficult to untie.

**6.** Separate the strands and run them around narrowest part of your partner's waist...

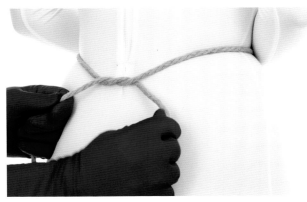

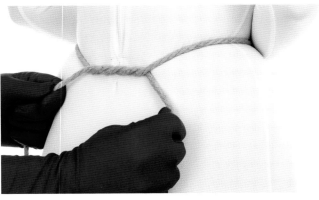

**7.** ...to their back. Then form the first half of a **Surgeon's Knot** by doing one twist, then...

**8.** ...adding a second twist. You need to pull this very tight as your partner may be able to work some slack free as they struggle.

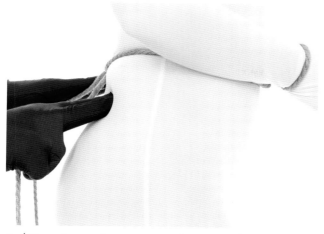

**9.** (Changing angles so you can better see.) Holding one tail in each hand, I push my partner forward just a little.

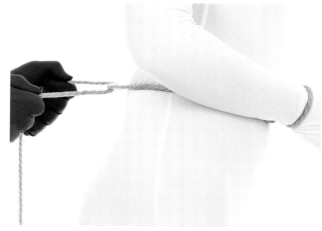

**10.** As they tip forward, pull on the rope to help them catch their balance and, at the same time...

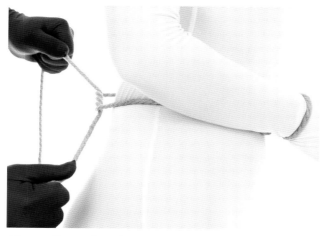

**11.** ...pull your hands apart...

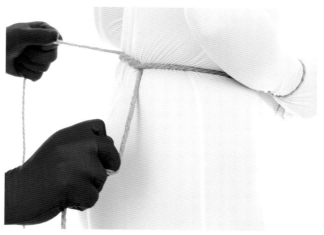

**12.** ...hard. This almost always results in being able to close this knot even tighter, resulting in a much more secure tie.

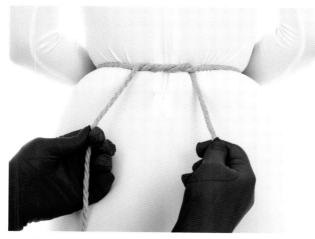

**13.** Keep tension on the ends as you bring them together so that you do not lose the tightness you just achieved.

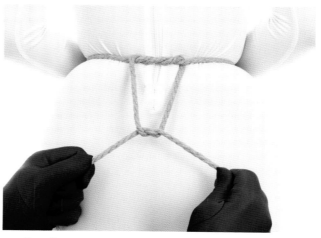

**14.** Finally, lock the belly chain by completing the **Surgeon's Knot** just as you would a **Square Knot**.

*continues...*

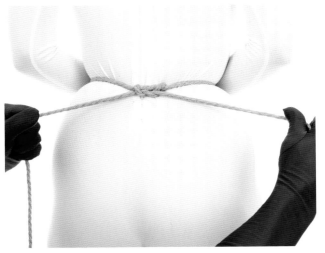

**15.** Again, snap it closed, very tightly.

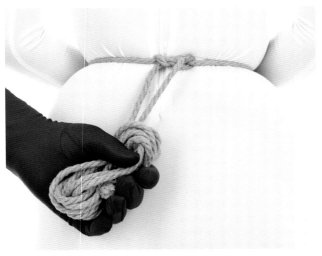

**16.** Use up any extra rope you have in any way you like, perhaps by attaching it to something else.

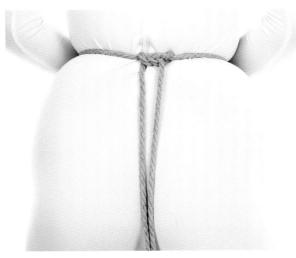

**17.** Completed from the back.

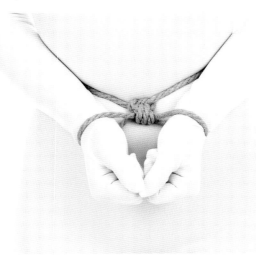

**18.** This is what is looks like from the front. You can see that, now that they have pulled on the tie a little, there is an appropriate amount of space in the cuffs. Make sure to check this!

# Untying the Knot

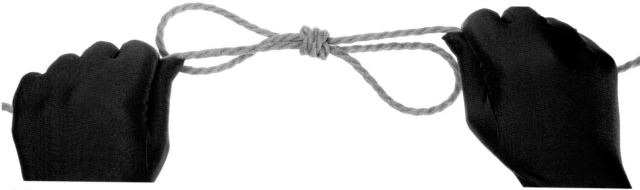

**1.** When you are done, first untie the knot to this point, then...

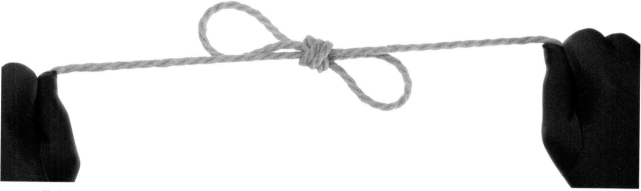

**2.** ...pull the tails in opposite directions.

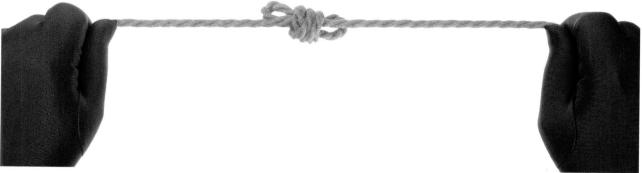

**3.** The loops will pull through and the knot will untie itself.

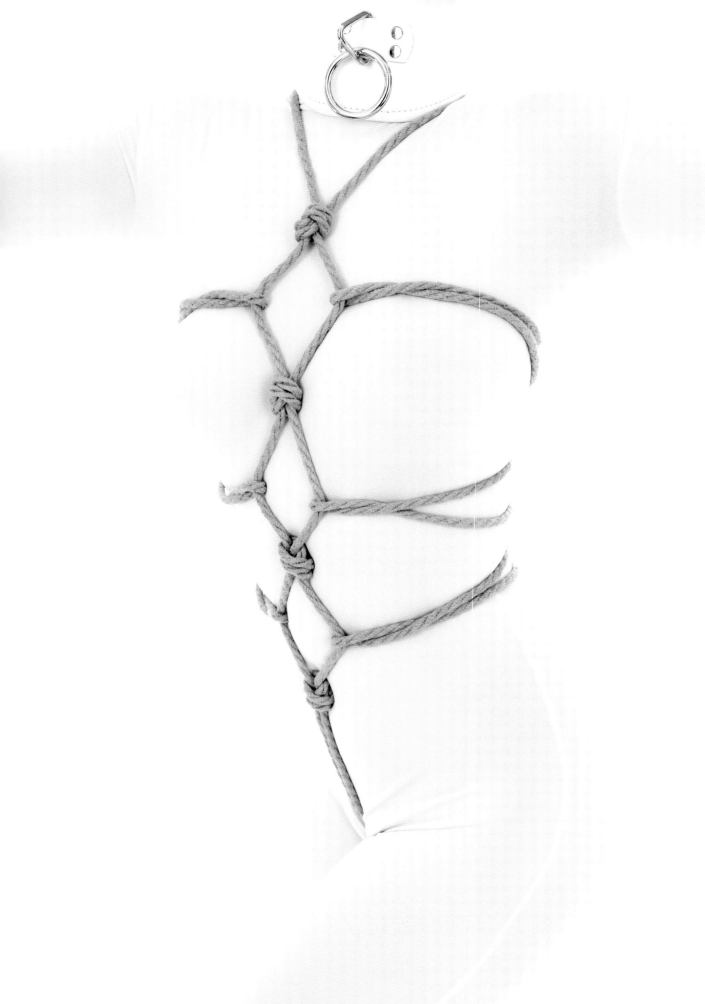

# 8

# More Rope Handling Techniques

Up to this point we have focused on techniques that can be done with a relatively short length of rope. Next, we will be getting into chest and hip harnesses. These harnesses are comprised of smaller building blocks to create larger, more complex ties and scenes.

This chapter will share techniques that will help you navigate these more complicated ties. We will be delving into junctions — when a rope crosses another — extending your rope, and using up leftover rope after your tie is complete.

These simple tricks and techniques are important when working with harnesses because the amount of rope needed varies depending on who you are tying. For each harness below, I will tell you how much rope I used to do that tie, but that information is only true for that particular bottom, who is 5 feet 5 inches and has an athletic build. If the person you are tying is smaller or larger than that, you will need a different amount of rope, which is why this chapter is important!

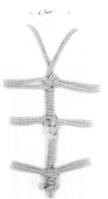

Wrapping around the stem.

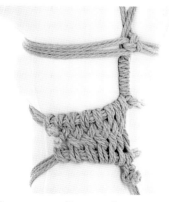

Weaving in a **Figure-8 Pattern**.

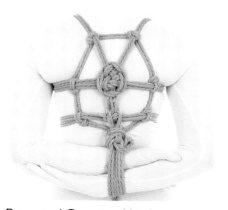

Repeated **Crossing Hitches**.

**269**

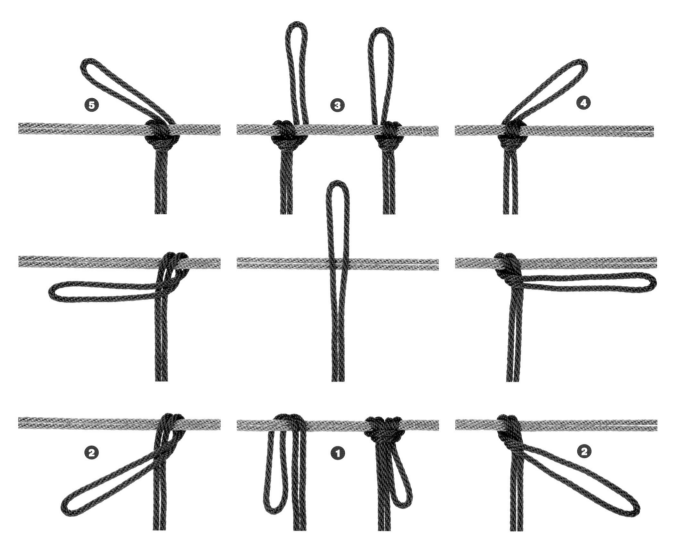

# Building Blocks: Junctions

One very common activity when rigging is deciding what to do when two ropes cross each other. Which direction do you want them to go as they move away from the junction?

This is something that you may not have thought about if you are always tying known patterns, but understanding these basic building blocks can be extremely helpful if you want to create your own.

Here are some common options when two ropes cross each other and how they are all related:

**❶** If you are coming straight back down, just fold the rope over or use a **Cow Hitch**.

**❷** If you are going down and to the left or right, just use a twist.

**❸** If you are going straight up, use a **Crossing Hitch** (a.k.a. "Munter Hitch" or "Nodome").

**❹** If you are going up and to the right, use a right-handed **Crossing Hitch**.

**❺** If you are going up and to the left, use a left-handed **Crossing Hitch**.

TheDuchy.com/building-blocks-junctions/

# To Explain Further

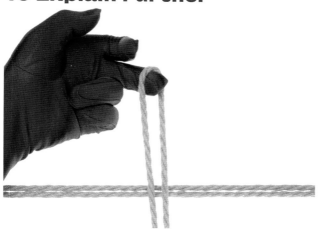

**1.** When one rope crosses another, you have several options. If you want the rope to continue moving upward and to be able to move freely over the other rope, you do nothing at all, like this.

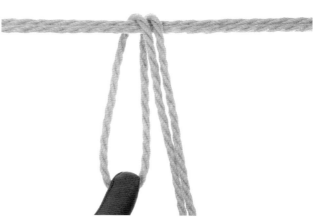

**2.** If you want the rope to come back down and be free to move with respect to the other rope, fold the tail over the crossing line.

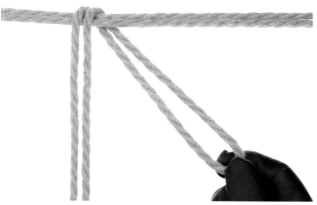

**3.** If you want it to go down and to the left, first fold the tail over the crossing line on the righthand side, then...

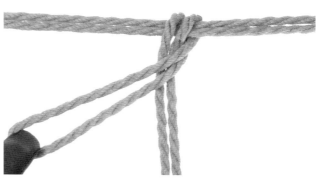

**4.** ...lay it on top of the incoming line. This gives you a small twist that helps keep the rope in place, especially if quite tight (under tension).

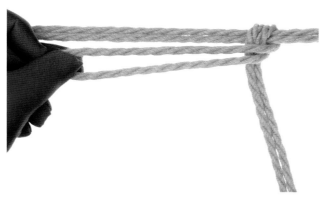

**5.** This is good for almost any direction you want to go in this quadrant even all the way to the left.

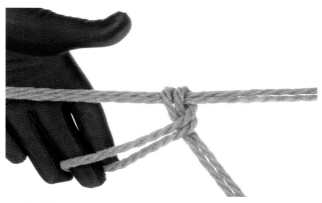

**6.** And if you want the rope to have a decent grip on the crossing line and continue to move upward (as opposed to Step 1 where it can move freely), you simply take the tail from this point... *continues...*

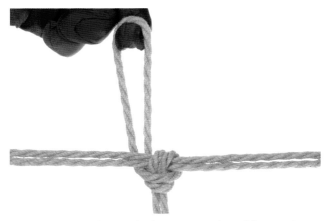

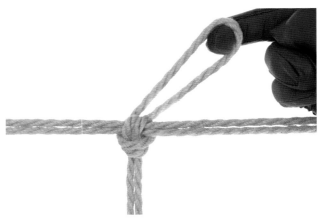

**7.** ...and go underneath the crossing line. You might recognize this as the **Crossing Hitch** or **Nodome**. It is also commonly called the **Munter Hitch**.

**8.** Now if you would like to come up to the upper right quadrant, you use this exact same technique. Just move the tail in that direction. Remember, at the beginning of this sequence, we did our first tail pull on the righthand side. From this we form the general rule for **Crossing Hitches: Do your first tail pull on the same side as the direction you want the tail to go when you are done!**

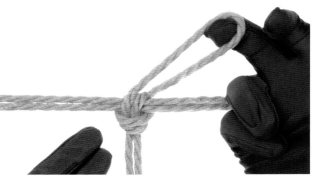

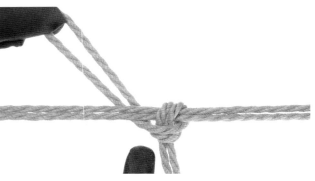

**9.** It is important which direction you make your **Crossing Hitch** when you have it go at an angle. If you do it like this, the tension on the cord moving away from the junction will tend to make the **Crossing Hitch** grip the other rope more tightly. This form is called a "closed" **Crossing Hitch**.

**10.** If, on the other hand, you position the cord at an angle like this, you can see that it tends to make the knot less tight — have a weaker hold. This form is called the "open" **Crossing Hitch**. Normally this is not what you want.

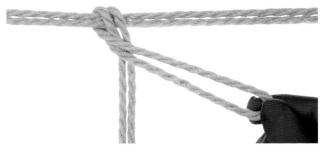

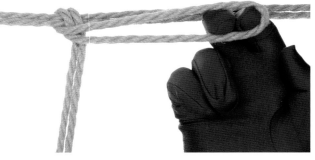

**11.** You can also do all this in reverse. If you want the rope to go to the lower right, do your first tail pull on the left and then lay it on top of the incoming line.

**12.** This is good all the way until it is going straight to the right.

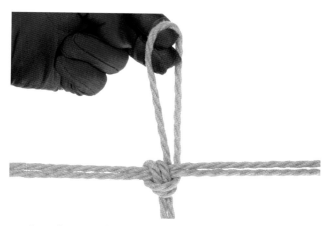

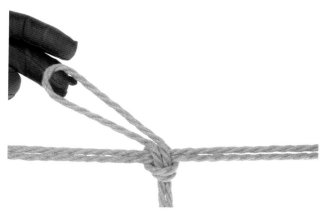

**13.** It is also good for a line moving straight forward. At this stage you have a **Crossing Hitch**.

**14.** Or for any angle in the upper *left* quadrant.

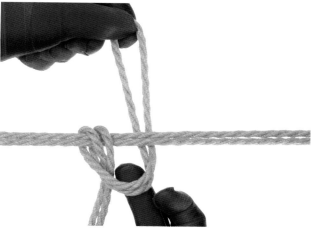

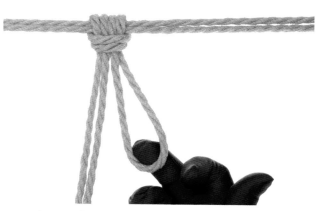

**15.** If you want the tail to go back the way it came, but to have a grip on the rope, start with either **Crossing Hitch**, then loosen the loop...

**16.** ...then pull the rope through and tighten.

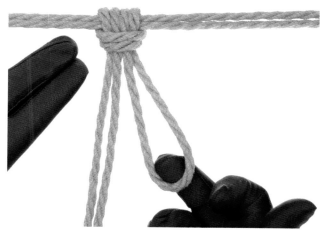

**17.** This is the **Cow Hitch**.

Structurally, this is the same as a **Lark's Head Knot**, but tied on instead of being created first. If you tighten this, it will grip firmly onto the crossing line and stay in place quite well.

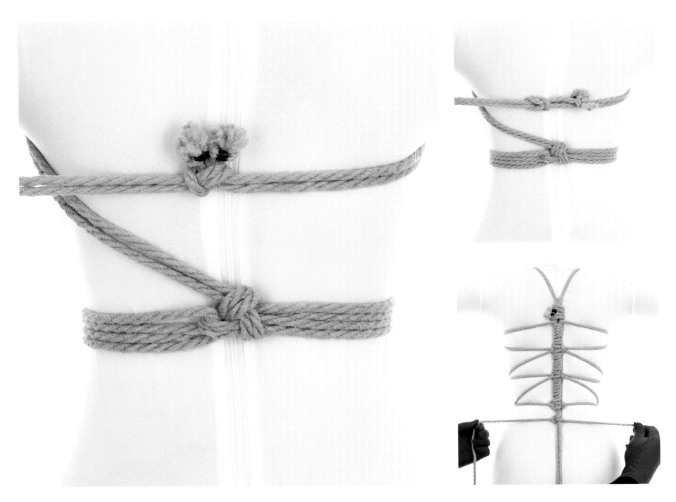

# Extending Rope

Many riggers only carry ropes of common lengths like 30 feet and 15 feet. These are useful for different purposes and are easy to handle. We do this because it saves us time when tying for a scene. Many common ties require you to pull the tail through multiple times. With shorter ropes, you can pull the tail through in one to three moves. But the longer your rope, the more moves (and more time) each tail pull will take.

However, there are many ties that require more than 30 feet of rope — many chest and waist harnesses, for example. You will either need a very long rope, or you can simply learn how to extend your rope when you need more! Once you understand these simple techniques, there is no need to use extra-long ropes for most cases. That said, some riggers still carry extra-long pieces for cases where they specifically want to have no rope joins, for example if doing a rope corset for a photo shoot.

　Here are three techniques that will allow you to simply extend your rope and continue.

TheDuchy.com/extending-rope/

# Alternative 1 — Knotted Ends

If the rope ends are knotted and even, simply use a **Lark's Head** to grab those knots and connect the ropes.

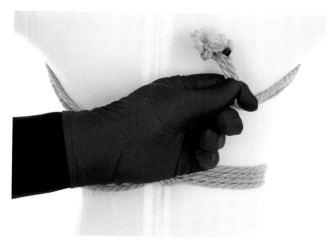

**1.** Keep tension on the first rope with one hand.

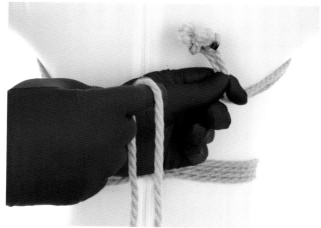

**2.** With the other, get a new rope.

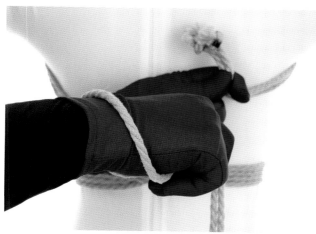

**3.** Drape the bight over your wrist. Grab the tail and shake the bight off to...

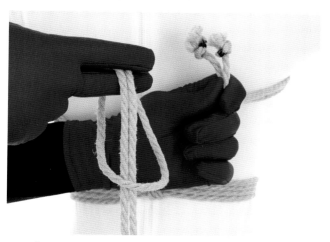

**4.** ...form a **Lark's Head Knot**.

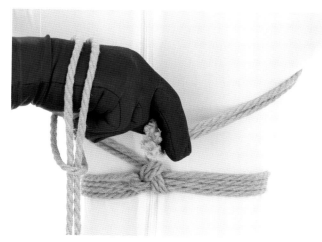

**5.** Reach through that **Lark's Head** and grab the knots on the first rope.

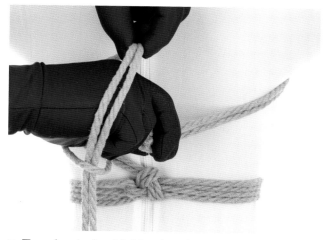

**6.** Transfer the **Lark's Head** to the first rope.

*continues...*

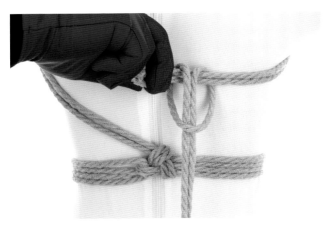

**7.** Like this.

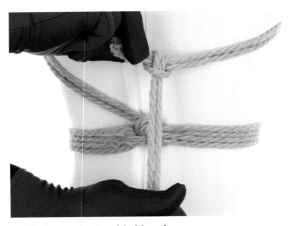

**8.** Tighten the **Lark's Head**.

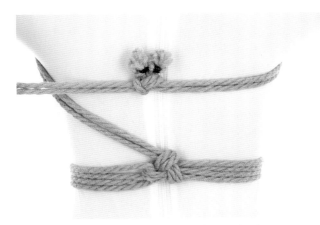

**9.** Slide it to the end where it will grip the knots. Continue your tie!

## Alternative 2 — Unknotted Ends

If the ends of your rope are *not* knotted, you can still use a **Lark's Head** by collapsing it into a **Square Knot**! This technique is also helpful if the two ends of your first rope are not even.

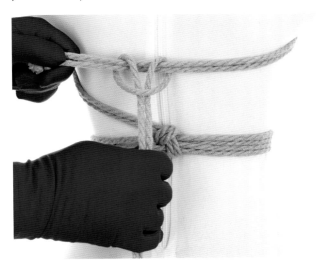

**1.** Do Steps 1-7 from Alternative 1.

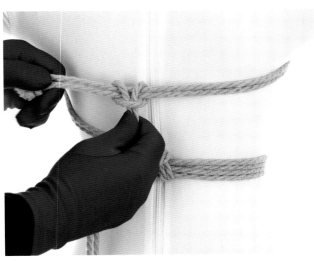

**2.** Run the old rope through 2 inches or so.

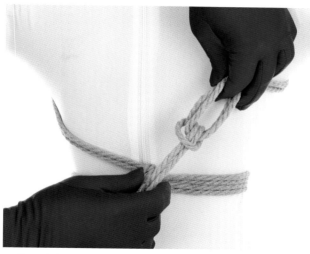

**3.** Bend the first rope back on itself, around the strands of the **Lark's Head**.

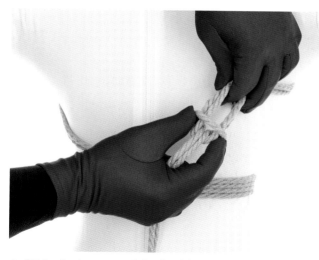

**4.** Slide the bottom of the **Lark's Head** over and onto the first rope.

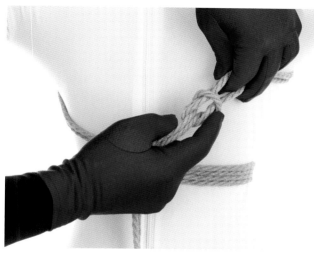

**5.** Like this. This has capsized the **Lark's Head** into a **Square Knot**!

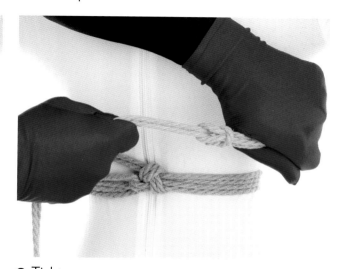

**6.** Tighten.

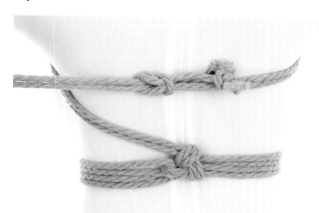

**7.** Your rope is now extended. (Optional) You can wrap the tails of the first rope around the line to keep them out of the way.

# Alternative 3 — Add New Rope to Stem

You can also completely end the first rope — use up extra rope and then tie off the end — and then add a brand-new rope to any line that is under tension, like the chest band, waist band, or stem.

In this example, we have completed a **Hishi Karada** (p. 358), used up the extra rope and tied it off. Now we want to add a new rope so we can do something different around the hips.

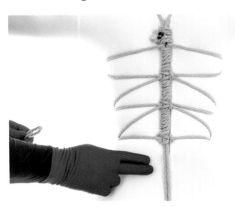

**1.** You can connect to any line under tension.

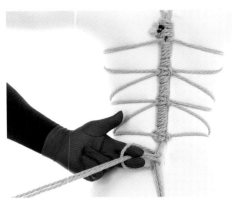

**2.** Run the bight under the line, then reach through it to hook the tail.

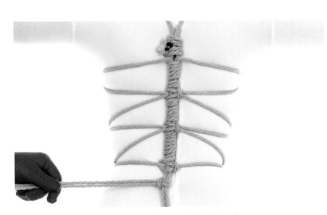

**3.** Tighten to complete the **Lark's Head.**

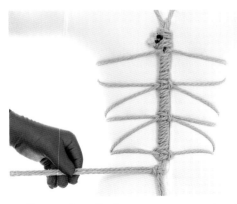

**4.** If your tie calls for your ropes to be doubled, you can simply continue your tie from here.

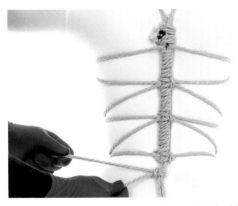

**5.** If not, as in this case with the **Hishi Karada**, you can separate the tails and...

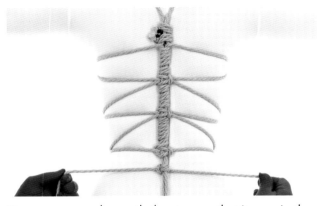

**6.** ...run one underneath the stem so that it goes in the opposite direction. Continue your tie!

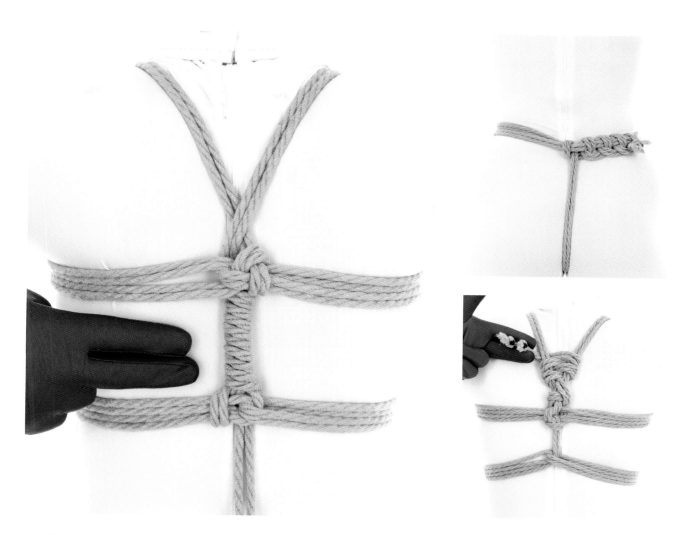

# Using Up or "Burning" Extra Rope

Every tie requires a different amount of rope. Also, the same tie will require a different amount of rope when put on a different person. You have learned to extend your rope when you need more, but what happens when you finish the tie and have rope left over? How do you use it up — "burn" it — preferably in a quick and attractive manner?

This is a set of skills you want to build. If you leave the ends of your tie flopping around uncontrolled, the tie will look unfinished. Your work will appear to be more skillful if the rope is attractively used up and the ends are locked so everything is a neat package.

Here are a few good options for short, medium, and long lengths of rope.

TheDuchy.com/using-up-rope/

# Short Tail

## Alternative 1 – Tuck Ends Under a Line

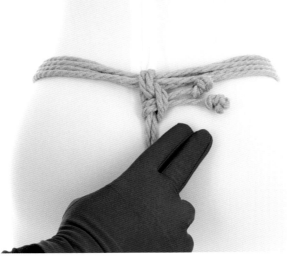

**1.** If you have only a little rope left after you have locked it off...

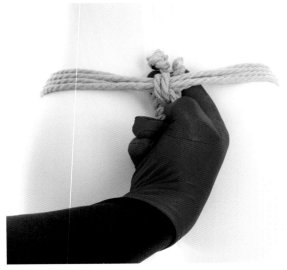

**2.** ...do not leave it hanging; tuck the ends under and out of the way.

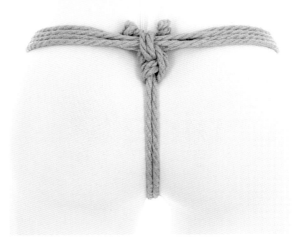

**3.** This is much more polished and looks more skillful.

## Alternative 2 – Wrap Tail Around Lines

Simply wrap the tail around any existing lines that are under tension, like the stem or band. When you run out of rope, lock with a Half Hitch, or tuck the ends between some of the tensioned lines.

### Example 1 – Wrap Around Waist band

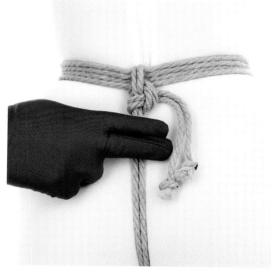

**1.** Here we have locked off with two **Half Hitches**, but we have more rope left than we can hide by tucking the ends under.

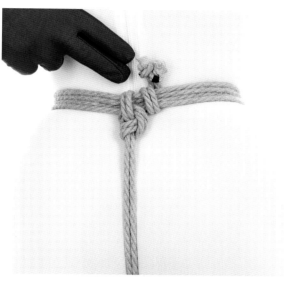

**2.** Wrap the rope around the waist band until you are almost out.

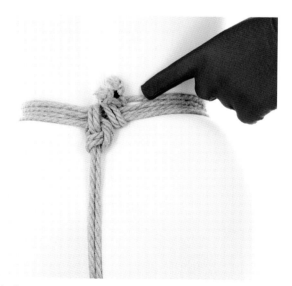

**3.** Tuck the remaining ends between two lines that are under tension.

**Example 2 – Wrap Around Stem (the center vertical line of a harness)**

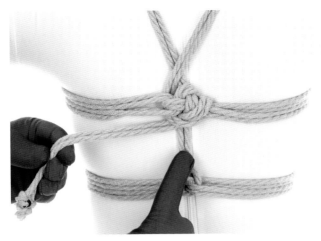

**1.** The stem is also a good place to wrap.

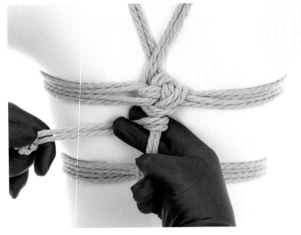

**2.** Reach behind to hook the tail...

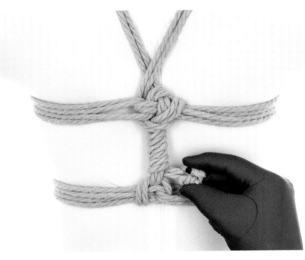

**3.** ...and wrap.

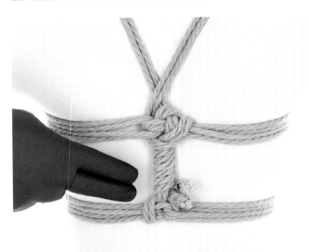

**4.** When you get to the end you can lock with a **Half Hitch**, or...

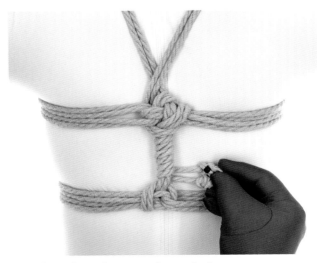

**5.** ...if you have knots in the end of your rope...

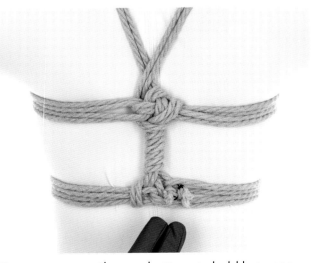

**6.** ...you can use them as buttons to hold between two strands under tension.

## Example 3 – Split the Tails and Wrap Around a Band on Each Side

This approach will take more time, but if you have plans for the stem or the stem has already been used for something, this approach is another way to get a nice, clean look.

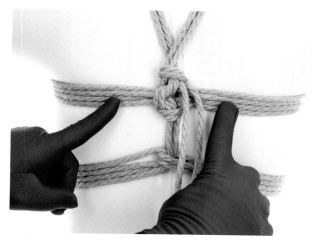

**1.** This time we want to wrap on both sides.

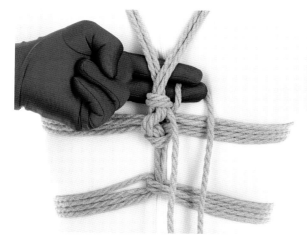

**2.** Reach under the stem and hook one of the tails.

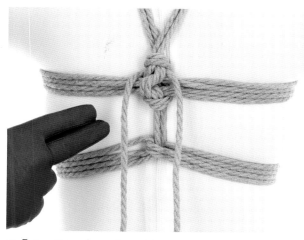

**3.** Bring it to the other side.

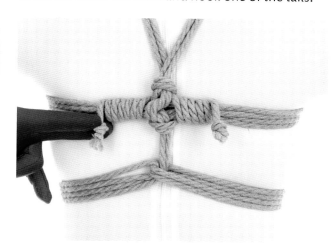

**4.** Wrap the tail around the band on each side.

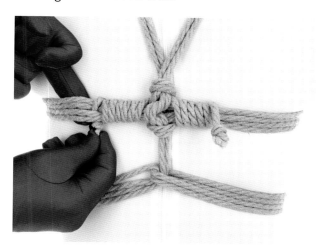

**5.** Lock with a **Half Hitch** or by tucking the ends between two strands.

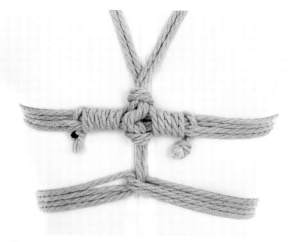

**6.** Done.

## Alternative 3 – Use Half Hitches

Lock with multiple **Half Hitches**.

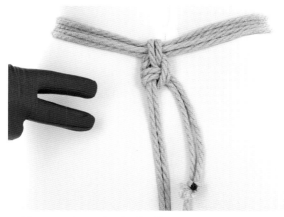

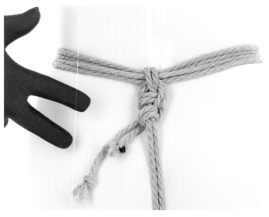

**1.** Here we have locked off with two **Half Hitches**, but we have more rope left than we can hide by tucking the ends under.

**2.** Just add another **Half Hitch**, or more if more are needed. When you have only a little rope left...

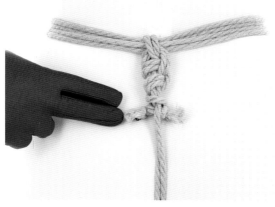

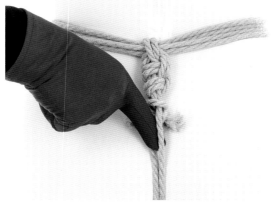

**3.** ...tuck the ends between other strands that are under tension.

**4.** If you have knots at the end of your rope, the tension in the strands will keep the ends in place.

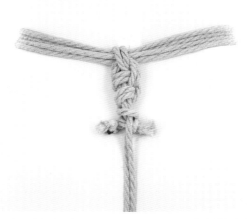

**5.** Again, this looks more attractive and skillful than leaving it at Step 2.

## Alternative 4 – Use Crossing Hitches

Weave at a T junction using repeated **Crossing Hitches**. This can be helpful when the tail is joining a band in a T junction where you have three elements coming together. This can be used for up to about 12-18 inches of rope or so, but much more than that and it becomes bulky and unattractive.

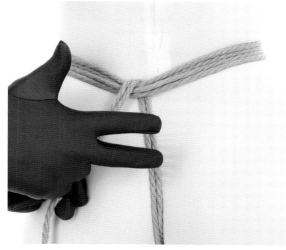

**1.** If you have three lines coming together, you can weave the tail.

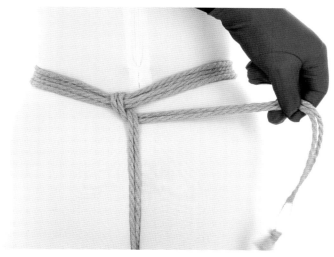

**2.** Start with a Crossing Hitch.

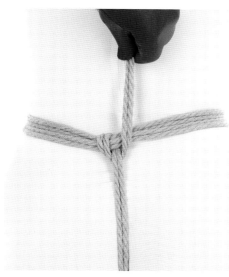

**3.** Like this.

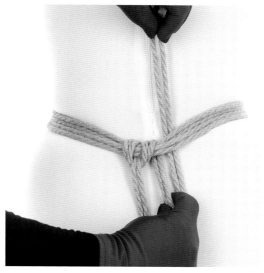

**4.** Then reverse tension...

*continues...*

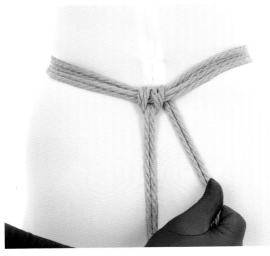

**5.** ...and repeat the pattern

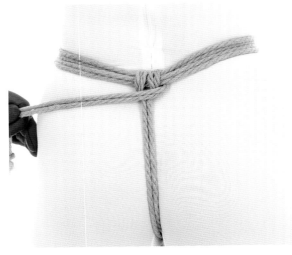

**6.** ...and repeat...

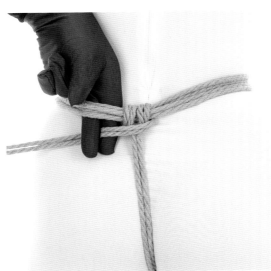

...and again...

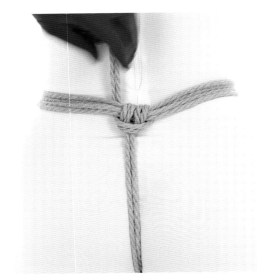

...again...

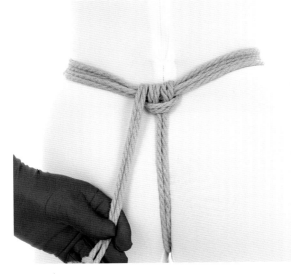

...continue to repeat...

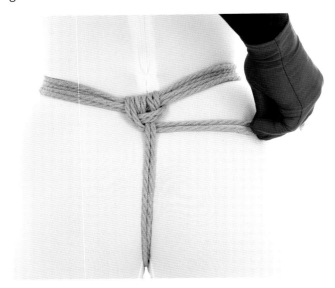

...and repeat...

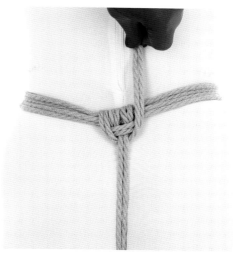

...keep repeating...

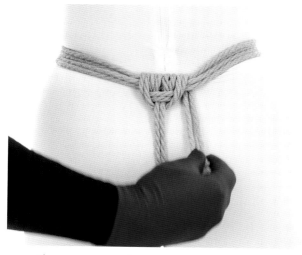

...until you run out of rope

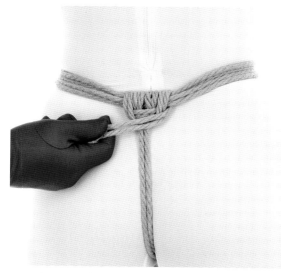

...in this case for a ninth time.

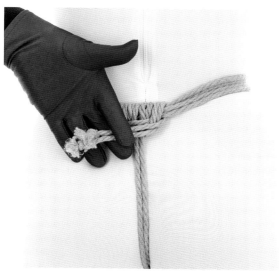

**7.** When you run out of rope...

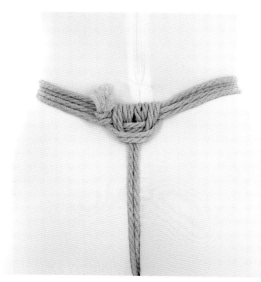

**8.** ...tuck ends under or lock off some other way that you prefer.

### Alternative 5 – Use Decorative Cored Square Knot

This can be used as one option for the crossing lines on the back of the **Hishi Karada** (p. 358). This option adds a bunch of additional friction and allows you to precisely control where that knot lies.

It can also be used as a decorative knot and can be extended to form the **Solomon Bar**, a decorative way to finish a tie.

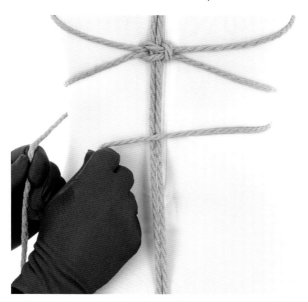

**1.** To do this, take Cord 1 and lay it over top of the center line.

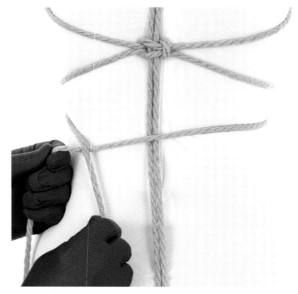

**2.** Lay Cord 2 over Cord 1.

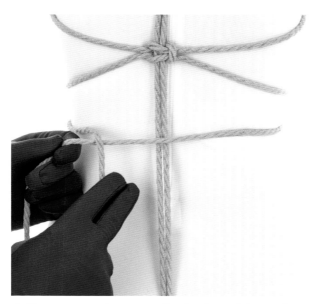

**3.** Now you need to move Cord 2 from this quadrant...

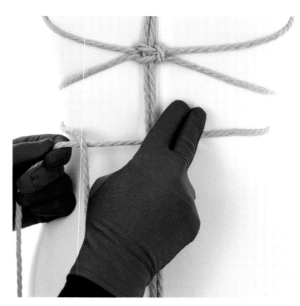

**4.** ...to this one.

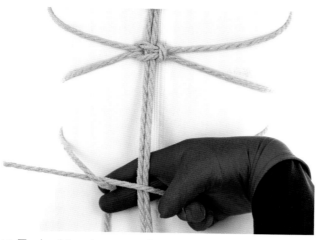

**5.** To do this, place your fingers behind the center line and Cord 1 and grasp Cord 2.

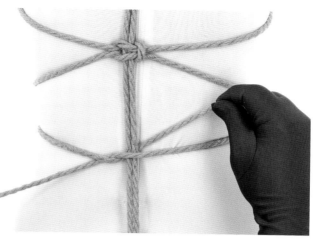

**6.** Pull it through.

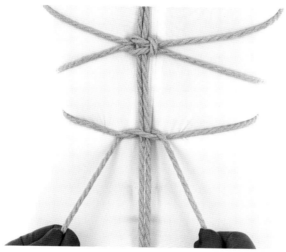

**7.** Bring it back down. The first twist is complete.

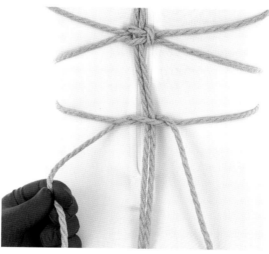

**8.** This rope is still Cord 1 (you can see it is the same one as is coming in from the right-hand side).

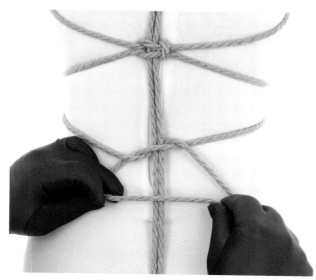

**9.** Do exactly the same thing you did before: place Cord 1 over top of the center line.

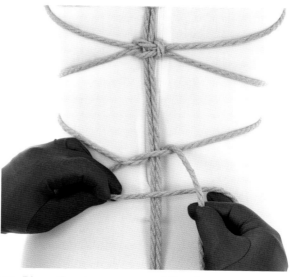

**10.** Place Cord 2 over top of Cord 1.　　*continues...*

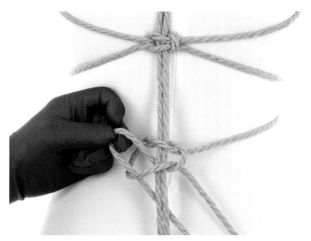

**11.** Reach through and pull Cord 1 from where it is to the opposite quadrant.

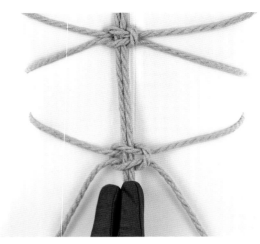

**12.** The form of the **Square Knot** is complete. Now you need to tighten it.

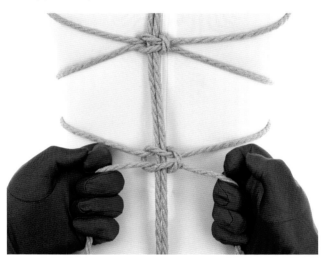

**13.** To tighten, grasp a cord in each hand.

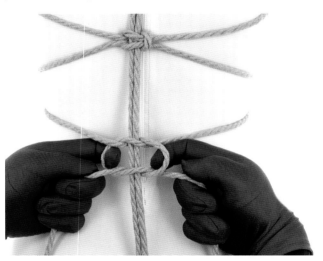

**14.** Hook your forefingers inside the bends of the **Square Knot**.

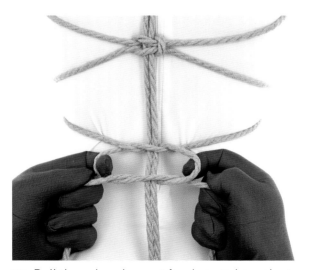

**15.** Pull those bends apart firmly to tighten the top twist, then...

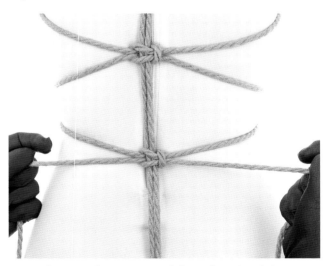

**16.** ...slip your fingers out of those bends while pulling the tails apart at the same time to "snap" the knot closed tightly.

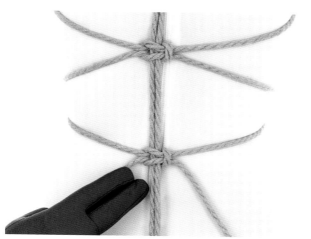

**17.** This is a **Cored Square Knot**. If you look at it, it is a **Square Knot** around a core: The stem.

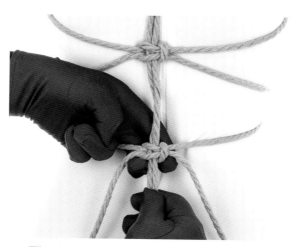

**18.** This knot will have a good grip on the stem, so you can adjust its location and it will stay in place.

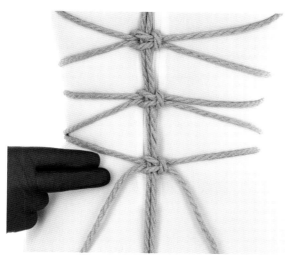

**19.** You can lock off a tie with this attractive technique.

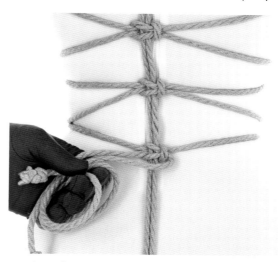

**20.** It is also useful for using up small amounts of extra rope!

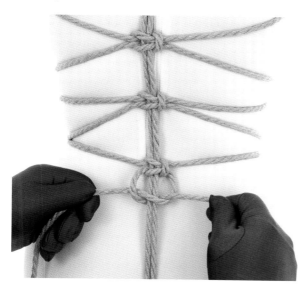

**21.** Just keep repeating that technique to add more twists...

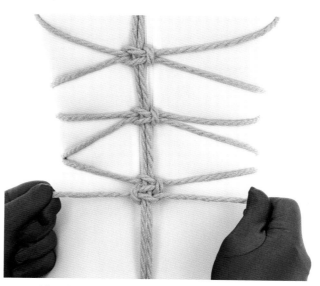

**22.** ...like this.

*continues...*

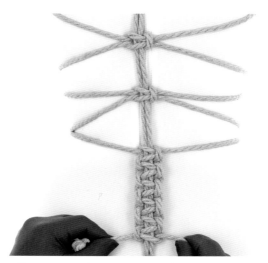

**23.** Repeat until you are out of rope. This pattern is called a **Solomon Bar**.

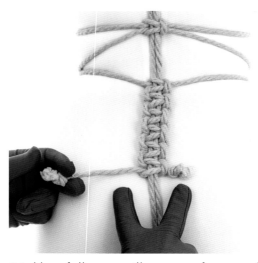

**24.** Hopefully, you will run out of rope on both sides at the same time...

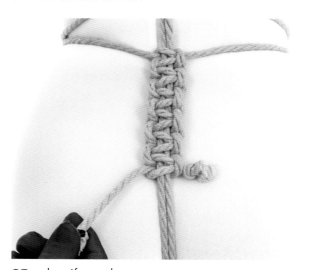

**25.** ...but if you do not...

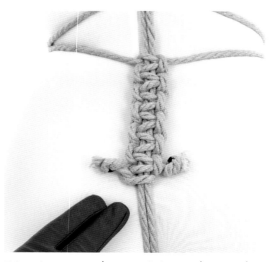

**26.** ...just wrap the remaining end around in one last **Half Hitch**.

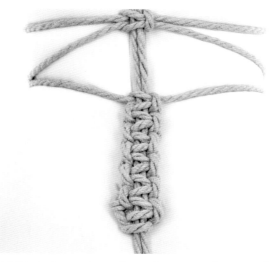

**27.** Tuck the ends under or between the strands of the stem. This makes the tie look much more refined.

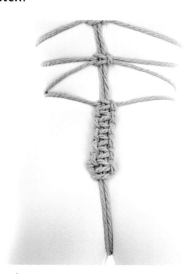

**28.** Done!

# Medium Tail

A medium tail is one that is too long to use one of the short tail techniques, but not long enough to go around your partner's body, in which case you should consider using one of the long tail techniques coming up.

## Alternative 1 — Figure-8 Pattern

A classic technique for burning rope. Take care to not pull the shoulder straps together when doing this. It is easy to do this, especially if you are trying to use up a longer length of rope.

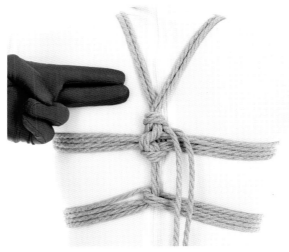

**1.** This is locked off and we will weave between these two straps.

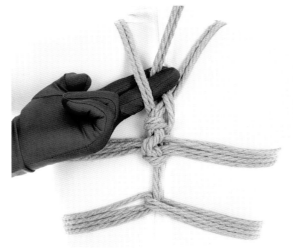

**2.** Place your finger under the other side of the rope from the outside.

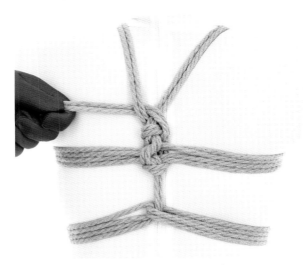

**3.** Hook the rope and pull it through.

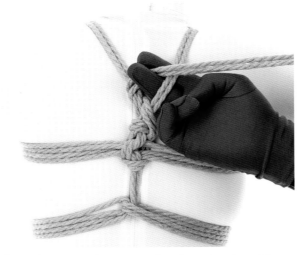

**4.** Now place your fingers under the other band from the outside. Hook the tail and pull through.

*continues...*

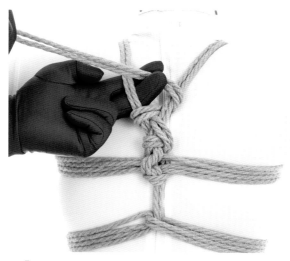

**5.** Repeat.

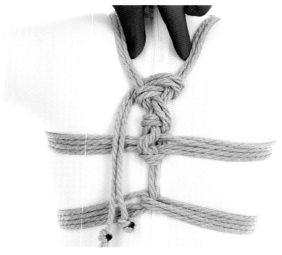

**6.** It is easy to pull these bands together while doing this. Make a choice if you want to do this.

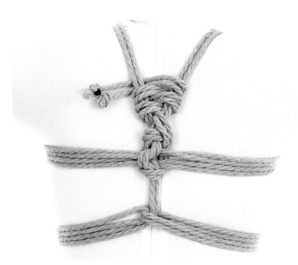

**7.** Continue.

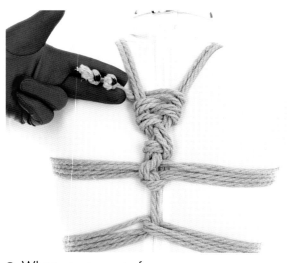

**8.** When you are out of rope...

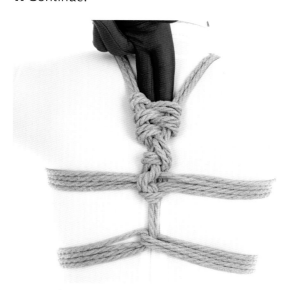

**9.** ...tuck the ends under the pad or lock off with a **Half Hitch**.

## Alternative 2 — Weave Tail Around Bands

Weaving a medium-length tail around bands makes a nice rosette-looking pattern that can be quite attractive. This works best if you have an odd number of lines to weave around, as is common for the upper node of a chest harness. This example comes from the **Pentagram Harness** (p. 350).

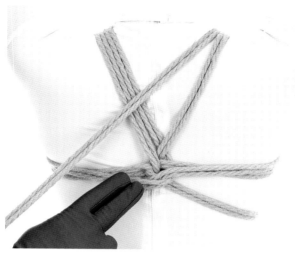

**1.** The tie is basically done, we just need to lock it off and use up any remaining rope here on the back. One way to do this is to weave the tail into all these lines to use up what remains.

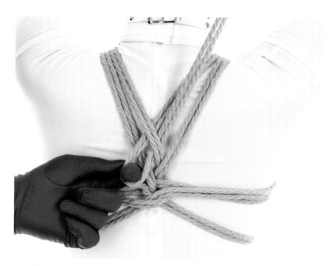

**2.** To do this, run the tail under one set of lines...

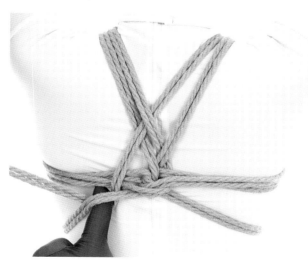

**3.** ...over the next and under the next...

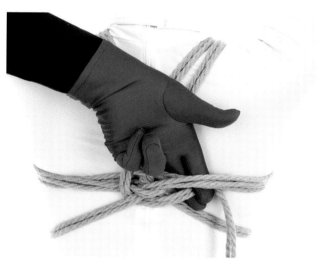

**4.** ...and over and under again.     *continues...*

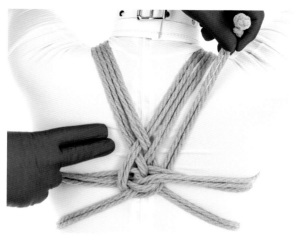

**5.** If you have more rope than this, you could use up the rope using a Figure-8 pattern around the shoulder straps (p. 293).

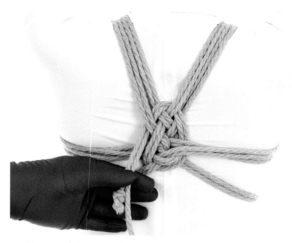

**6.** But, as I have only a small amount left, I will just continue weaving.

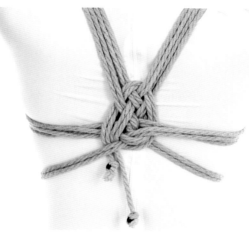

**7.** At this point I am out of rope. The ends are uneven because I have been going around a circle here on the back. This is not a problem!

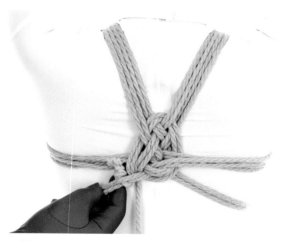

**8.** You can lock off the shorter end on one side...

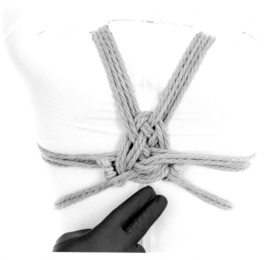

**9.** ...and continue weaving the other end until it is done, then lock it off as well.

## Alternative 3 — Use Half Hitches

Similar to the short tail alternative, you can use a series of **Half Hitches** around a band to make a "bunting" look. This adds an attractive flair and is highly flexible.

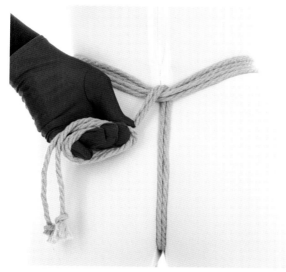

**1.** Reverse tension.

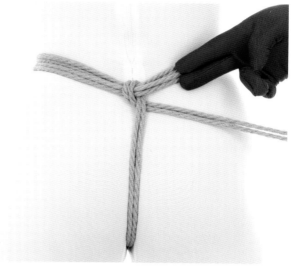

**2.** Run the tail under the stem to the other side.

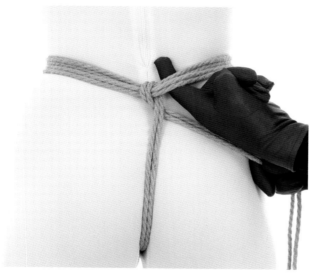

**3.** Now just make a series of **Half Hitches**. Place your finger on top of the tail and under the band.

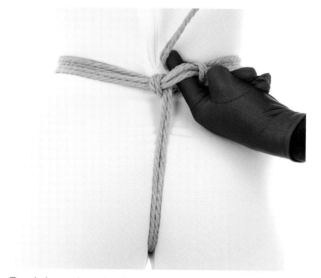

**4.** Feed the tail to the finger. *continues...*

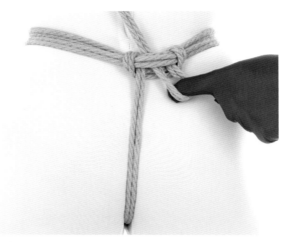

**5.** Hook the tail under and through.

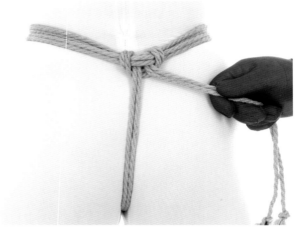

**6.** Tighten.

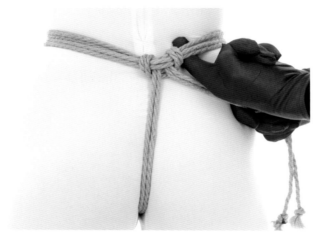

**7.** Repeat.

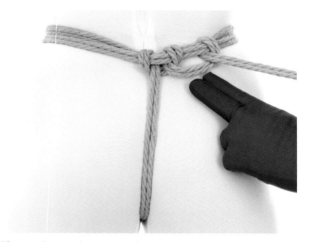

**8.** If you do not have much rope to use up, you can leave a gap.

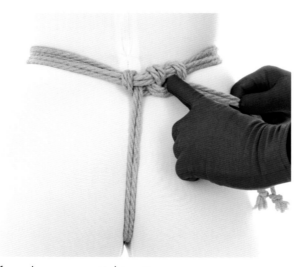

**9.** If you have more, tighten it up.

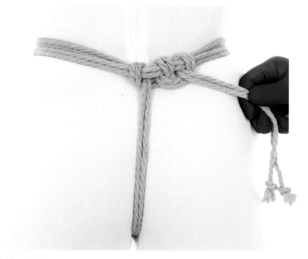

**10.** Like this.

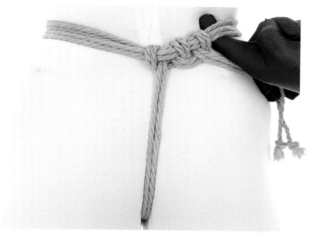

**11.** Repeat.

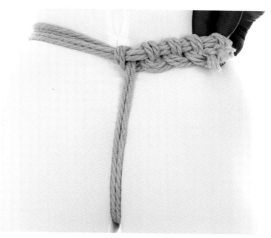

**12.** When you run out of rope, lock off.

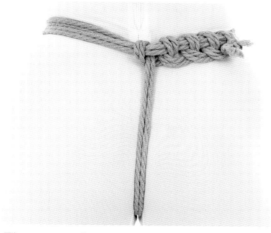

**13.** This creates this nice bunting pattern.

................................................................

**Variations for Different Amounts of Leftover Rope**

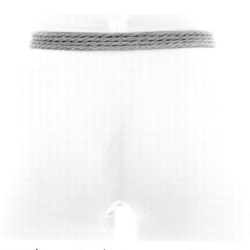

**1.** Here we have a simple strap around the waist...

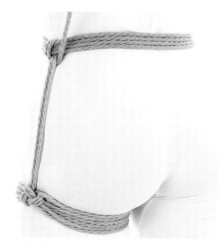

**2.** ...to which we have added a **Lark's Head Single Column** around the thigh to make a garter look. We then connect the tail to the waist strap with a **Crossing Hitch**.

*continues...*

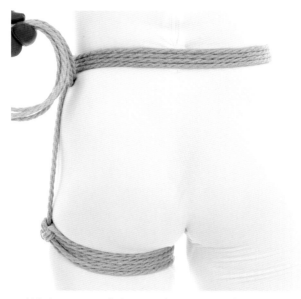

**3.** We have rope left over that we need to use up.

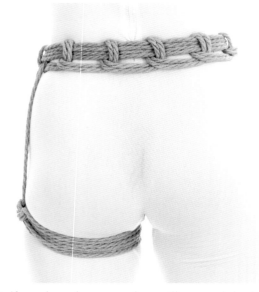

**4.** If you have less rope, but still wanted the bunting to cross the whole back, space the **Hitches** out.

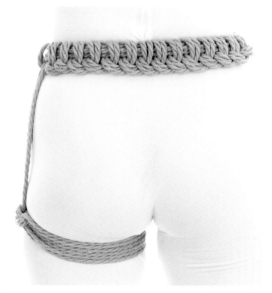

**5.** If you have more rope you need to use up, place the **Hitches** closer together.

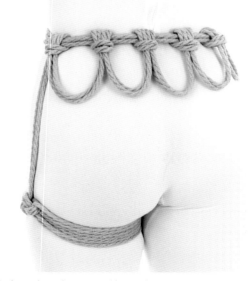

**6.** Related technique: If you have even more rope, you can use **Cow Hitches** instead of **Half Hitches** and drape the rope more dramatically.

........................................................................................................................

## Alternative 4 — Add Extra Knots While Tying

If you know that you will have rope left over — perhaps you have done this tie on this person before, or perhaps you are nearing the end and can see that you have more rope than you need — you can add optional knots that consume more rope. For example, instead of connecting one rope to another with a twist like we show in Steps 21-23 of the **Hishi Karada** (p. 363), you could choose a **Cow Hitch** (p. 273). This can convert a medium length of leftover rope to a small length, which is easier to burn at the end.

# Long Tail

A long tail is one that can go around your partner's body more than once.

## Alternative 1 — Add Extra Wraps and Bands

If you have a long tail left over, you can simply add extra wraps or bands around the body or limb at the end of the tie. Making long runs like this is a great way to quickly use up lots of rope. Important: This band is not a functional part of the original tie. This is its own new element that does not add additional security to the original tie.

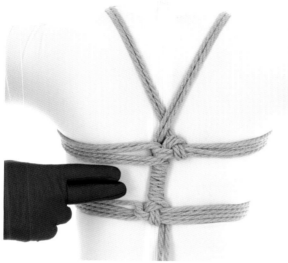

**1.** I wanted the tail to be below the rest of the tie before adding the band so I wrapped it around the stem.

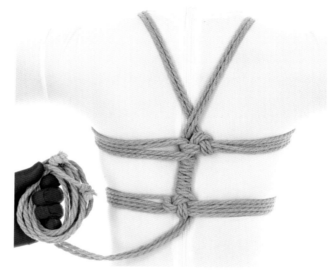

**2.** There is enough rope left over to wrap around the body twice.

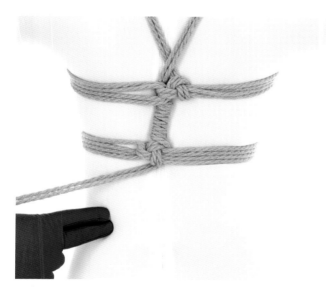

**3.** Let us do that around the waist.

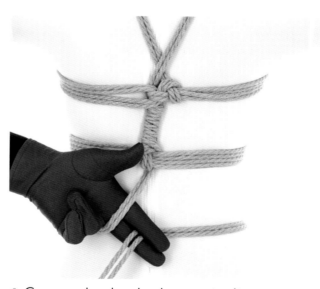

**4.** Go around and under the outgoing line.

*continues...*

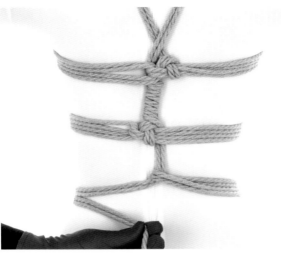

**5.** Reverse tension and go around again.

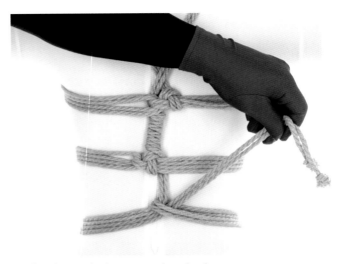

**6.** Go through the secondary bight.

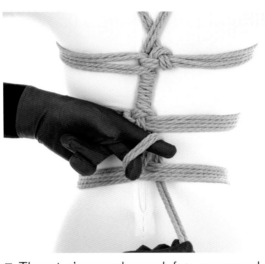

**7.** There isn't enough rope left to go around again so lock off with a **Half Hitch** as usual.

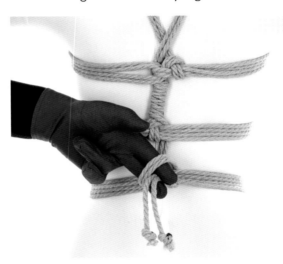

**8.** ...

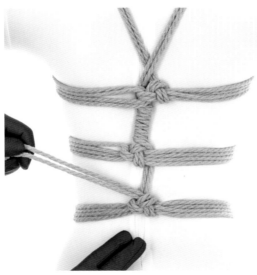

**9.** As is shown in the **Lark's Head Single Column** tutorial (p. 181).

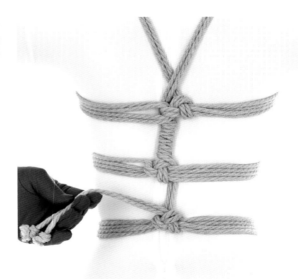

**10.** There is still some rope left.

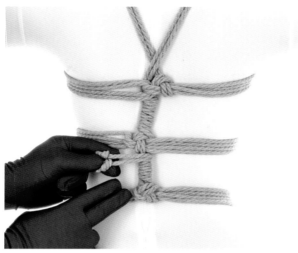

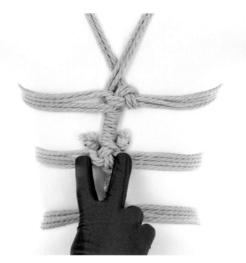

**11.** Use one of the short or medium techniques. This time I will just wrap it around the stem...

**12.** ...and tuck the ends under the band.

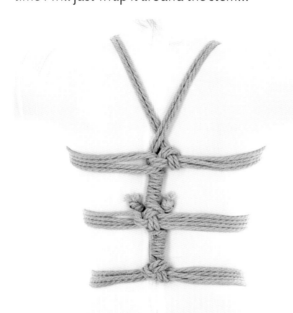

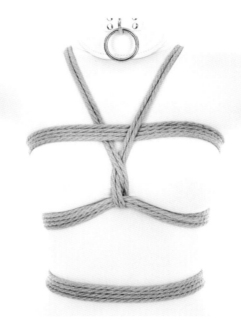

**13.** Finished from the back.

**14.** Finished from the front.

## Long Tail

### Alternative 2 — Add Extra Wraps While Tying

If you know from the beginning that you will have extra rope, you can burn some rope during the main tie instead of waiting until the end.

This example modifies the **Shinju** (p. 345), adding an extra wrap to the upper chest band.

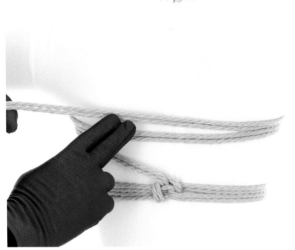

**1.** Make two wraps before reversing tension instead of one.

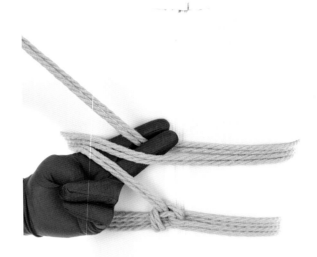

**2.** Then reach under both to hook the tail.

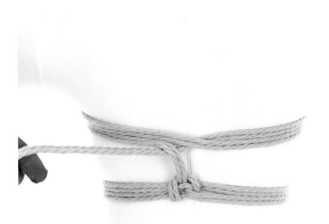

**3.** Pull through. From here everything progresses as usual...

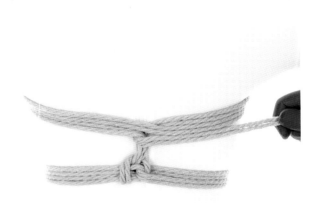

**4.** ...reverse tension...

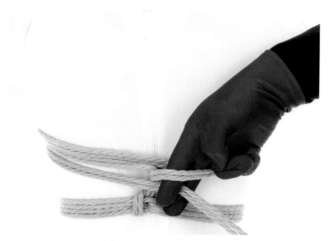

**5.** ...wrap around below the other wraps.

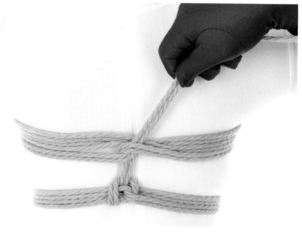

**6.** Pull through.

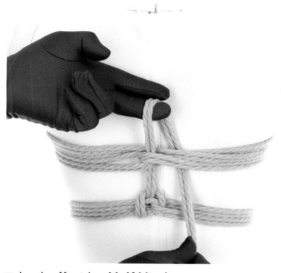

**7.** Lock off with a **Half Hitch**.

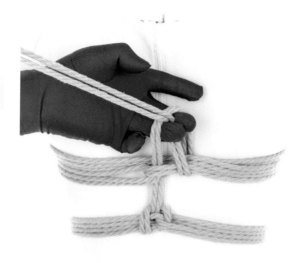

**8.** ...

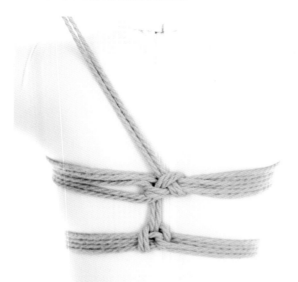

**9.** Modified band complete, continue as usual.

Long Tail

## Alternative 3 — Use Crossing Hitches

This approach is often seen at the end of **Gote Shibari**/(TK) type chest harnesses.

(See TheDuchy.com/gote-shibari/ for more about those ties.)

When the tie has multiple bands, the tail can be attached to those bands with a series of **Crossing Hitches** (p. 271). This adds a lovely decorative element to the tie while also consuming extra rope.

In this example, we are creating a simple **Box Tie** (p. 397) and have a lot of rope left to use up.

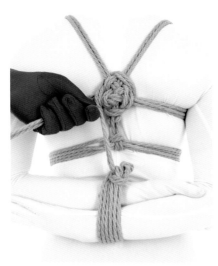

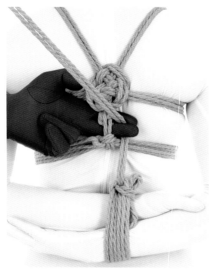

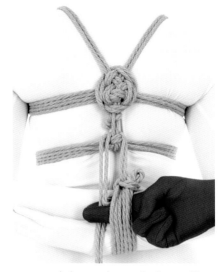

**1.** There is a **Shinju** on the chest and a **Slipped Somerville Bowline** around both wrists.

**2.** First, connect the wrist tie to the chest tie by running the tail up to the lower chest band, behind the stem...

**3.** ...and down through the cuff.

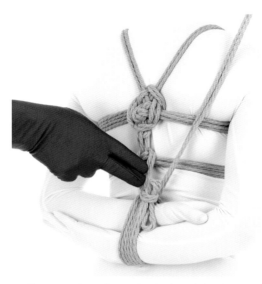

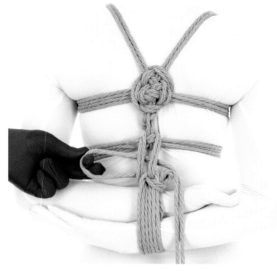

**4.** Be sure that the tail is behind the knot of the **Somerville Bowline**. This is important. You need to keep that knot clear, or you will not be able to use it for emergency release.

**5.** Bring the tail around to the other side again.

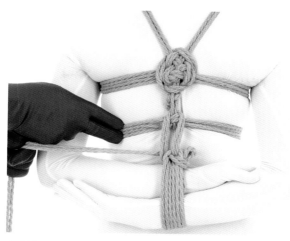

**6.** We are now going to put a series of **Crossing Hitches** in place, going around the back, starting with this band.

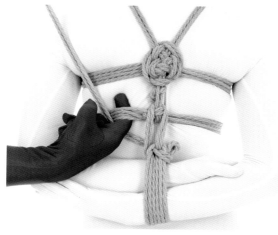

**7.** For all of these **Crossing Hitches**, do the first tail pull on the side closest to the center of the body.

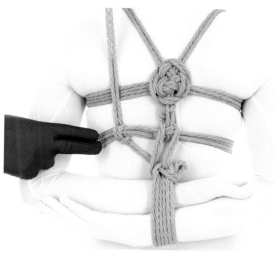

**8.** Then complete. This makes sure that you are using a closed version of the **Crossing Hitch**, which will have a better grip.

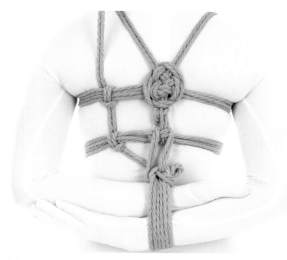

**9.** Now just repeat going around all the bands.

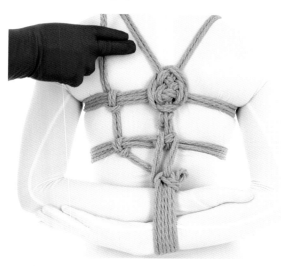

**10.** Continue.

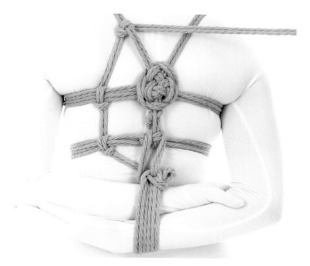

**11.** …

*continues…*

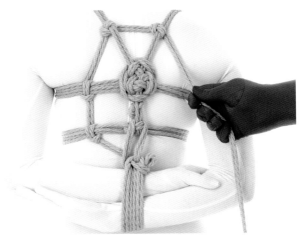

**12.** ...

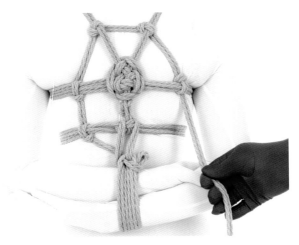

**13.** ...

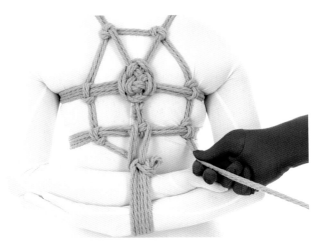

**14.** ...

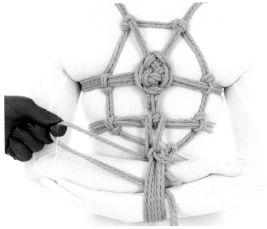

**15.** When you get back to the cuffs, run through them again. Again, make sure it is behind the quick release of the **Somerville Bowline**.

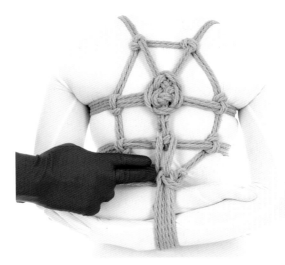

**16.** Finish using up the rest of the rope. If you have enough rope, you can keep going. Make another round of **Crossing Hitches** inside of the first one! If not, use up the rest some other way and lock off.

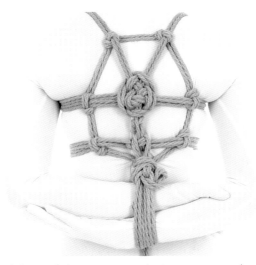

**17.** Many of the gorgeous designs you may have seen on various ties are simple things like this that are added just to use up rope! Surprise!

## Long Tail

### Alternative 4 — Trace an Existing Element

Go back the way you came or repeat something you did before! Here we have finished a **Shinju** (p. 345) but have a lot of rope left over. This time let us double up on the shoulder strap!

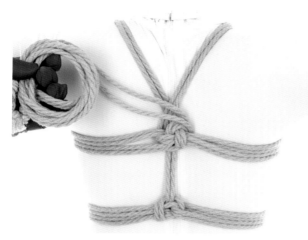

**1.** We have enough rope to double the shoulder straps.

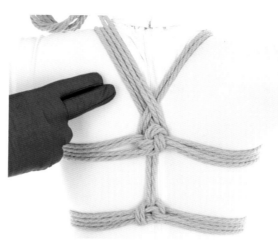

**2.** Just follow the path of the first one.

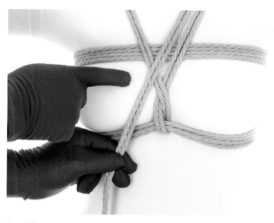

**3.** Always stay on the same side, not letting the new line cross the old.

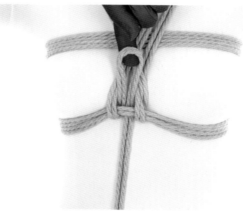

**4.** Repeat the same steps you used to create the first shoulder band.

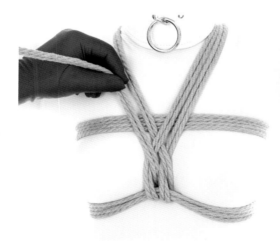

**5.** ...

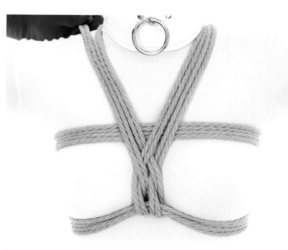

**6.** ...

*continues...*

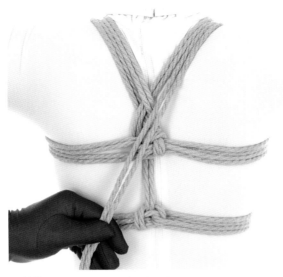

**7.** When you get to the back...

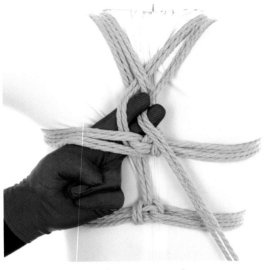

**8.** ...weave the tail in as seems best.

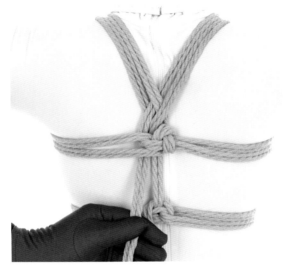

**9.** ...

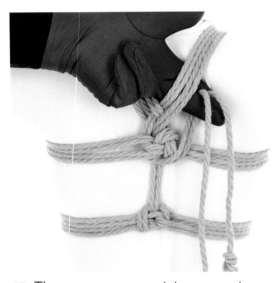

**10.** Then use up any remaining rope using some other technique and lock off as desired.

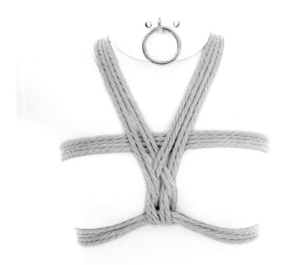

**11.** Done!

## Alternative 5 — Connect Tail to Other Ties

Connecting the tail to another element of bondage can make your scene look more organized and intentional. Here is just one of many possible examples. In this example, we have a lot of rope left after tying a **Shinju** (p. 345).

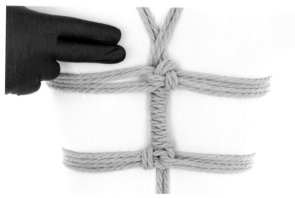

**1.** For this **Shinju**, I wanted an extremely clean look. So, instead of locking off with a **Half Hitch** as usual...

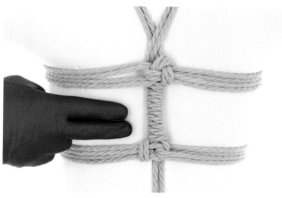

**2.** ...I wrapped the tail around the stem.

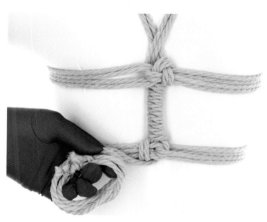

**3.** The tail is now at the bottom of the **Shinju** and needs to be used up. Here is where you might consider connecting it to some other bondage element.

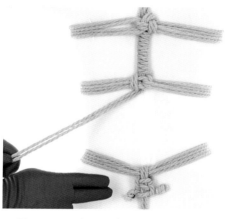

**4.** For example, perhaps you also have a **Crotch Rope** in place.

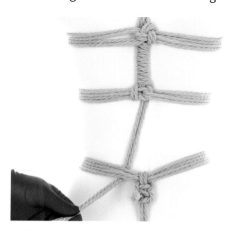

**5.** Bring the tail down under the waistband...

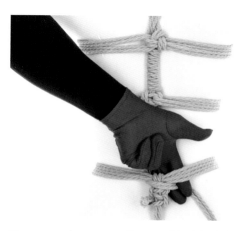

**6.** ...over the center line and behind the waistband on the other side.

*continues...*

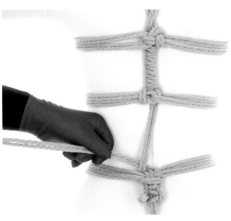

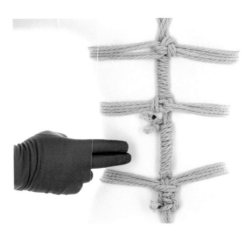

**7.** You can run it up and down once or twice to use up more rope, but when you have only 12-18 inches remaining, begin wrapping it around the new stem you created.

**8.** Like this.

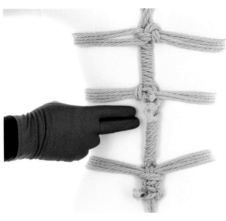

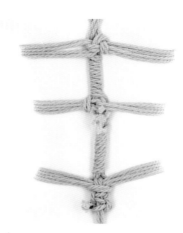

**9.** When you run out of rope, run your tails between the strands of the stem. If you have a knot at the end of your rope, that will lock them off. If not, add a **Half Hitch** to complete.

**10.** Done!

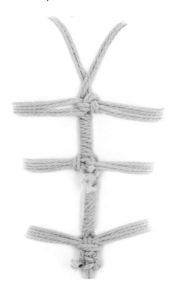

**11.** This gives the finished tie a clean, attractive look.

## Alternative 6 – Figure-8 Pattern

The medium tail alternative shows how to do a Figure-8 pattern between shoulder bands (p. 293). Another option is do this between the upper and lower chest bands of the chest harness itself. But let's take what we learned from the previous method and try something different.

**Example 1 – Wrap Asymmetrically**

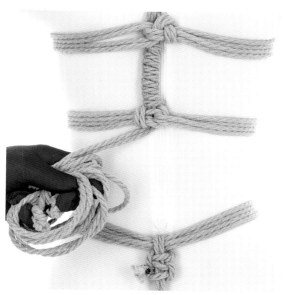

**1.** Rope to be used up from the **Shinju**.

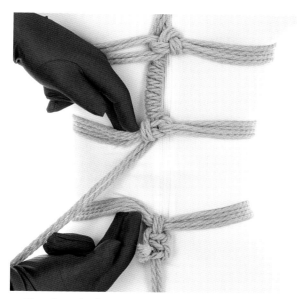

**2.** Two bands, lower chest band and waist band.

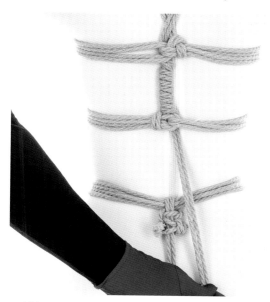

**3.** We are going to do this pattern on the left side, but I want something to anchor it in place, so I will do my first **Hitch** on the right.

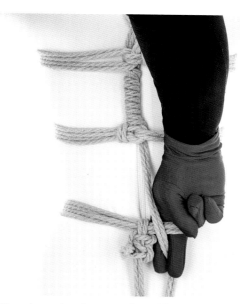

**4.** Reach under the waistband from above and hook the tail.

*continues...*

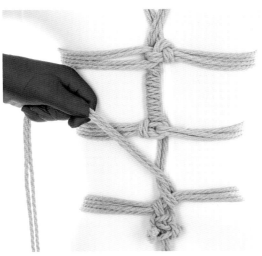

**5.** Pull the tail up and through, then lay it on top of the incoming line.

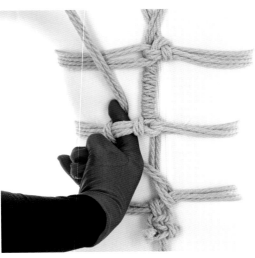

**6.** Lay it on top of the upper band. Reach under the band from below and hook the tail.

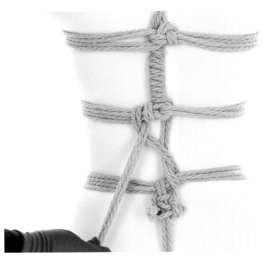

**7.** Pull it down and through. Lay the tail on top of the lower band.

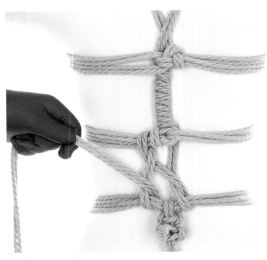

**8.** Repeat the pattern...

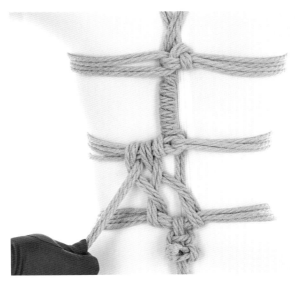

**9.** ...

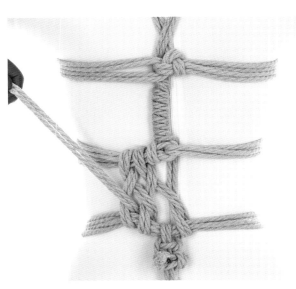

**10.** ...

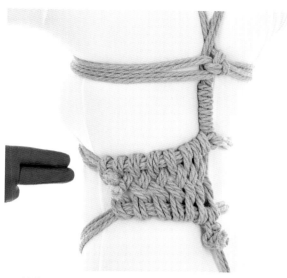

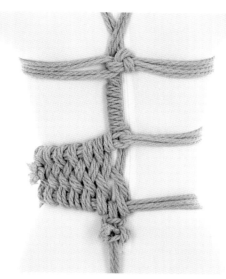

**11.** When you run out of rope, lock off.

**12.** Done!

But some people do not like the asymmetric look, so here is how to do this symmetrically.

### Example 2 – Separate the Lines and Wrap Symmetrically

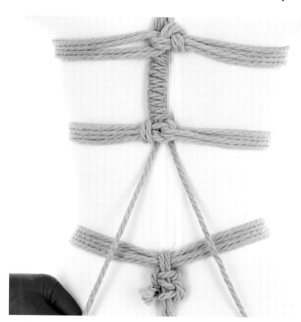

**1.** Separate the lines of the tail.

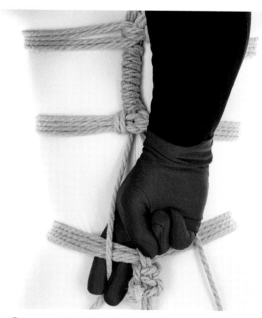

**2.** On one side, lay the strand on top of the lower band, then put your fingers under that band from above on the incoming side. *continues...*

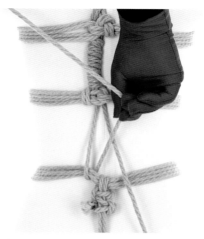

**3.** Hook the tail and pull it up and through.

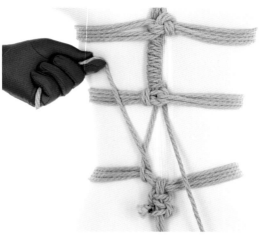

**4.** Lay the tail on top of the incoming line and on top of the upper band.

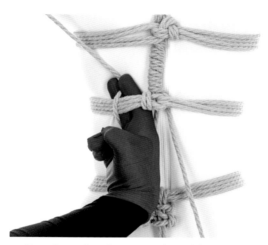

**5.** Reach under the upper band from below, on the incoming side.

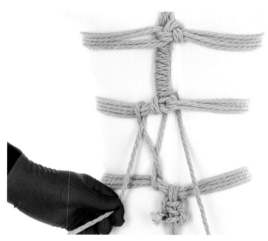

**6.** Hook the tail and pull it through. Then lay it on top of itself and the lower band.

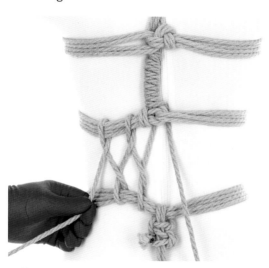

**7.** Repeat this pattern. You can space it out instead of weaving them tightly as in Example 1. This will conserve rope if you wanted to move the rope over and do something else with the tail! See p. 318 for an example.

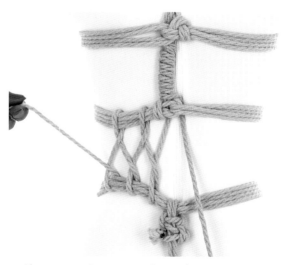

**8.** If you are planning to have the rope move away from this layer to do something else, lock if off here first by...

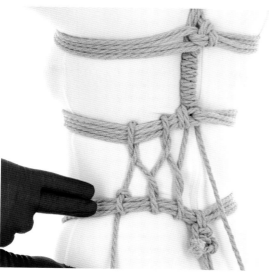

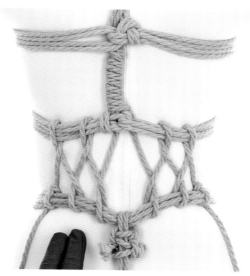

**9.** ...adding a **Crossing Hitch**. If you are out of rope entirely, lock off in some more solid way like with a **Cow Hitch** or by wrapping the tail around the band and tucking the ends between some of the strands, etc.

**10.** Since we want this to be symmetric, make sure that whatever you do to one side...

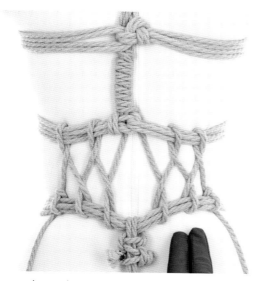

**11.** ...you do to the other.

If you made the choice to have some rope left over like I have done in this example, see the next page for one idea of what you could do with it!

### Alternative 7 – Add More Elements and Ties

You can use that tail to add a whole new layer of bondage! There are many ways to do this. In fact, this is all that is happening to turn a **Lark's Head Single Column** (p. 181) around the waist into a **Crotch Rope** (p. 370)! We simply run the tail between the legs and tie it off.

You can exercise your creativity to add other fun elements. Let's just invent here. This example begins where the example on the previous page leaves off.

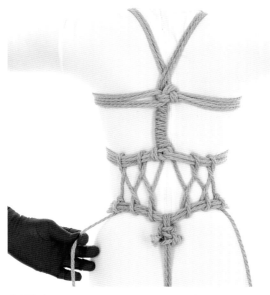

**1.** We have yet more rope to use!

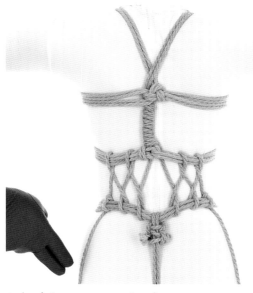

**2.** Let's invent some simple garters.

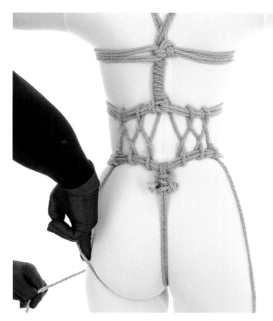

**3.** Bring the line down the hips, under the butt cheek, between the legs, and across the front of the thighs.

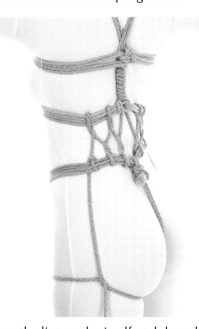

**4.** Run the line under itself and then down.

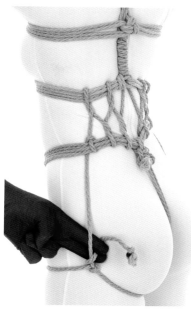

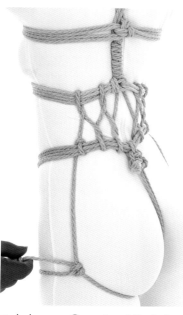

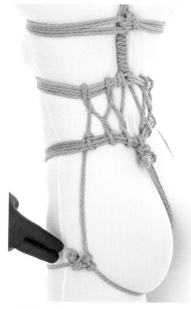

**5.** We are now almost out of rope, so lock off with a **Crossing Hitch** or **Cow Hitch**.

**6.** I chose a **Crossing Hitch** for no particular reason.

**7.** Wrap the remaining line around itself and tuck the knotted end under or add a **Half Hitch** to lock off.

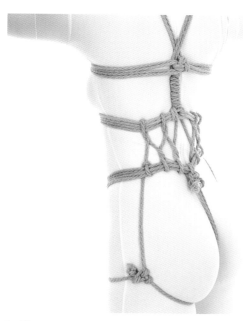

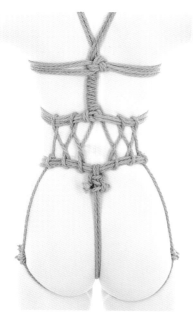

**8.** Done.

**9.** Repeat on the other side. We have just invented a fun, flirty look in our quest to use up extra rope. Fun, right?

This is just one of *many* ways to add elements. For other fun ideas and patterns, join TheDuchy.com and check out these members-only tutorials:
- **Gingham Thigh-highs**: TheDuchy.com/gingham-thigh-highs/
- **Loop-chain Evening Dress**: TheDuchy.com/loop-chain-evening-dress/

## Long Tail

### Alternative 8 — Connect Tail to Something Else

So, you have rope on your partner and what basically amounts to a leash leading from it. This can be wonderfully useful in tying them *to* something, so they do not wander off. Perhaps to a chair or a bed or a strong post or beam!

There are a myriad of ways to do this. We won't even try to cover them all. Many of the ideas in this book lend themselves to this. But we will cover one technique that can be useful for anchoring multiple bands to something.

In this example, you are anchoring your partner to a post using the tail from a chest harness and a **Square Lashing** or, as in this case, a series of **Square Lashings**:

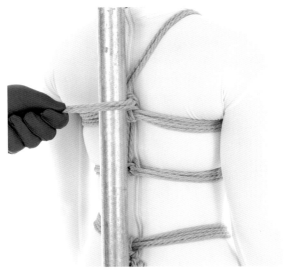

**1.** Bring the tail around the column...

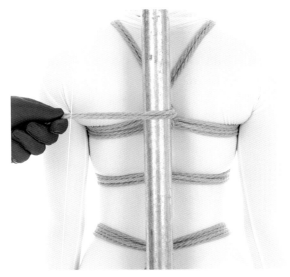

**2.** ...to the other side.

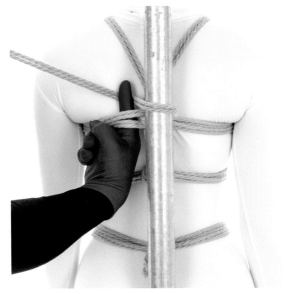

**3.** Run the tail under the upper band on the other side of the column.

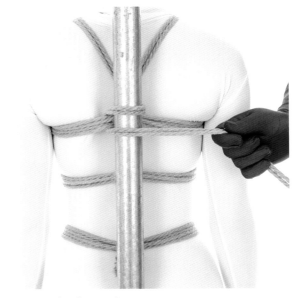

**4.** Return to the first side.

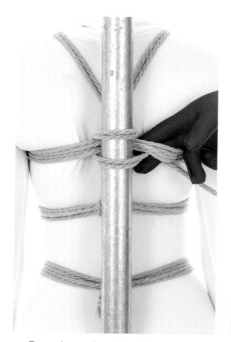

**5.** Run the tail under the band.

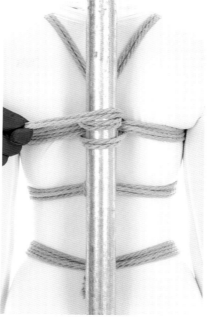

**6.** Wrap the tail around the pole.

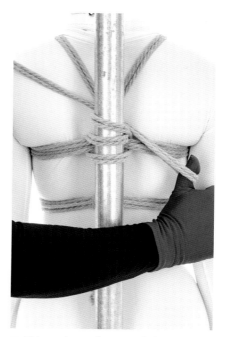

**7.** Wrap the tail around the strands of the lashing.

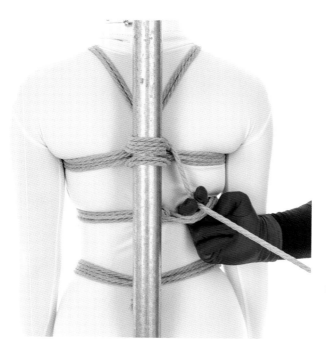

**8.** Now bring the tail down to the next band and hook the tail under it.

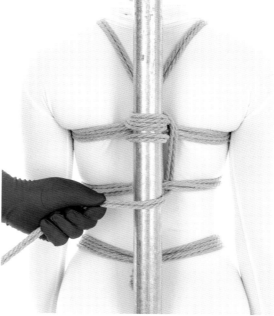

**9.** Repeat the process to make another **Square Lashing** around the column. *continues...*

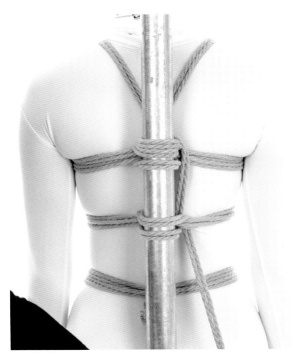

**10.** …

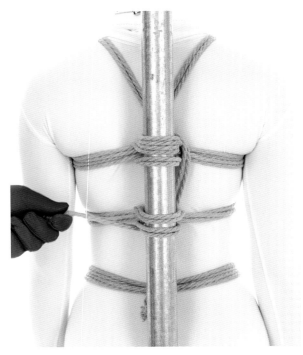

**11.** …

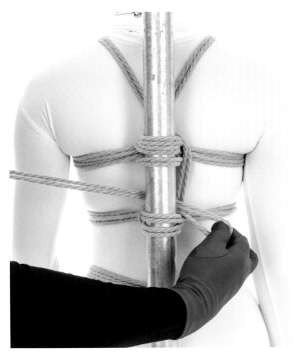

**12.** …

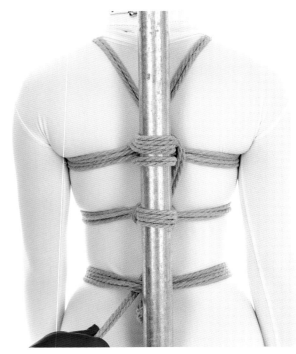

**13.** Bring it down and under the next band. Note that it does not matter which side you start this on. This time I crossed under the pole and started from the other side. This may hide the lines better and some may prefer it. Structurally, it makes no difference.

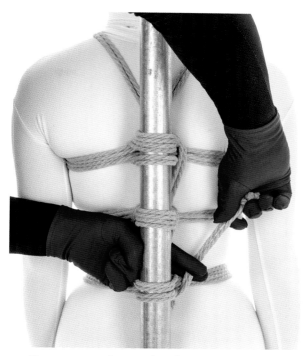

**14.** Repeat to make another **Square Lashing**.

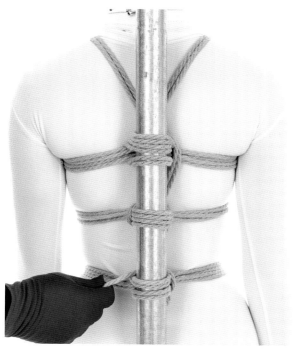

**15.** When you run out of rope (whether at this point or before), tie it off.

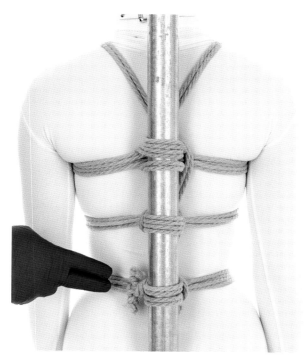

**16.** In this case, I separated the strands of the tail, put one on each side of the lines of the **Square Lashing**, and tied off with a **Square Knot**.

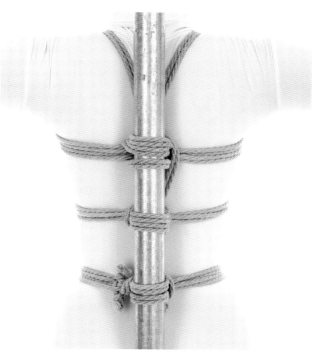

**17.** Done! Now they will stay put as you consider what to do to them next.

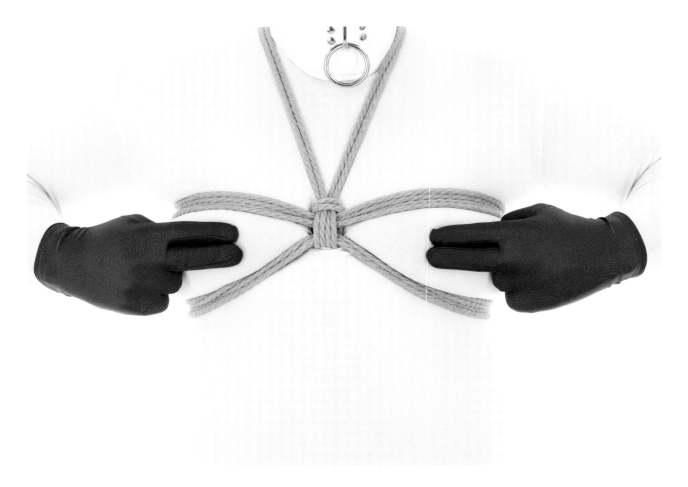

# Body Type Considerations

Most pictures in this book show ties applied to Kajira Blue, a person with one particular body type. They happen to be one of your authors, which made it easier to get all these pictures! But there are lots of different body types and, as we have said, rope is for every body and anyone who is interested in tying or being tied.

Interest in shibari is found in every demographic. Every gender, orientation, identification, body type, and level of physical capability.

The nice thing is that there are a few relatively easy techniques that will allow you to modify any tie in this book for virtually any need. Let's look at:

• Considerations when tying someone with no breasts.
• Considerations when tying someone with a penis.
• Considerations when tying someone with softer flesh or skin that is sensitive to pressure.

TheDuchy.com/body-type-considerations/

# Tying Someone Without Breasts

Some people assume that chest harnesses can only be tied to people with breasts. In reality, it is rare that a chest harness requires breasts. It may include considerations that allow it to be tied on without putting undue pressure on breasts, but most chest harnesses work equally well without them.

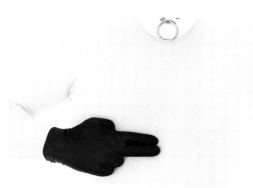

**1.** The position of the bands remains the same, the lower band goes just over the lower part of the sternum.

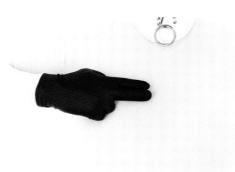

**2.** The upper band over the sternum, on or just above the mid-point, typically about even with the armpits.

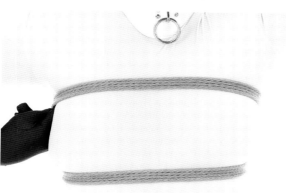

**3.** Make sure the bands are quite tight. The rope should be sunk about halfway into the skin on their sides. This helps keep the rope in place. Do not go too tight though; you still need to be able to slip at least two fingers under that rope.

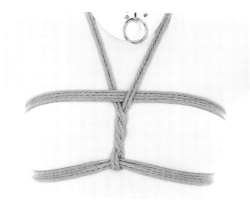

**4.** You can also help the bands stay in place by adding extra twists to help keep the bands apart.

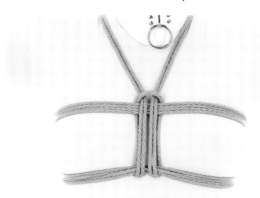

**5.** OR you can do the complete opposite of that and use a technique like the **Cow Hitch**...

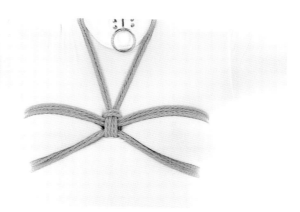

**6.** ...to give your partner breasts even if they do not usually have them!

# Tying Someone With a Penis

The only time this issue typically arises is when you want to run rope down between the legs, directly over where the penis is. There are several ways to handle this, but the easiest is to...

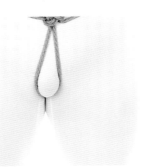

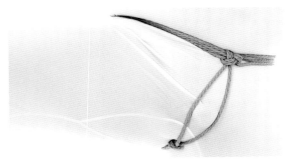

**1.** ...simply run one strand on one side and the other strand on the other side of the shaft. Be sure the strands are next to the skin and not on top of or between the testes.

**2.** You can still even put in a happy knot if you like. It goes just behind the balls on the perineum or on the anus, or both.

**You can also convert it to a strap-on:**

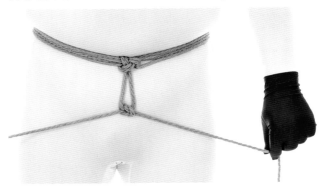

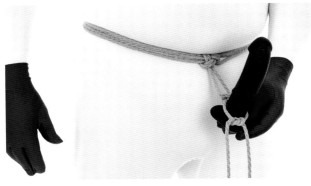

**1.** If you put a knot in the right place above...

**2.** ...and below a dildo that has a base...

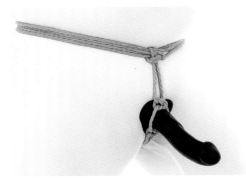

**3.** ...you can replace your partner's equipment with a substitute. Or give them a second one (not pictured).

This technique is suitable for many kinds of ties with rope between the legs and it will work well for the **Hishi Karada** (p. 358) and **Simple Crotch Rope** (p. 370).

# Tying Someone with Softer Flesh

An important technique to know when tying someone with softer flesh or more sensitive skin is how to lower the pressure of a band on the skin.

It is important to manage the amount of force rope places on the body.

That management starts with how tight the ropes are when you tie them. Making sure you can get two fingers between the rope and the skin helps you confirm the rope is not too tight for most people. But what if it is still pressing too firmly and is uncomfortable for your partner? Perhaps their skin is particularly sensitive to certain kinds of touch or pressure.

Even if the rope feels fine to them when you tie it, it is still possible for the pressure of that rope to change later. If they move into a different position, the internal parts of their body move relative to each other and a band that previously felt fine might become uncomfortably or even dangerously tight. This is why we advise that you put someone in the general position they will be in before you tie them.

If the rope is tied to some other object, the pressure might change.

## Risks of Increased Tension

No matter the reason, if the tension of or on the ropes increases, the risk of injury also increases. As the tension increases, the pressure of the band and force of the rope against the skin increases; the ropes will dig more deeply into a person's skin and press more firmly onto what is beneath — nerves, blood vessels, muscles, and bone — increasing the risk of damage.

When a person's flesh is softer, the rope will have more ability to press more deeply into them. This means that muscles, nerves, and veins can be moved further relative to each other. This means that the risk of nerve damage, by pressing on a nerve too hard or by stretching that nerve too far, can be greater.

There is yet another consideration: Comfort and pain. Our body is sensitive to forces on it. Too much force is not comfortable.

There is a single solution that can help in any of these cases: Make wider bands. Spread the force over a wider area. This reduces the pressure on the skin and the forces on things under the skin.

You can make wider bands by using thicker rope, or with more wraps, or by employing both of these techniques.

## Body Type Considerations

### Use Thicker Rope
Keeping all else the same, thicker rope will mean wider bands.

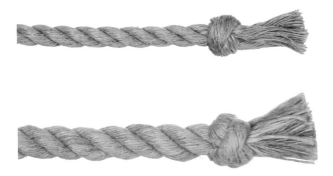

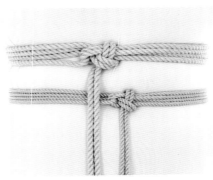

**1.** You might simply use thicker rope. Above is a ¼-inch compared to ⅜-inch.

**2.** The band created by the ¼-inch is about 1 inch wide. The one created by the ⅜-inch is about 1½ inches.

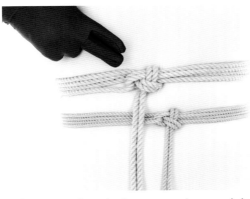

**3.** Be aware that the knots are also much bulkier.

### Pinching Hazard

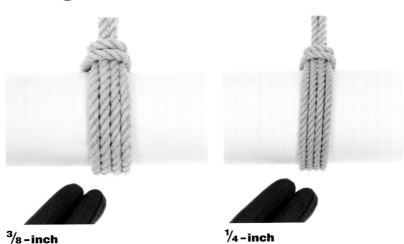

**⅜-inch**            **¼-inch**

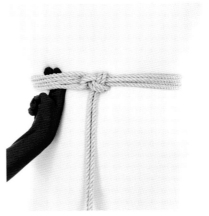

Also, there is a larger gap between strands of rope in the two different band sizes. Some people find that it is easier to get their skin pinched between the strands when those strands are larger.

One thing you can do to help with this is to run your fingers under each band when it is complete. This helps settle the rope evenly on top of the skin and can reduce the risk of pinching for some people.

## Add More Wraps

Adding more wraps also widens the band. There are limits to this. If you add too many wraps, it can make the band bunch up too much at the knot and make it difficult to keep all strands parallel and at the same tension at points where the rope puts pressure on the skin. It is usually possible to do three to four wraps for a total of six to eight strands; more wraps can take more work to get right.

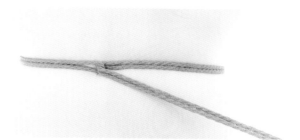

**1.** Complete the **Lark's Head** as normal.

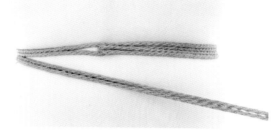

**2.** Make your first wrap, but this time...

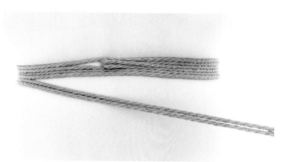

**3.** ...keep going and make a second wrap.

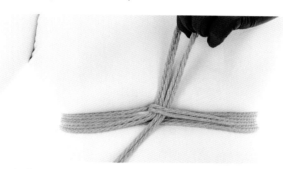

**4.** NOW go through the secondary bight...

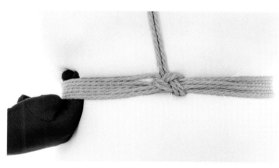

**5.** ...and lock off with a **Half Hitch**. Run your fingers under the band to better settle the lines on the skin.

### Another Helpful Solution: Make More Bands!

Another way to distribute force over a larger area is to add entirely new bands.

This applies more when combining multiple techniques or when doing more advanced ties, so we will leave this to explore later.

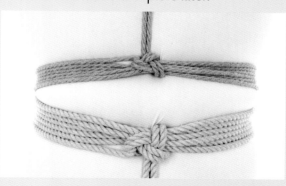

You can also combine both, use larger rope *and* more wraps.

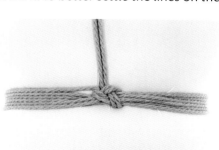

**6.** Done!

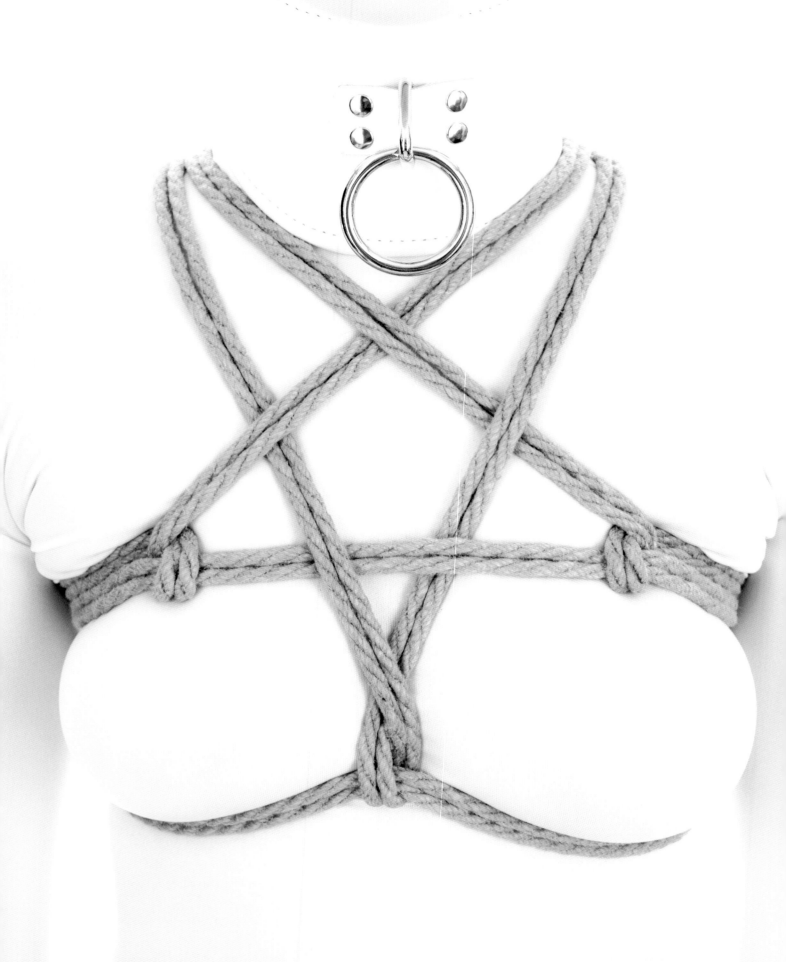

# Chest Harnesses

Chest and body harnesses can feel amazing! They act as restraints or as a frame to which you can attach other layers of bondage. For example, you can add a cuff to each wrist then connect them to a chest harness. Or you can attach a new rope to a chest harness then tie that harness to a chair, headboard, or vertical beam to keep your partner in place.

There are many wonderful chest and body harnesses out there. We will cover four ties:

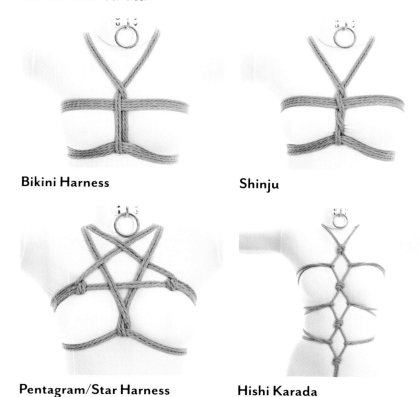

**Bikini Harness**

**Shinju**

**Pentagram/Star Harness**

**Hishi Karada**

For more, check out **TheDuchy.com/tutorials/** and select "Chest" from the **Categories** drop-down box.

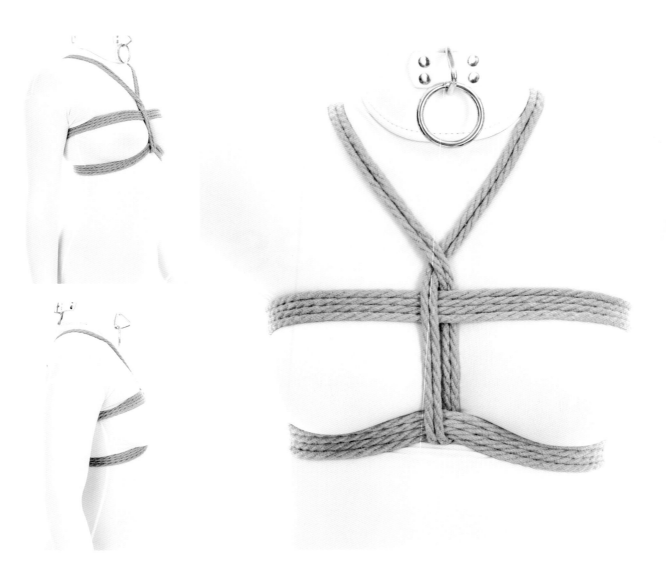

# Bikini Harness

This simple harness is a good first layer upon which to build additional bondage. It is very similar to the **Shinju**, but each chest band is not locked. This makes it fast to put on and a fine choice for floor work, but not suitable for suspensions.

You can tie the bands while standing behind your partner; you do not need to move around them. With practice, even the front (starting with Step 27) can be done from behind, but most people move to the front or have their partner turn at that point to make it easier.

You can make this quite tight without significant risk, but do not place tight bands around both the chest and the waist at the same time. Your partner needs one of the two to breathe! If you tightly constrict them both, you increase the risk of asphyxia. See the discussion on p. 49 of the *Reducing Risk* chapter for more.

TheDuchy.com/bikini-harness/

For this tutorial, I used one 30 foot piece of ¼-inch rope. Remember, the amount of rope you need will vary depending on the build of your partner and other factors. It is easy to extend your rope (p. 274) if you need more!

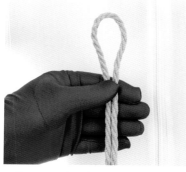

**1.** Start with a long rope, folded in half.

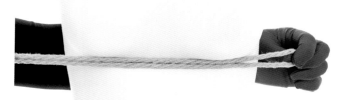

**2.** Run the rope around your partner's body. The rope should run across the lower part of your partner's sternum, just under the breasts if your partner has breasts.

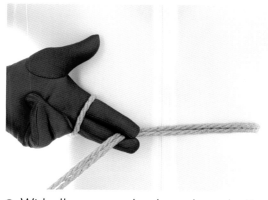

**3.** With all wraps you lay down, keep the lines flat to your partner's skin with no twists. Bring the tail to the back. Reach through the bight and hook the tail.

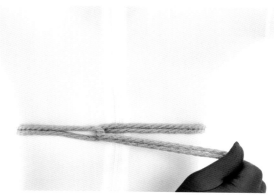

**4.** Pull the tail though and reverse tension.

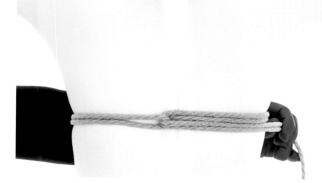

**5.** Wrap the rope around across the lower chest a second time. Place this new wrap below the first.

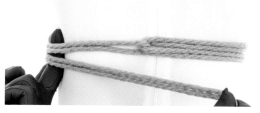

**6.** As you lay down the new wrap, remember to keep it flat, with no twists. Also, keep it parallel to and touching the first wrap, and confirm it has the same tension.                    *continues...*

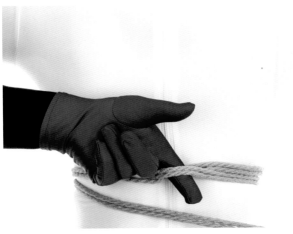

**7.** Run your finger down through the new bight you just formed...

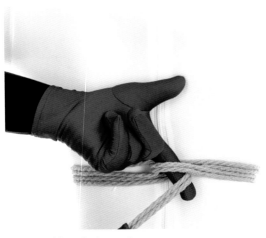

**8.** ...and hook the tail.

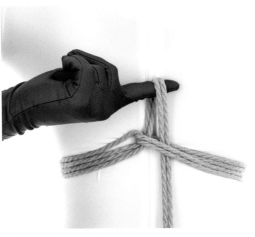

**9.** Pull it up, and...

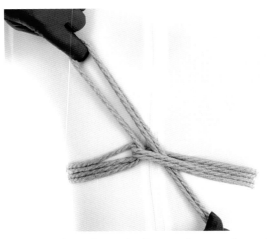

**10.** ...guide it through. Remember to place the part of the rope that is moving in the larger hole so it is moving through the path of least resistance, not rubbing against the bight (p. 158).

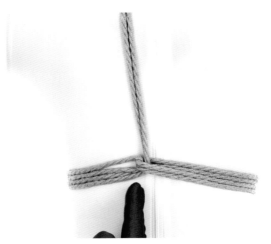

**11.** You want the node to be close to the center, but not directly on the spine. This is just a little to the left of where it should be.

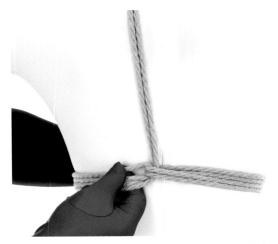

**12.** If you need to move the node, grab all the strands in the front and the back and then slide them around as needed.

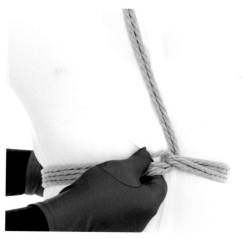

**13.** Like this.

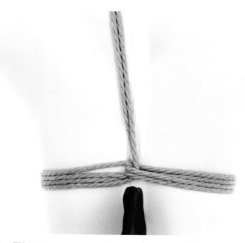

**14.** This is now positioned correctly.

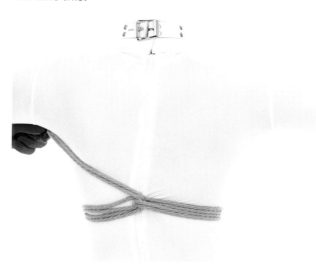

**15.** Reverse tension and begin going around the body the opposite way.

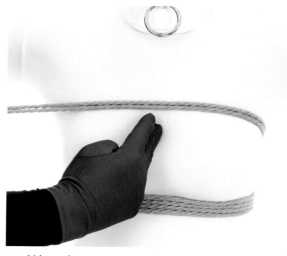

**16.** Wrap the rope around your partner again, this time over the mid-chest, above the breasts if your partner has breasts.

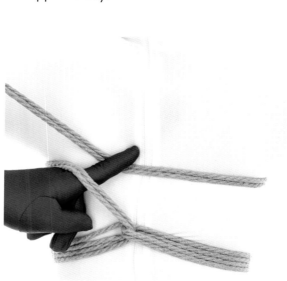

**17.** Run your finger under the stem and hook the tail.

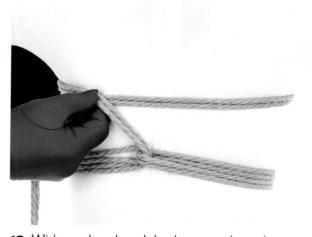

**18.** With one hand, grab both ropes where they cross. With the other hand, grab that band in the front.

*continues...*

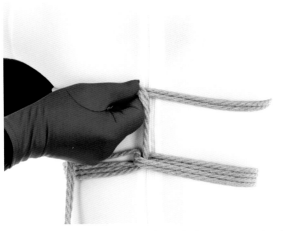

**19.** Slide the band around until the stem — the line that connects the two bands — is vertical.

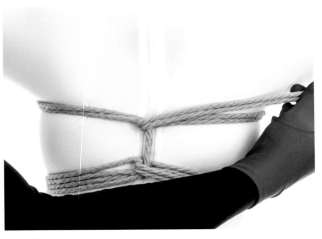

**20.** Reverse tension.

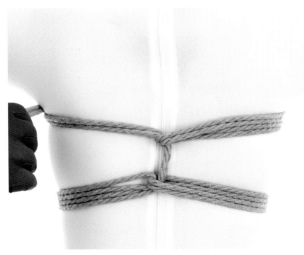

**21.** Wrap the rope around your partner's upper chest again. For this tie, this second wrap can be above or below the first wrap.

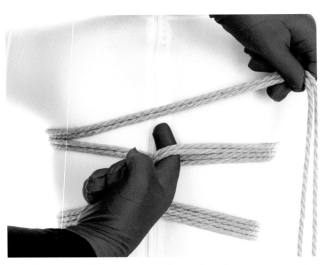

**22.** Run your fingers through the last bight you made.

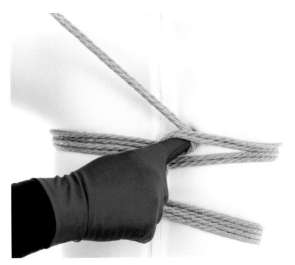

**23.** Hook the tail.

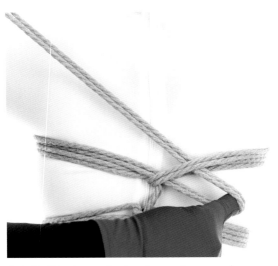

**24.** Pull it through. Again, make sure the rope is traveling through the path of least resistance.

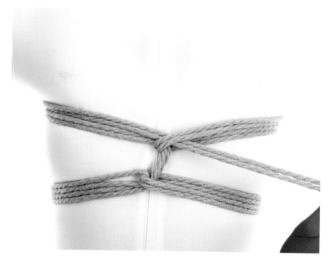

**25.** Pull it through, then...

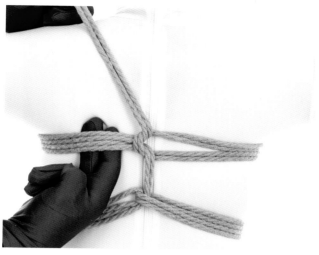

**26.** ...reverse the tension. Test the upper band. Make sure the lines are parallel and have even tension.

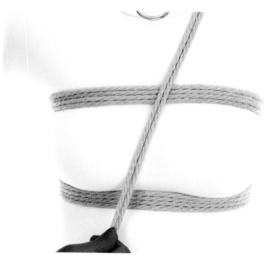

**27.** Run the tail over your partner's shoulder to the front. Lay the tail on top of both bands. There are *many* ways you can do the front. Here is one.

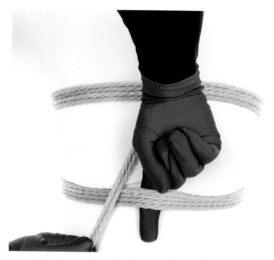

**28.** Reach under the lower band from above, on the same side of the tail as the shoulder you just came over from.

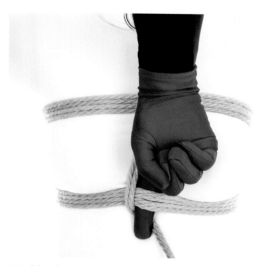

**29.** Hook the tail.

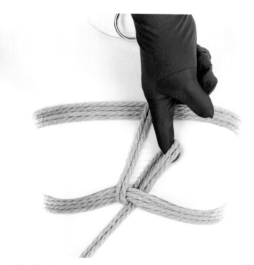

**30.** Pull the tail up and through.     *continues...*

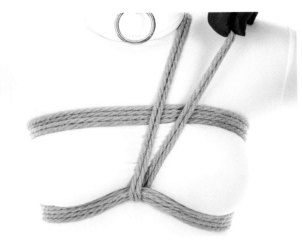

**31.** Like this.

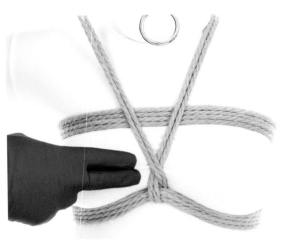

**32.** Now move the tail to the other shoulder. In doing so, you will create this twist.

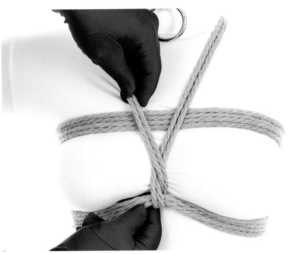

**33.** You can adjust the tightness by pulling up on the tail. If you do so, hold the strands of the lower band so they do not twist.

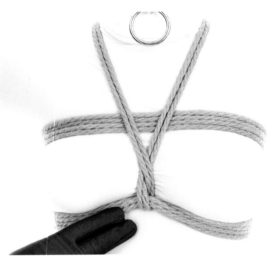

**34.** You want them to remain parallel and orderly. If you tighten this a lot, they may bunch up a little, though this is not usually an issue.

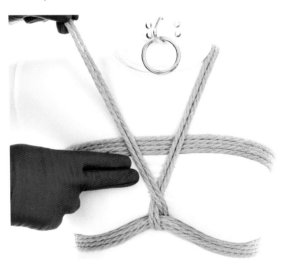

**35.** Here you can choose to run the tail over or under the upper chest band.

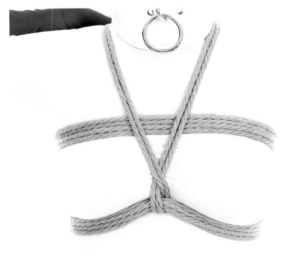

**36.** Bring the tail over the opposite shoulder, making sure the tension on both shoulders is the same.

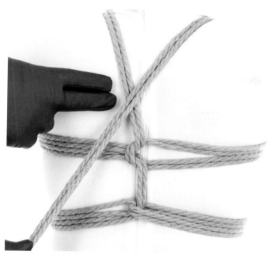

**37.** On the back, weave the tail around the upper node before locking it off. To do this, lay the tail on top of the opposite shoulder band...

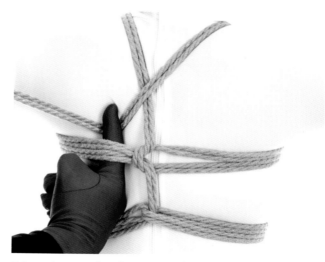

**38.** ...then under the upper chest band.

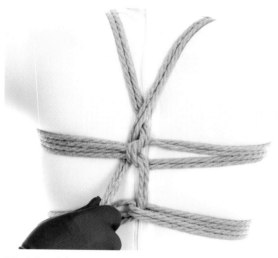

**39.** Like this.

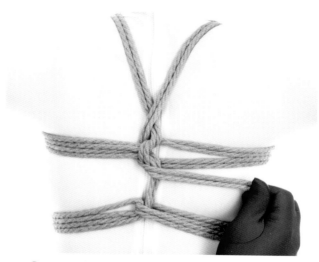

**40.** On top of the stem...

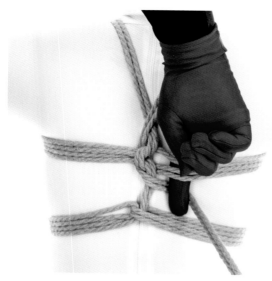

**41.** ...and under the upper chest band.

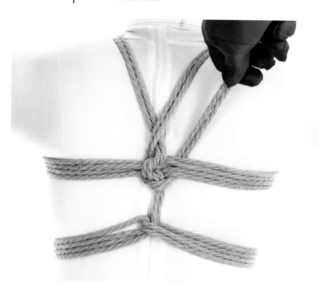

**42.** Like this.

*continues...*

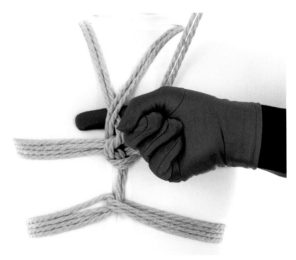

**43.** Now lock it off however you wish. Here I will do so using a **Half Hitch** around the stem.

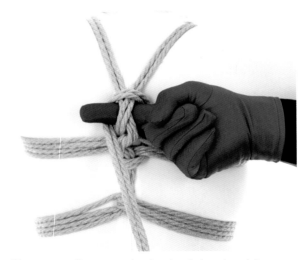

**44.** Place your finger under both of the shoulder bands, then lay the tail on top of them and hook it around your finger.

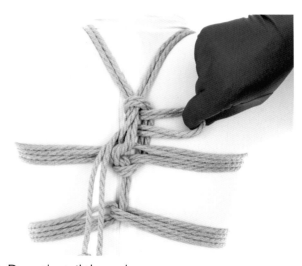

**45.** Draw the tail through.

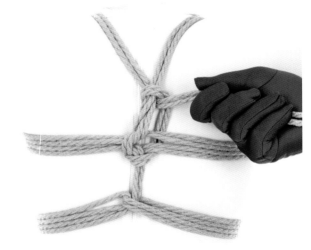

**46.** Hold the tail, then...

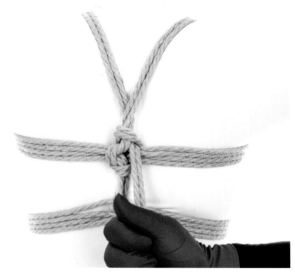

**47.** ...pull down to lock the **Half Hitch**.

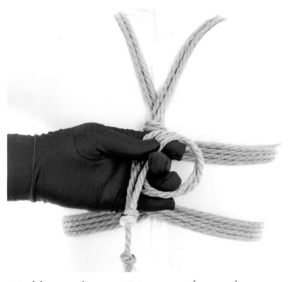

**48.** Use up the remaining rope (p. 279).

# Variations for the Front

There are many ways to do the front. They all result in different appearance and qualities. Here are a few ideas.

### Alternative 1 – Expand the Twist on Chest Strap

For this alternative, place a twist around both bands instead of just the lower band.

This creates a nice straight vertical line in the center of the chest that can make a nice handle. It can also be cinched quite tightly if you like. This can add some fun breast bondage if your partner has breasts... or can give the illusion of breasts to your partner if they do not!

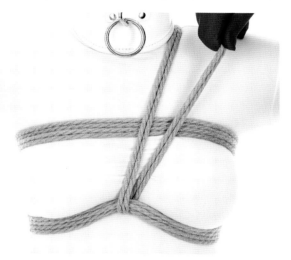

**1.** Starting with Step 31 (p. 338)...

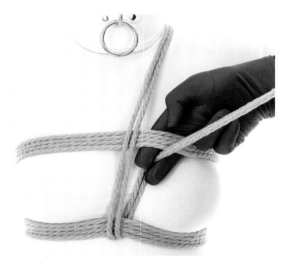

**2.** ...stay on the same side for a moment and run the tail under the upper band, too.

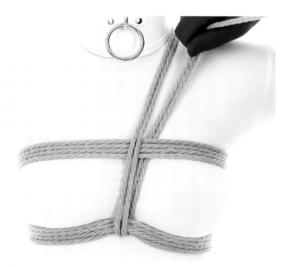

**3.** Like this.

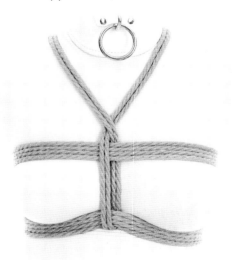

**4.** Then bring it to the other shoulder.

## Alternative 2 – Add Extra Twists on Stem

For this alternative, add extra twists as you move up the center band.
This will also add support for the upper chest band.

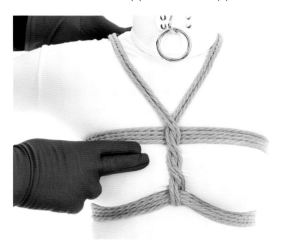

**1.** Option 1: You can simply add more than one twist if you like.

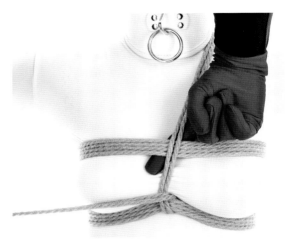

**2.** Option 2: While adding the twist, you can run the rope behind the upper band...

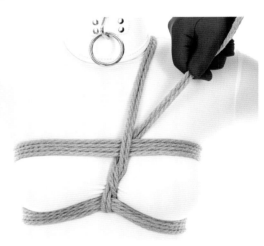

**3.** ...like this.

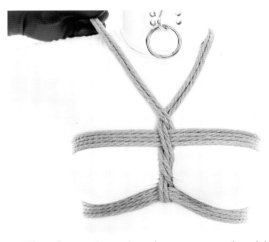

**4.** Then bring the tail to the opposite shoulder.

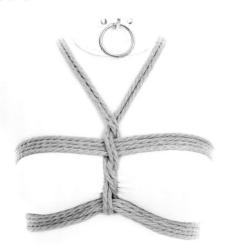

**5.** This adds support to the upper band, so it does not easily migrate up or down.

## Alternative 3 – Add a Cow Hitch

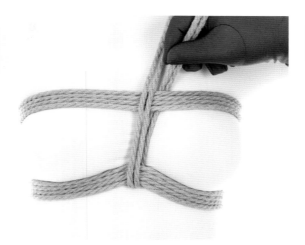

**1.** Bring the tail up on the same side and under the upper chest band.

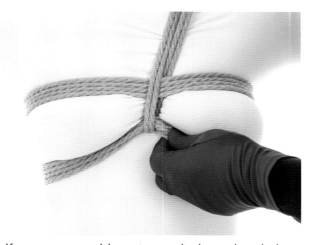

**2.** If you want to add tension to the lower band, do so now.

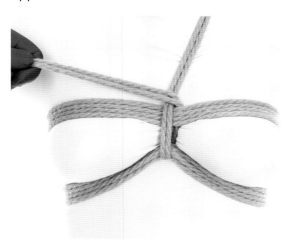

**3.** Lay the tail on top of the shoulder band.

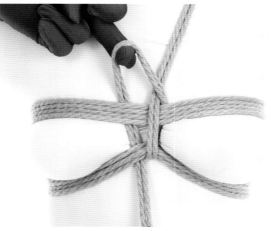

**4.** Run the tail under both chest bands on the opposite side. Do not pull it all the way through. Protect a little loop with your fingers.

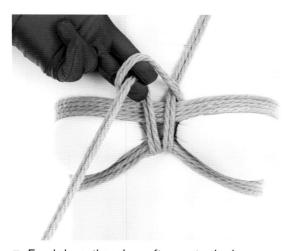

**5.** Feed the tail to those fingers in the loop.

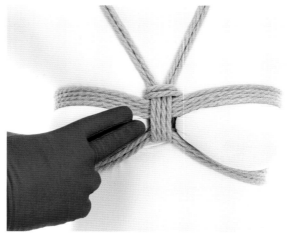

**6.** Pull through and tighten, then take the tail to the back and complete the tie.

# Bikini Harness

**A View of Bikini Harness Alternative 3 From Various Angles**

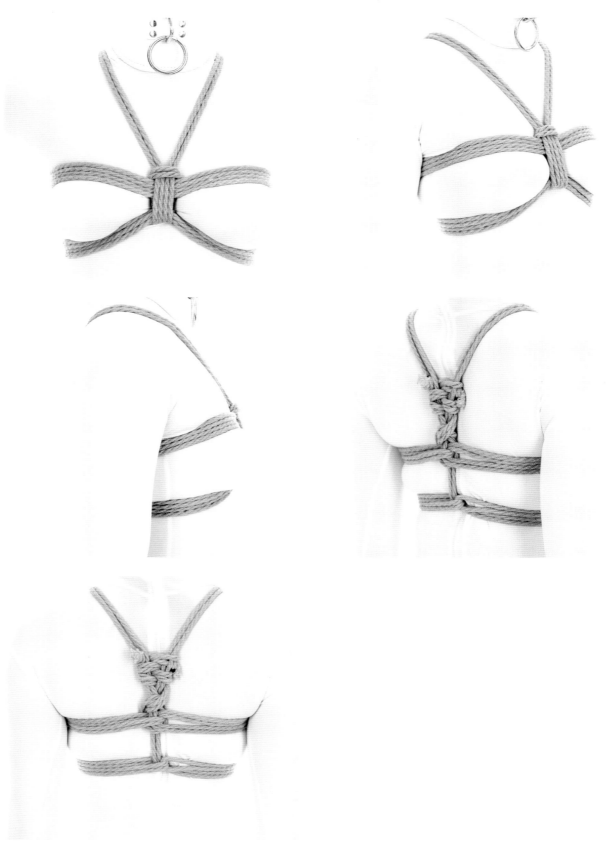

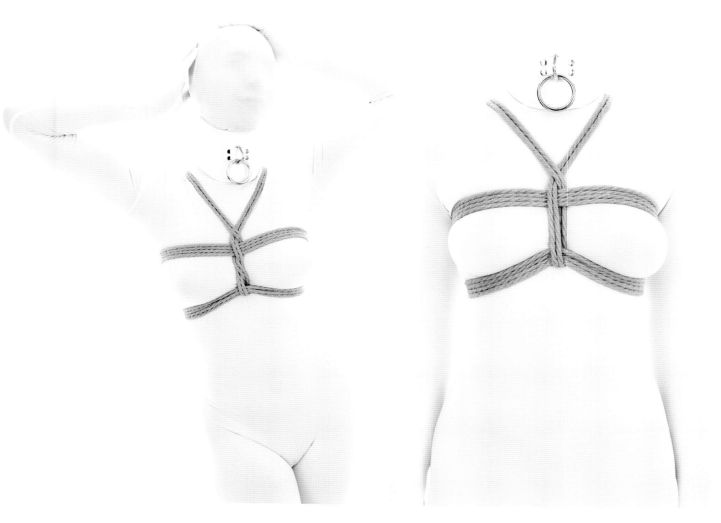

# Shinju

This classic chest harness is known and practiced by riggers throughout the world. It is simple, secure, and can be used for suspension when applied properly. But suspension is its own topic; there are many important things to know before you try it, things that we will not cover in this book.

This tie can also be used for breast bondage, by making the upper and lower bands very tight to the chest, then using the line that goes between the breasts to cinch the upper and lower chest bands together, thereby trapping and accentuating the breasts, as seen on the previous example.

Also: Surprise! When you learned the **Bikini Harness** (p. 332), you were also learning the **Shinju**!

The primary difference between the two is that with the **Shinju**, you lock off each band with a **Half Hitch** and you specifically choose a front option that holds the bands apart, like the *Front Alternative 2* (p. 342) shown in the **Bikini Harness** tutorial.

Locking off the bands improves their stability, making them more

TheDuchy.com/shinju/

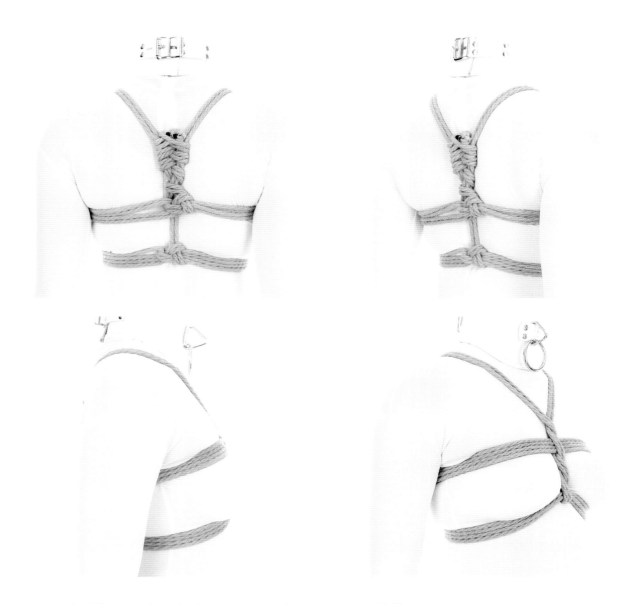

trustworthy. That is, when the band is put under tension, the **Half Hitch** helps keep all the stands together, so they work as a team and distribute the force over the wider area of all four strands. It helps prevent individual strands from tightening or loosening and thus putting pressure on a smaller area. This is not typically a big concern for floor bondage, but it can become one if you are planning to connect other elements to the chest harness, thereby putting the ropes under external tension.

Also, choosing a front that keeps the two separate bands from collapsing into one serves a similar function. This helps prevent the bands from migrating together, keeping them as two bands, thereby helping distribute force across a larger area. This also helps protect anyone that may have flesh or breasts between those two bands so that they do not get pinched too much.

Generally, if the harness will be on its own, the **Bikini Harness** is fine. But if you plan to tie other things to the bands of the harness, take the extra few moments to tie it as a **Shinju**.

This tutorial used one 30-foot piece of ¼-inch rope.

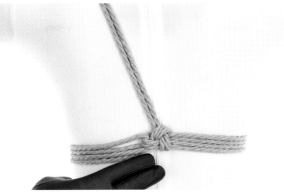

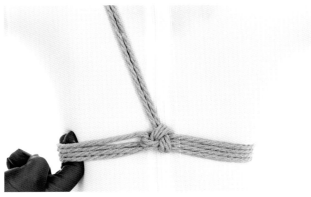

**1.** Tie a **Lark's Head Single Column** (p. 181) around the middle of your partner's chest with the tail leading upward. I chose to lock off the strap with a **Half Hitch** on the forward tension side, but that is only a personal preference.

**2.** Ensure you can fit a finger or two under the band so it is not too tight.

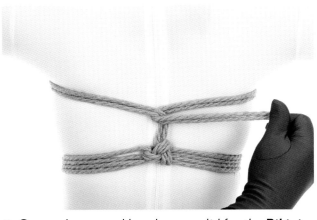

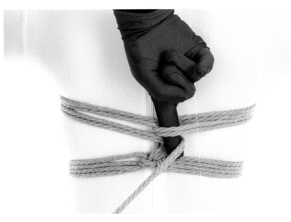

**3.** Create the second band as you did for the **Bikini Harness**. Place the second wrap *below* the first wrap so the tail will naturally flow upward once locked.

**4.** Reach through the new bight and hook the tail.

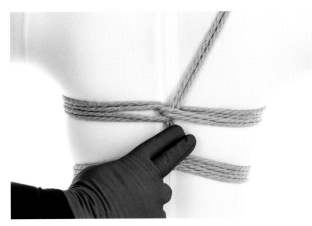

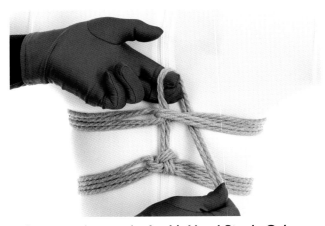

**5.** Pull the tail through.

**6.** Just as with a regular **Lark's Head Single Column**, run the tail behind the band, protecting a loop of the tail with your fingers, then... *continues...*

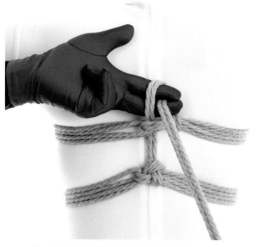

**7.** ...feed the tail to those fingers in the loop.

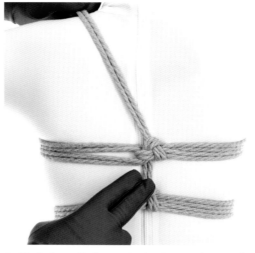

**8.** Pull the tail through the loop, then tighten.

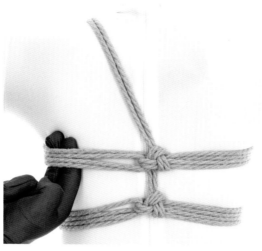

**9.** Again, this band should be quite tight, but you should still be able to slip two fingers under it.

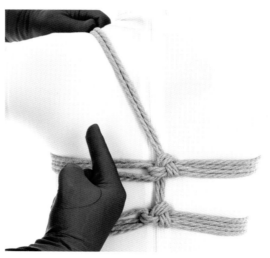

**10.** The tail is naturally flowing in this direction, so run it over that shoulder.

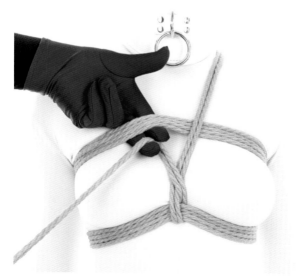

**11.** Complete the V in the front, then either run the tail under the upper chest band...

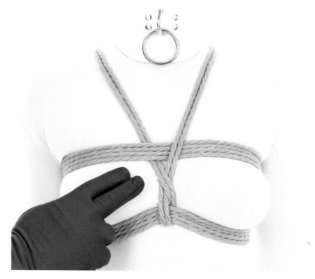

**12.** ...thereby creating a little shelf for the upper band to sit on if it tries to migrate downward, or...

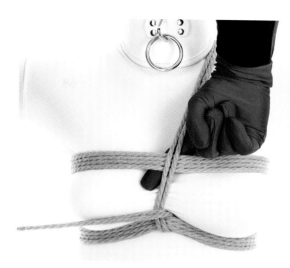

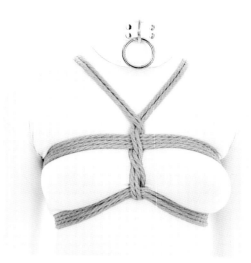

**13.** ...take another approach that will keep the bands apart. One option being Alternative 2 shown for the **Bikini Harness** (p. 342).

**14.** Complete the tie as shown in the **Bikini Harness** tutorial. Completed from the front.

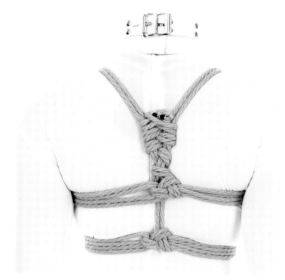

**15.** Completed from the back.

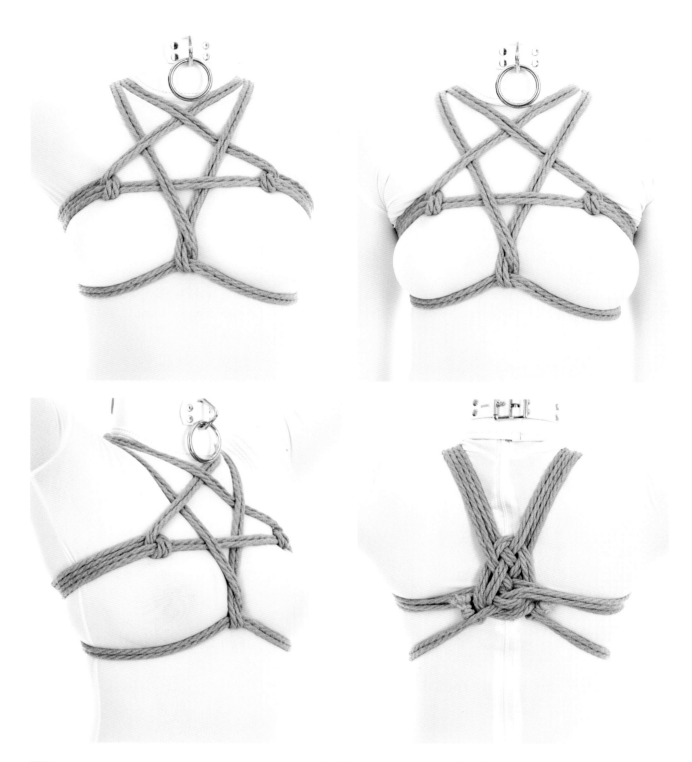

# Pentagram/Star Harness

This attractive harness can serve as a great anchor for other layers of bondage.
If you like religious- or occult-themed scenes, this can be a fun binding for your
favorite witch!

TheDuchy.com/pentagram-harness/

This tutorial used one 30-foot piece of ¼-inch rope.

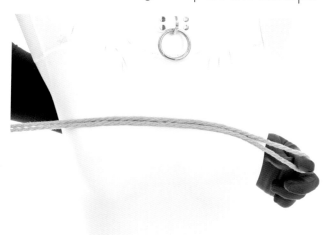

**1.** Start with a long rope folded in half. Run the rope across the upper chest.

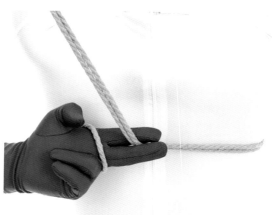

**2.** Bring the bight to the back. Reach through the bight and grab the tail.

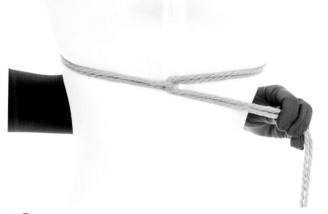

**3.** Reverse tension.

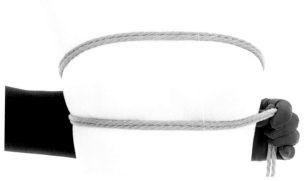

**4.** Run the tail across the lower chest, just below the breasts, if your partner has breasts.

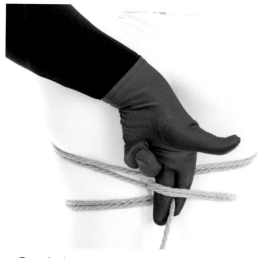

**5.** Reach through the secondary bight, the one you made in Step 3. Hook the tail and pull it though.

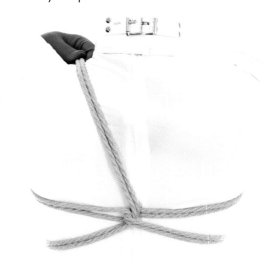

**6.** Run the tail up over the shoulder.     *continues...*

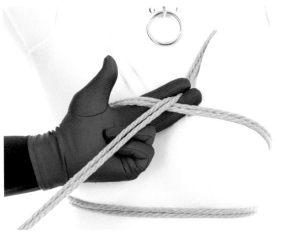

**7.** Reach under the upper chest band and hook the tail.

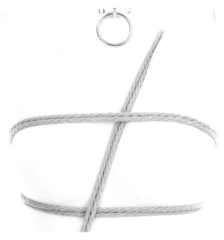

**8.** Run the tail down the middle of the chest, laying it on top of the lower chest band.

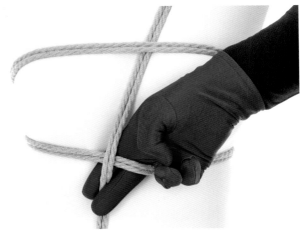

**9.** Place your finger under the chest band on the same side the rope came from. Hook the tail.

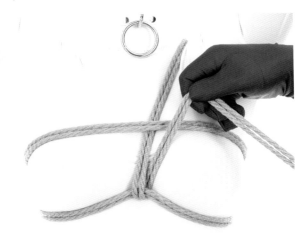

**10.** Pull the rope up and through. If you wish, you can pull the chest band upward a little to raise and support the breasts.

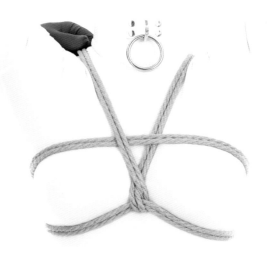

**11.** Now bring the tail to the other side, forming a nice decorative twist on the lower chest band. Once you get the hang of it, you can do Steps 9-11 in a single deft move for style points.

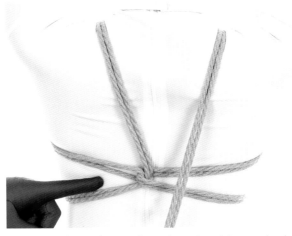

**12.** Bring the tail over the other shoulder to the back. You want to route the tail to this location, so...

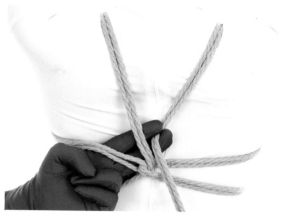

**13.** ...place your fingers under both bands on the other side like this and hook the tail.

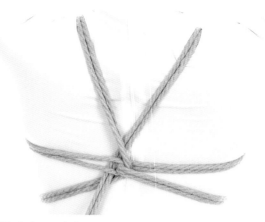

**14.** Pull the tail through.

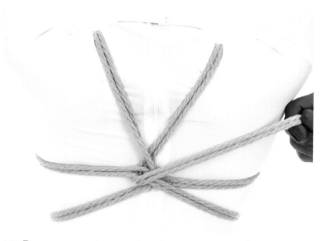

**15.** Reverse tension again, this time toward the armpit on the other side.

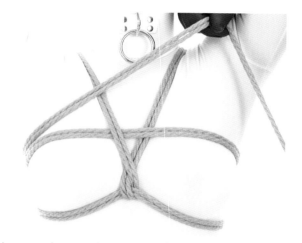

**16.** Now you have a choice to make. You can either run the tail directly to the shoulder on the opposite side like this, or...

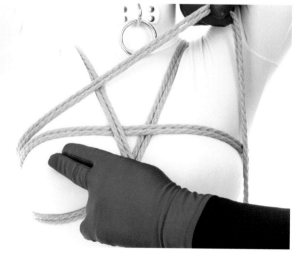

**17.** ...(optional) you can add a **Half Hitch** here first. The benefits of doing this are that it helps keep the rope from riding into the armpit and it makes the pentagram/star pattern more regular.

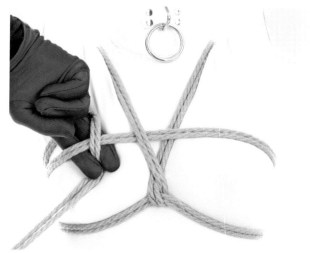

**18.** To do this, place your finger on top of the tail and under the upper chest band. Lay the tail on top of the upper chest band, then hook the tail.

*continues...*

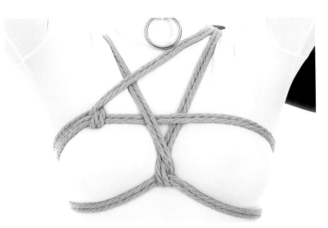

**19.** Pull the tail through, then lay the tail on top of the shoulder band (shoulder band on the left in this picture) and bring it to the opposite shoulder.

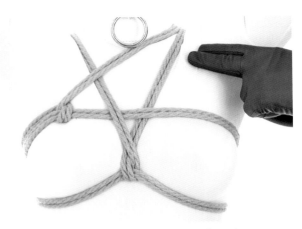

**20.** Place the tail close to the neck so that the two sets of lines lay next to each other and not on top of each other. This avoids creating a pressure point, spreading the pressure across a greater area and making it more comfortable.

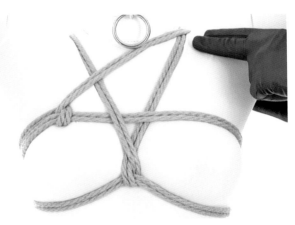

**21.** Another option: For a sharper point to the star, lay the line on top of the shoulder band. This looks cool, but comes with the trade-off of possibly creating a pressure point.

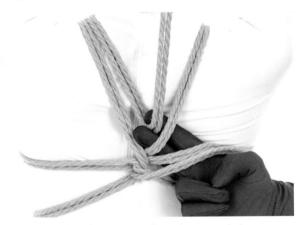

**22.** Reach under the upper chest lines and the shoulder line on the other side to hook the tail.

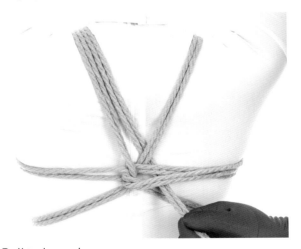

**23.** Pull it through.

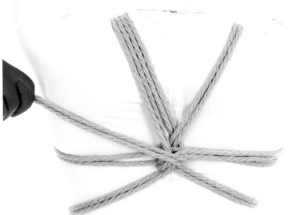

**24.** Reverse tension again, running the tail toward the armpit on the other side.

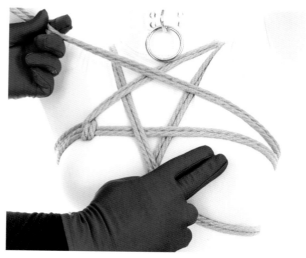

**25.** Again, you have the choice of adding a **Half Hitch** here or not.

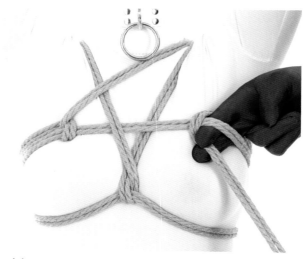

**26.** Mirror whatever you did on the other side.

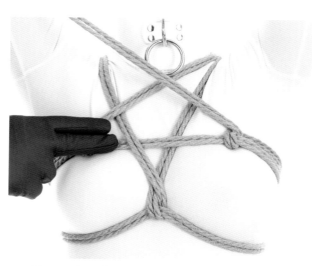

**27.** Notice that the way we have been laying the lines so far has naturally resulted in a woven pattern.

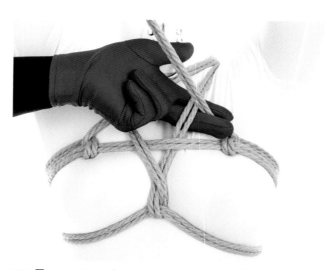

**28.** To continue the pattern, run the tail under the first shoulder band...

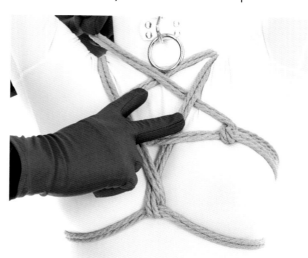

**29.** ...and then lay it on top of the second.

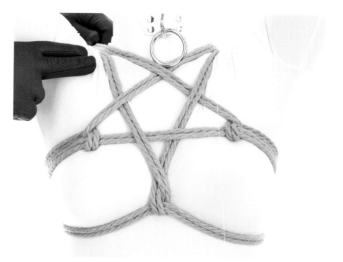

**30.** Run the tail over the shoulder, mirroring the choice you made on the other side. *continues...*

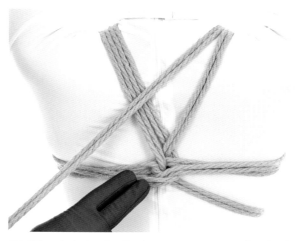

**31.** The tie is basically done, we just need to lock it off and use up any remaining rope here on the back. One way to do this is to weave the tail into all these lines to use up what remains.

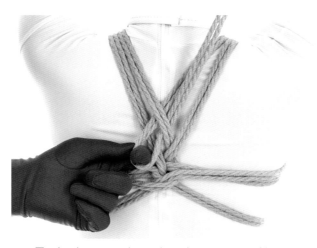

**32.** To do this, run the tail under one set of lines...

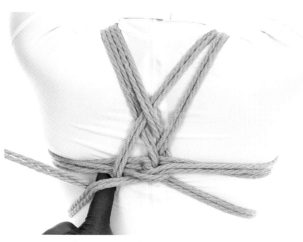

**33.** ...over the next and under the next...

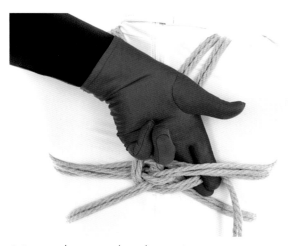

**34.** ...and over and under again.

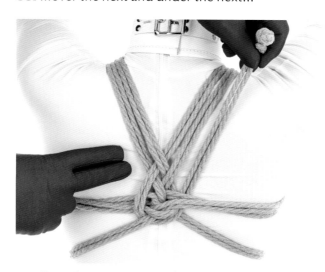

**35.** If you have more rope than this, you could use up the rope using a Figure-8 pattern around the shoulder bands (p. 293).

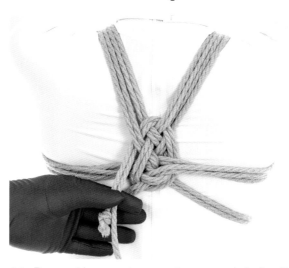

**36.** But, as I have only a small amount left, I will just continue weaving.

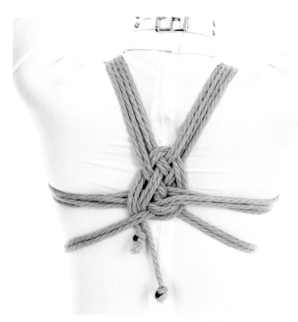

**37.** At this point I am out of rope. The ends are uneven, but this is not a problem!

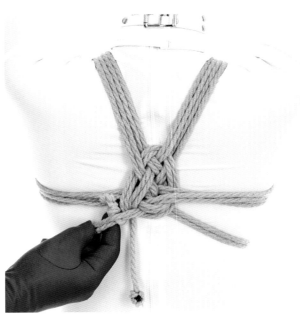

**38.** You can lock off the shorter end on one side...

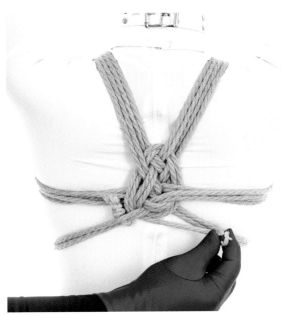

**39.** ...and continue weaving the other end until it is done, then...

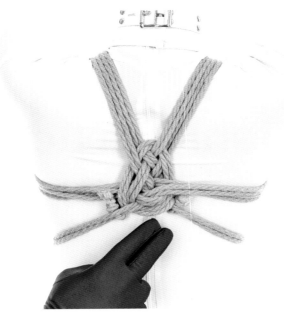

**40.** ...lock it off as well!

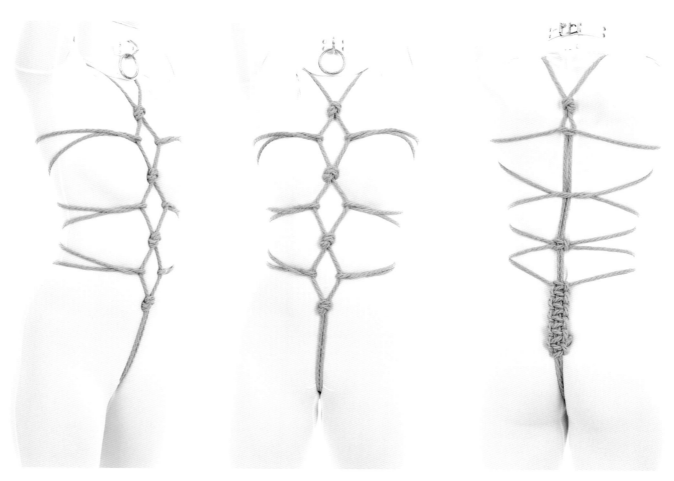

# Hishi Karada

The diamond pattern and tight lacing of the **Hishi Karada** (Diamond Body) is lovely and stimulating. It can be worn safely for quite a long period (note the caution below). It can also be worn under clothes for a bit of surreptitious bondage when out in public and when you take it off, you can enjoy the beautiful rope marks for a little while. You can also add an optional "happy knot" as shown in the **Crotch Rope** tutorial (p. 370) as a cool extra feature.

Caution: If laced too tightly, this tie can restrain both chest and waist at the same time. Because of how this tie is structured, it rarely causes any issue, but it is important to be sure that your partner does not have any trouble breathing. Review the discussion on asphyxia (p. 58) for important information about tight bands around the chest when combined with tight bands around the waist.

TheDuchy.com/hishi-karada/

For this tie, I used one 30-foot piece of ¼-inch rope, but the amount you will need will vary depending on the build of your partner and other factors. Remember, you can *Extend Your Rope* using technique 3 (p. 278) if you need more!

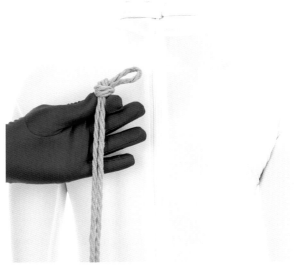

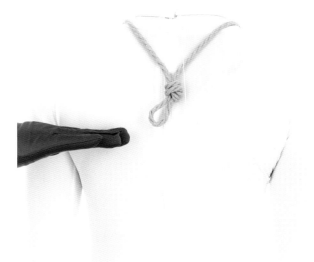

**1.** Start with a long rope folded in half. Put an **Overhand Knot** (p. 124) just a little below the bight so that you have a small (1-inch) loop at the end as shown here. This adds a little bit more stability to the tie later on.

**2.** Place the bight between your partner's shoulder blades. Position it so that the loop is at the level of the armpits. Run the tails over each shoulder.

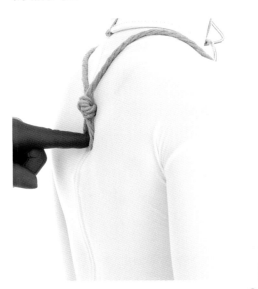

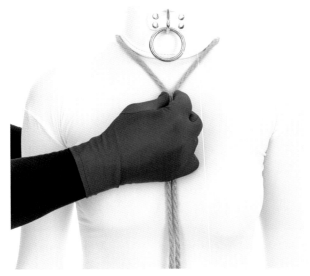

**3.** In a moment, you are going to put an **Overhand Knot** on the upper chest. Be sure to properly position the loop in the back before you decide where to place the knot in the front.

**4.** Continuing to hold the bight in the correct position (Step 3), grab the rope just below the clavicle. This is where you will make the first **Overhand Knot**. *continues...*

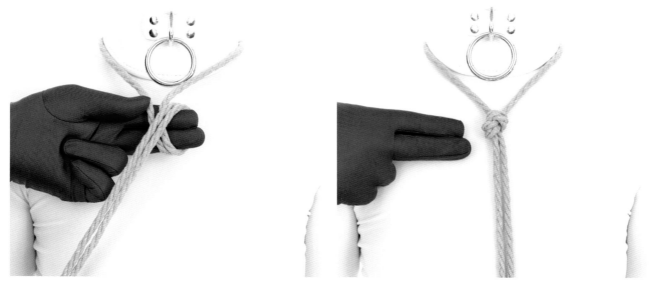

**5.** Add an **Overhand Knot**. See *Tying Overhand Knots Consistently When Rigging* (p. 129) for a technique that will help you make them all look the same.

**6.** Tighten the **Overhand Knot**. Note: You can also choose a different knot for a different look. Some people use **Cow Hitches**, some **Double Coin Knots**\*, for example. These add decorative flair, but take longer to tie.

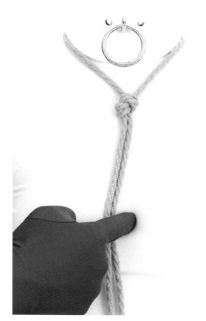

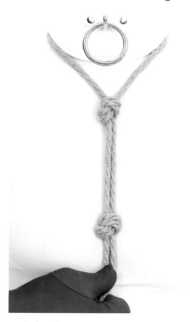

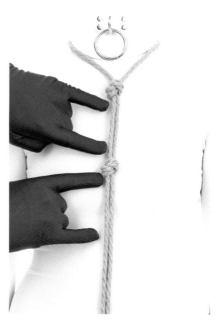

**7.** Again, make sure that the bight on the back is in the correct position. The second **Overhand Knot** should go directly on top of the middle of the sternum, between the breasts, if your partner has breasts.

**8.** Like this.

**9.** Now that you have the second knot, you can see the space between them.

\*If you are interested in the **Double Coin Knot**, it is not taught in this book but can be found on TheDuchy.com/double-coin-knot/.

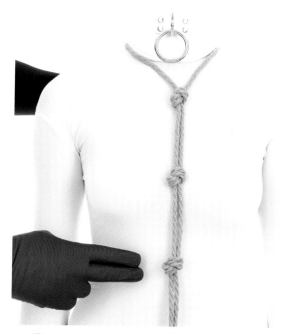

**10.** To have diamonds be the same size, all the knots need to be the same distance from each other, so place the third knot at that same distance.

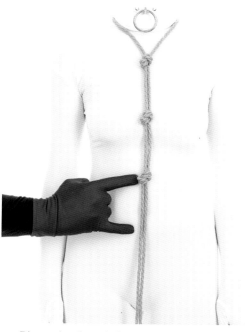

**11.** Place the fourth knot equidistant from the third.

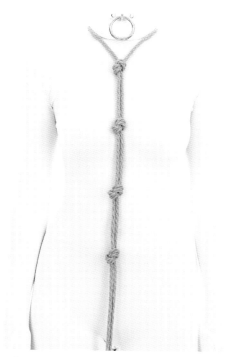

**12.** Four knots are usually enough, but you might need a fifth if your partner is tall or has a long torso.

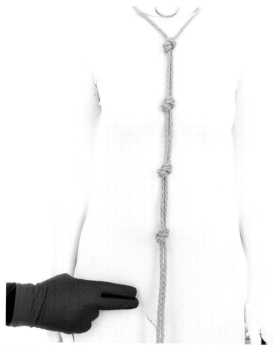

**13.** Optionally, you can add a happy knot. This is an **Overhand Knot** positioned so that it places pressure on your partner's clit or perineum, so it teases them as they move around. See the **Crotch Rope** tutorial (p. 370) for more.  *continues...*

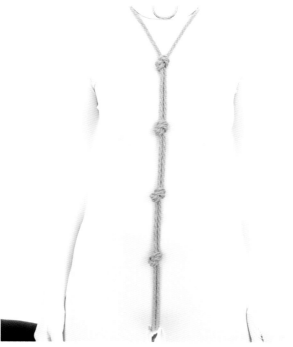

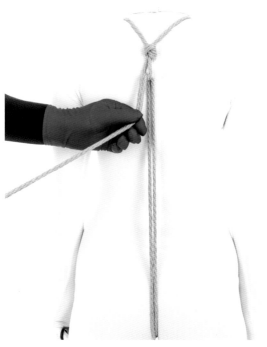

**14.** Run the tail between the legs to the back. Note: If you are going to run rope so that it touches someone's sexual organs or anus, that rope must now be reserved just for them; it is almost impossible to fully sanitize a rope. Alternatively, use barrier methods to protect your rope: Wrap plastic wrap around those parts of the rope that will make such contact.

**15.** Run the tail up your partner's back and through that small loop you formed in Step 2.

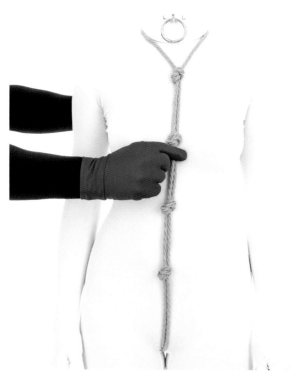

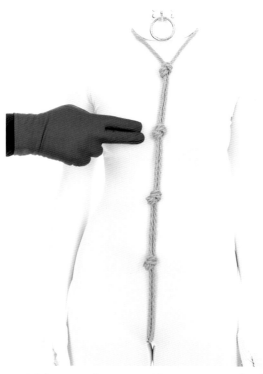

**16.** Before continuing, adjust and straighten the position of the rope.

**17.** Make sure this second knot is properly placed over the sternum.

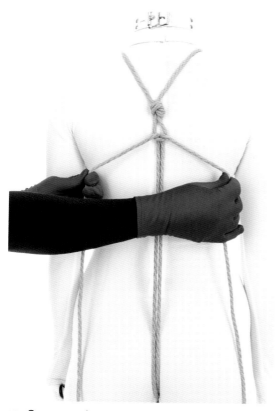

**18.** Separate the strands of the tail.

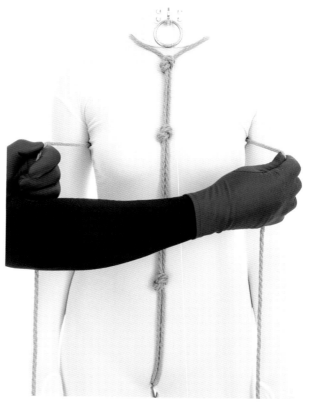

**19.** Bring them to the front.

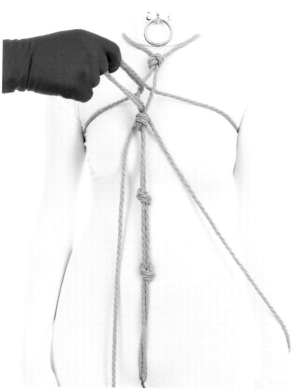

**20.** Run them through their respective sides of the upper diamond.

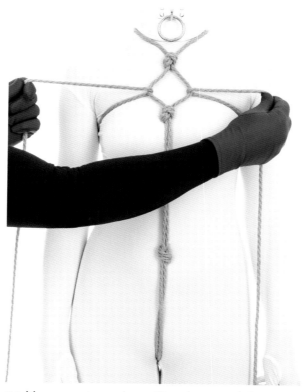

**21.** You are going to be pulling the strands back the way they came to separate the strands of the center line and thereby create this attractive diamond shape.

*continues...*

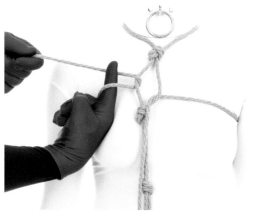

**22.** (Optional) You can add a little twist. This adds additional friction and a decorative flair. To do this, run your fingers underneath the incoming strand, hook the outgoing strand and pull through.

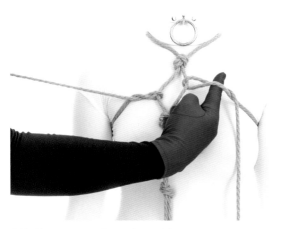

**23.** Repeat on the other side.
You can do this on both sides at the same time.

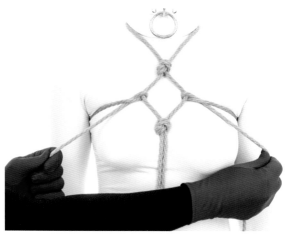

**24.** When done, your upper diamond should look like this.

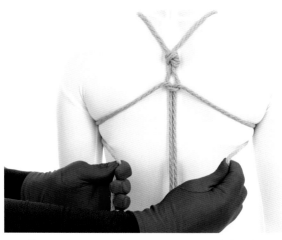

**25.** Bring the strands to your partner's back.

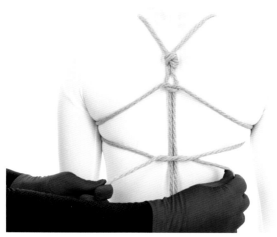

**26.** Cross them. Optionally, you can add a twist here. I almost always do because it adds a little friction and stability to the tie. Another great option is the **Cored Square Knot** (p. 288).

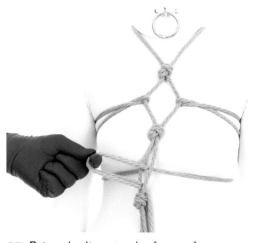

**27.** Bring the lines to the front of your partner and through the second diamond.

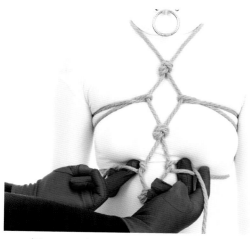

**28.** (Optional) Add the decorative twist if you wish.

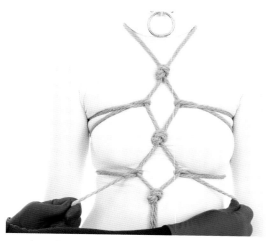

**29.** It will look like this.

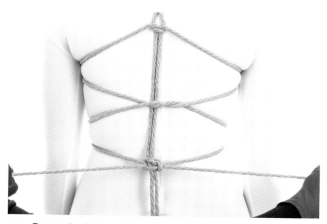

**30.** Bring the lines to your partner's back again and again cross them using any of the three choices we discussed. This time I will use the **Cored Square Knot** as it adds even more stability and control.

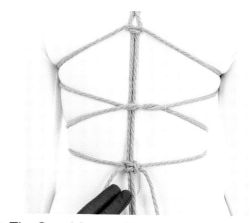

**31.** The **Cored Square Knot** locks your tails around the stem.

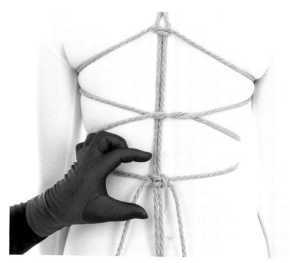

**32.** It has enough friction that you can then adjust the position of this knot in a range, and it will stay where you place it!

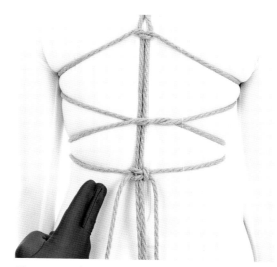

**33.** For example, I am going to slide this node up a little so that the rope lies in a nice consistent pattern on the front. *continues...*

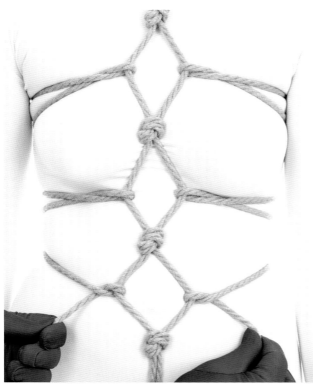

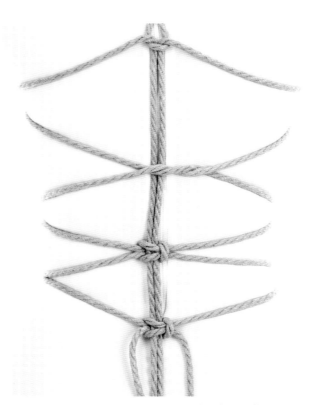

**34.** Repeat. Bring the tails to your partner's front and through the third diamond...

**35.** ...and again, to your partners back. I will again choose the **Cored Square Knot** because it has another cool feature! (See Step 37.)

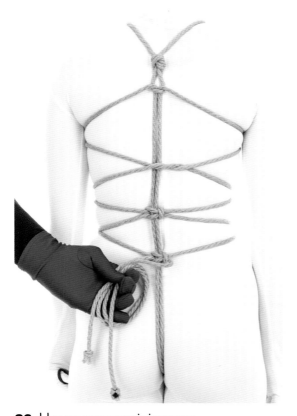

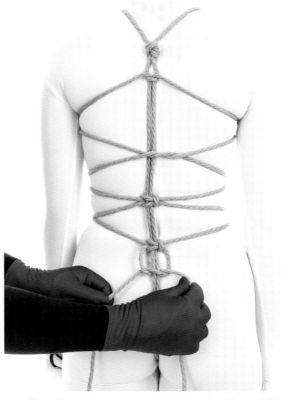

**36.** Use up any remaining rope.

**37.** One fun option is to continue the **Cored Square Knot**, repeating the pattern...

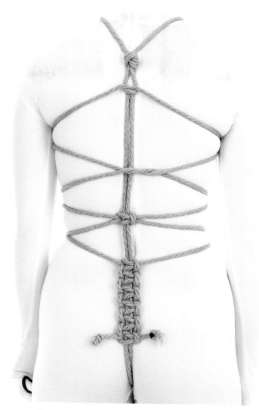

**38.** ...until you run out of rope!

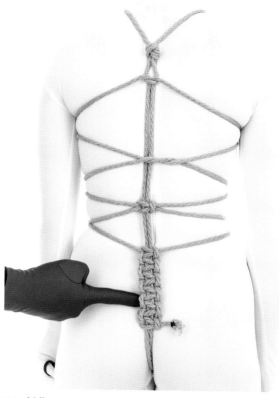

**39.** When you get to the end, just tuck the ends under.

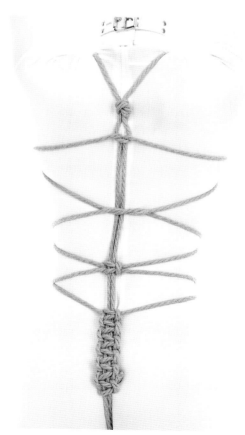

**40.** Completed from the back.

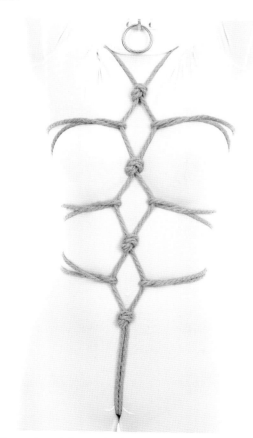

**41.** Completed from the front.

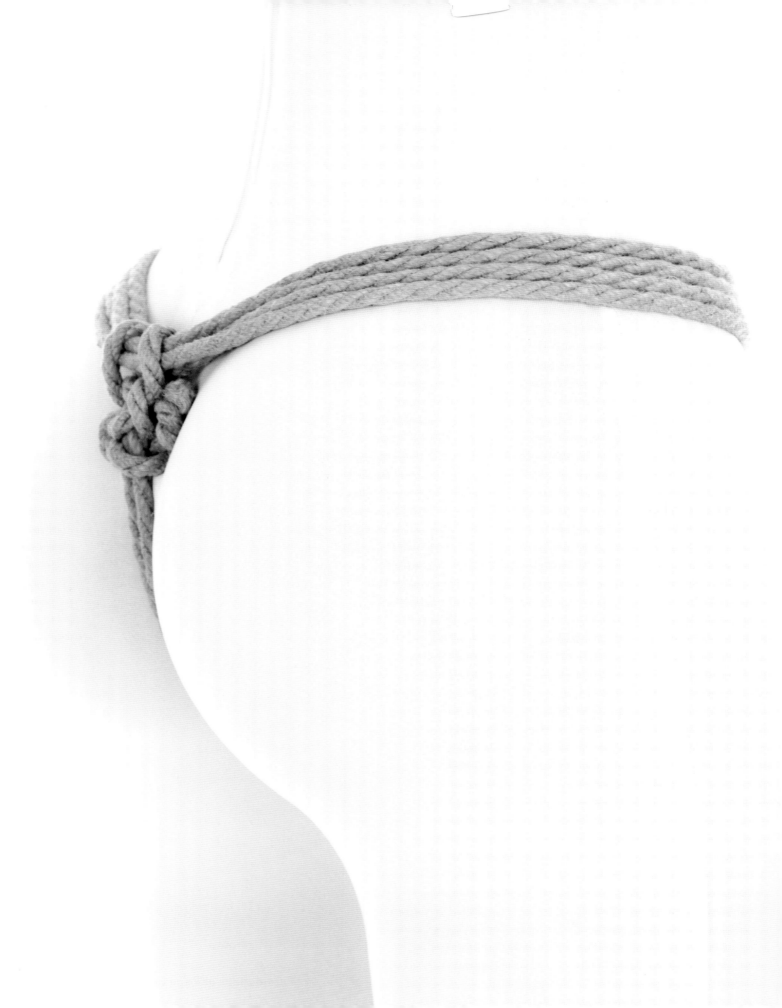

# 10

# Hip Harnesses

Hip harnesses are also wonderfully useful! Not only do they accentuate the hips and ass, but they can also provide an additional set of grips or anchor points that can be used to attach your partner to a chair, bed, post, or something to which you can connect other layers of bondage!

There are many wonderful hip and waist harnesses out there. We will cover two fun, simple options:

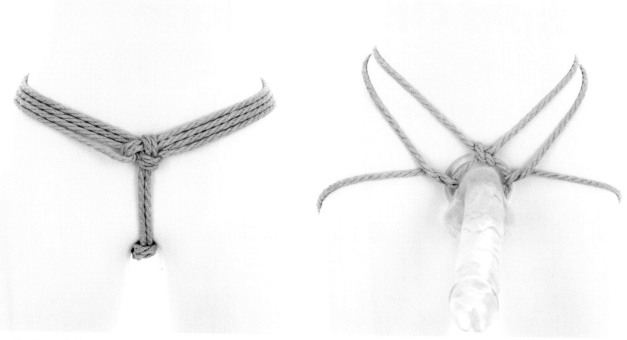

**Simple Crotch Rope, aka Unchastity Belt**

**Redmayne Strap-On**

For more, check out **TheDuchy.com/tutorials/** and select "Waist & Hips" from the **Categories** drop-down box.

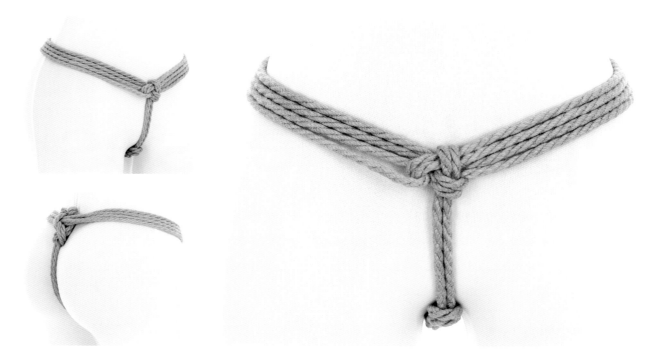

# Simple Crotch Rope

This simple hip harness is commonly known by the awful name "Crotch Rope." Ugh. This is really nothing more than a belt made from a **Lark's Head Single Column** and a clever use of the tail.

Optionally, you can add a fun little teasing feature called a "happy knot" if you like! A happy knot is a knot that puts pressure on the clit or the perineum (the area between the base of the penis and the anus). As the person moves, the knot moves on those sensitive areas. For some people, this teases them and can make them quite aroused. Think of it as an unchastity belt made from rope! This can be done on people with or without penises.

   You can also do a simple variation that will let you add a dildo to your partner like a strap-on.

**Important Safety Tip**
If you put this on the hips, it can be put on quite tightly and still pose little risk. But if you put this on a person's waist and also have a chest harness on them, it is important that at least one of them is not too tight. See asphyxia (p. 58).

**Important Health Tip**
This tie runs a rope directly between your partner's legs. If they are going to be naked and that rope is going to touch their sexual organs or anus, that rope is now theirs. It is virtually impossible to fully sterilize rope. If you do not want to dedicate a piece of rope to a person, ensure that rope fibers do not come in contact with bodily fluids by protecting them with a barrier method like plastic wrap around the rope where it goes between their legs or not having them naked.

TheDuchy.com/crotch-rope/

This tutorial used one 15-foot piece of ¼-inch rope.

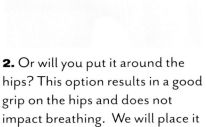

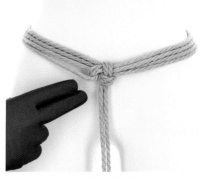

**1.** Choose: Will you put this around the soft waist?
If you do, you can optionally cinch it a bit tight and add some waist training to the session, but if you do so, make sure you do not also constrain the chest. Doing both at the same time can make it difficult to breathe.

**2.** Or will you put it around the hips? This option results in a good grip on the hips and does not impact breathing. We will place it around the hips in this example.

**3.** Start with a **Lark's Head Single Column** around the waist. Remember that for the **Lark's Head Single Column**, we wrap in the opposite direction that we want the tail to naturally run at the end, so do the second wrap above the first wrap.

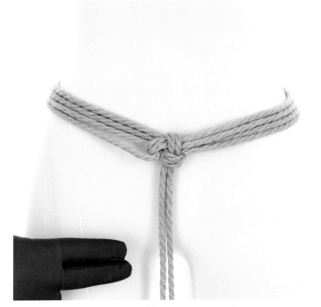

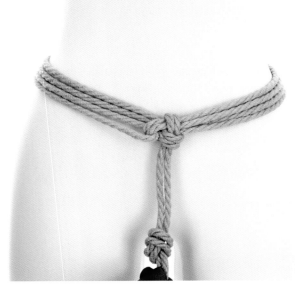

**4.** Bring the tail down. If your partner has a penis, run one strand on each side of the base, behind the balls.

**5.** (Optional) Add a happy knot — an **Overhand Knot** (p. 124) positioned so that it will press on something sensitive. Perhaps the clit, the perineum or on the anus. *continues…*

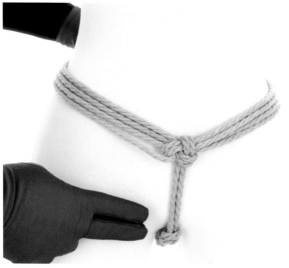

**6.** Confirm the placement of the happy knot and then bring the tail between the legs.

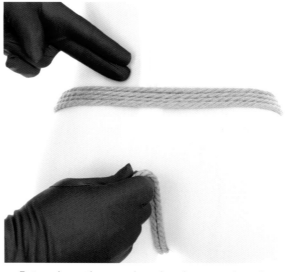

**7.** Bring the tail up and under the waist band.

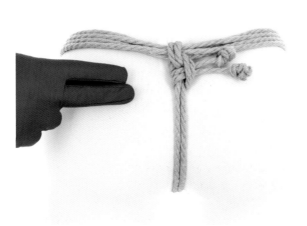

**8.** Lock off however you wish (p. 168). Here I have done so with two **Half Hitches**.

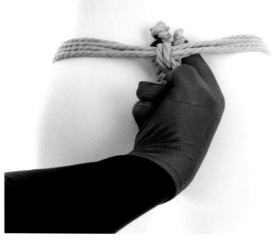

**9.** Use up any remaining rope (p. 279). Here, I have almost none, so I just tuck the ends under.

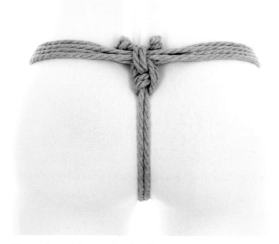

**10.** Completed from the back.

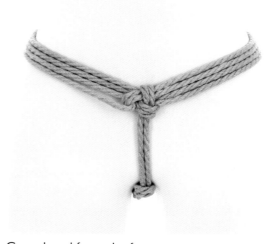

**11.** Completed from the front.

# Turn Into a Strap-On

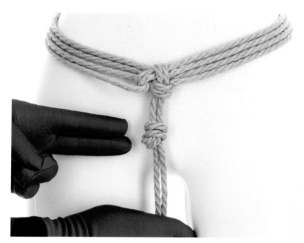

**1.** Add an **Overhand Knot** or **Square Knot** just above where you want the dildo to be.

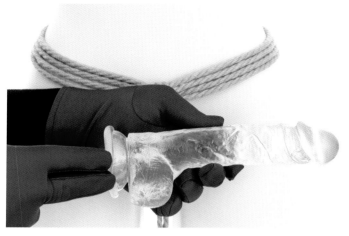

**2.** You will need a dildo with a base.

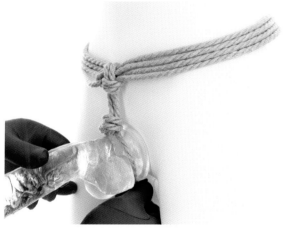

**3.** Place the dildo under the knot, between the strands. Make sure it is positioned were you want it. Adjust the knot, if needed.

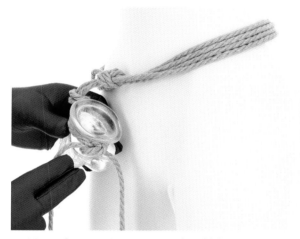

**4.** Use a **Square Knot** to tie the dildo into the band.

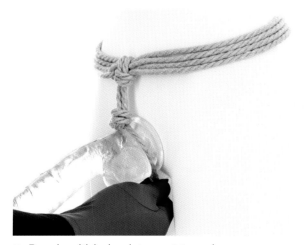

**5.** Put the dildo back in position, then...

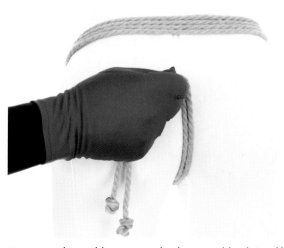

**6.** ...run the tail between the legs and lock it off to the waist band however you wish.

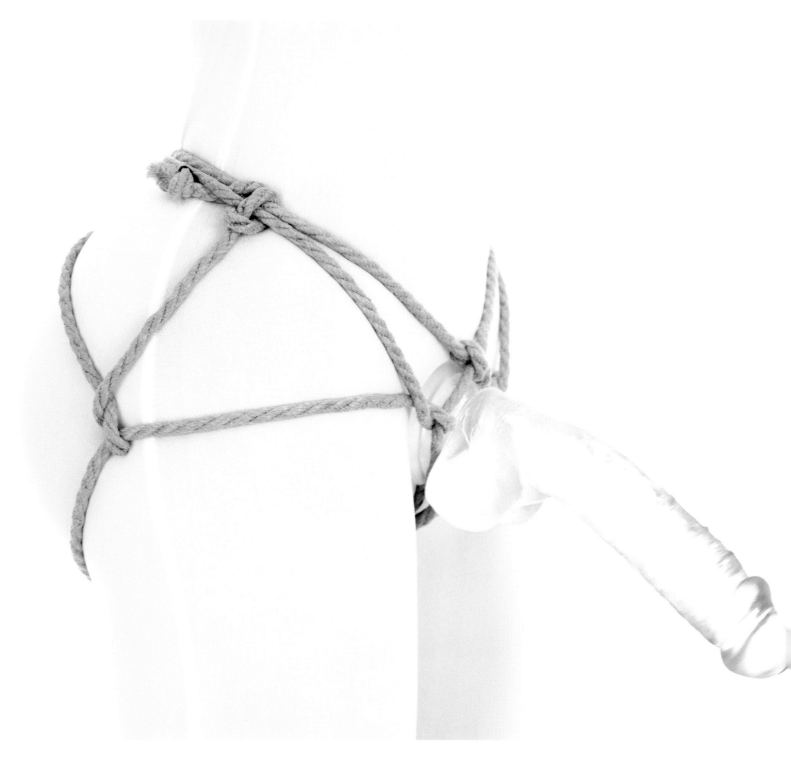

# Redmayne Strap-On

Here is one method for creating a custom-fitted strap-on harness with rope.
You will need a dildo with a base.

TheDuchy.com/redmayne-strap-on/

This tutorial used one 15-foot piece of ¼-inch rope.

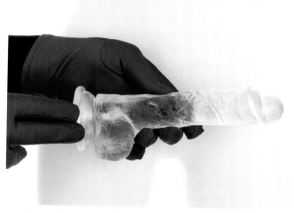

**1.** You will need a dildo that has some form of base.

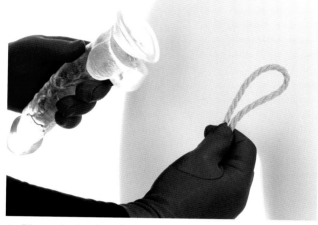

**2.** Place the bight of your rope...

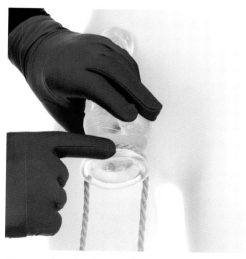

**3.** ...under the base of the dildo.

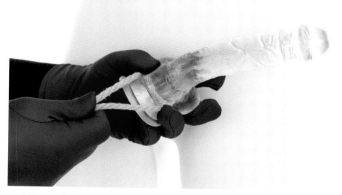

**4.** Wrap the rope ends around the dildo (not too tight).

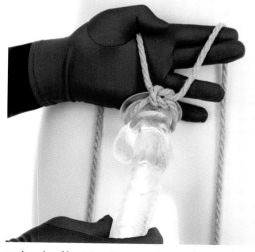

**5.** Lock off with a **Square Knot** (p. 149).

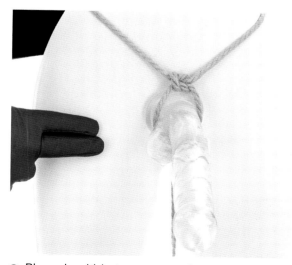

**6.** Place the dildo in position, then run the rope around your partner's waist to the back. *continues...*

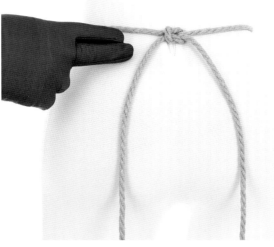

**7.** Confirm the placement of the dildo and tie off the ends with a **Square Knot** or **Surgeon's Knot**.

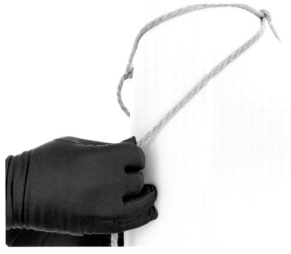

**8.** Bring the ends back to the front on each side.

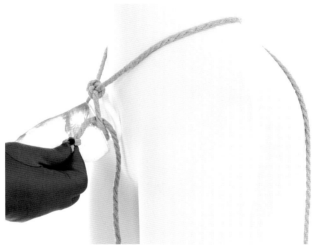

**9.** Run the ends under the rope ring.

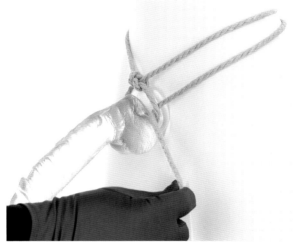

**10.** Pull the rope through.

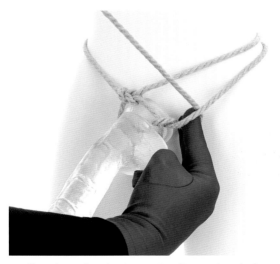

**11.** Reach under the incoming line to hook the tail...

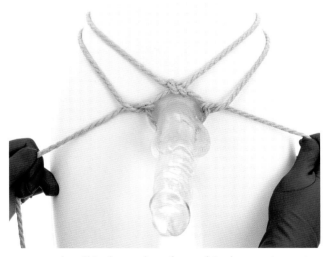

**12.** ...and pull it through to form this decorative twist (which also adds more friction and increases the stability). Do the same thing on the other side.

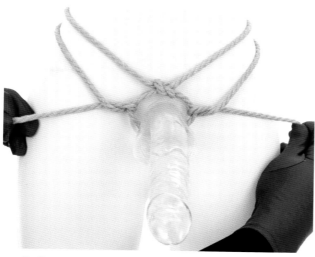

**13.** Pull the strands tight.

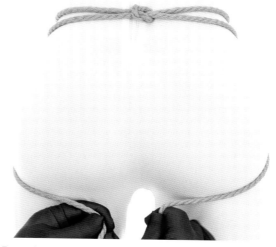

**14.** Run the tails around the hips to the back...

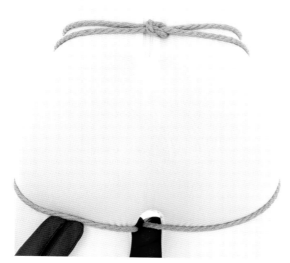

**15.** ...tightly underneath the butt cheeks...

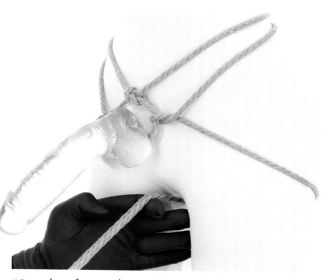

**16.** ...then forward again between the legs.

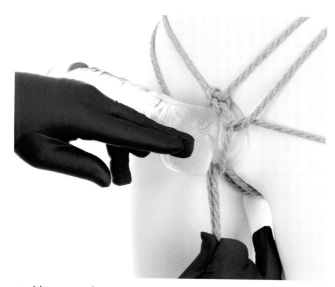

**17.** Now run the strands through the ring again.

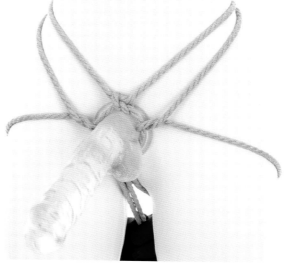

**18.** Run the strands back between the legs again.

*continues...*

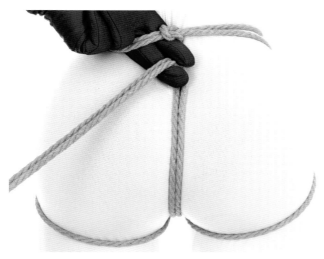

**19.** Reach under the waist band and grab the tail.

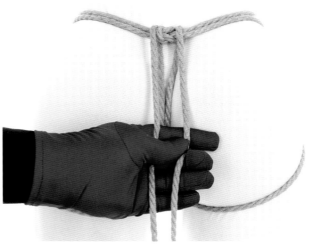

**20.** Pull the tail through and down to set the tension, then lock off however you wish (p. 168).

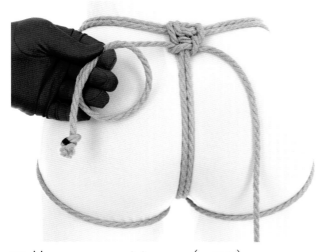

**21.** Use up any remaining rope (p. 279).

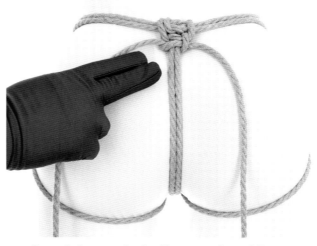

**22.** Since I chose to lock off using a **Cored Square Knot** (p. 288)...

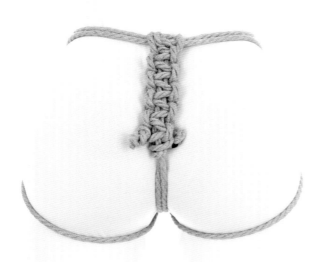

**23.** ...I will simply continue it to use up the rope.

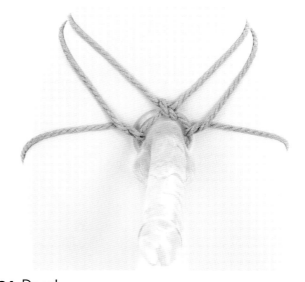

**24.** Done!

# Alternative Ways to Use Up Rope
## Example 1 – Wrap Tails Around Waist Band

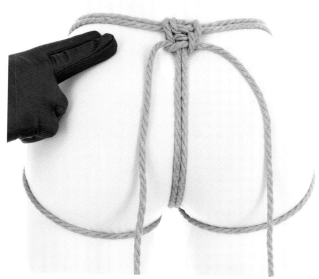

**1.** Use up the rope on the waist band instead.

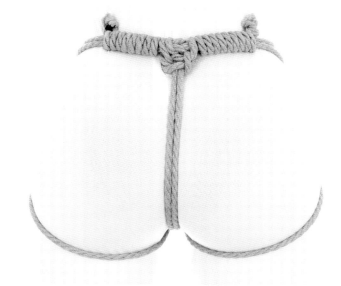

**2.** Wrap the tails around the waist band on their respective sides, then lock off by placing the ends between the strands.

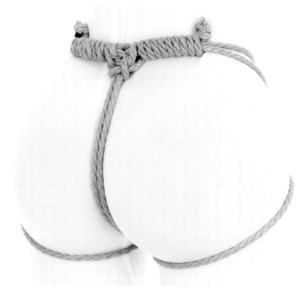

**3.** Done.

## Example 2 – Run Tails Between Lines Under Tension

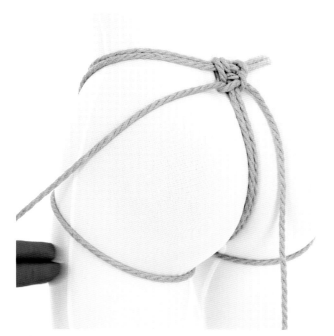

**1.** Bring the tail down to the leg.

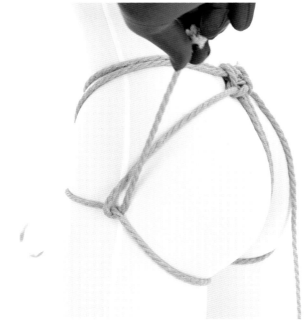

**2.** Run the tail under that line...

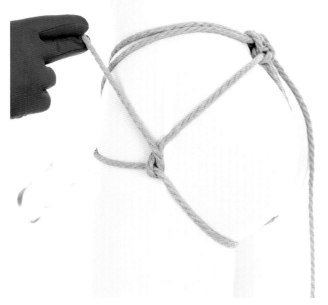

**3.** ...to form a twist.

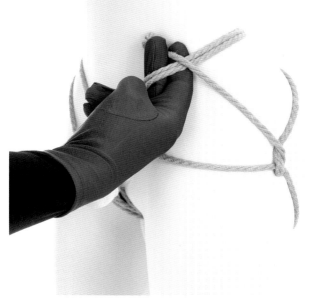

**4.** Bring the tail up to the waist band.

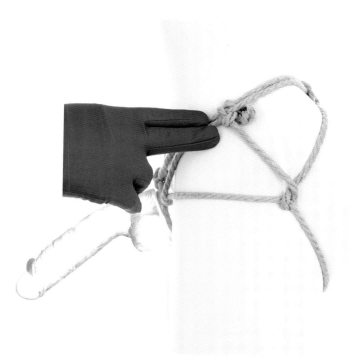

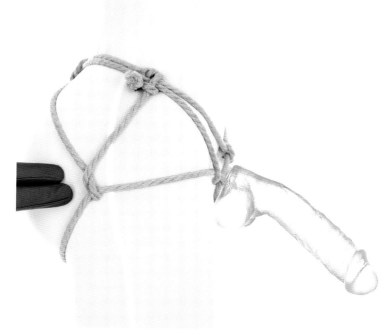

**5.** Lock it off to that band. In this case, I used a **Crossing Hitch** to connect, then tucked the remaining end between the strands of the waist band.

**6.** Repeat on the other side.

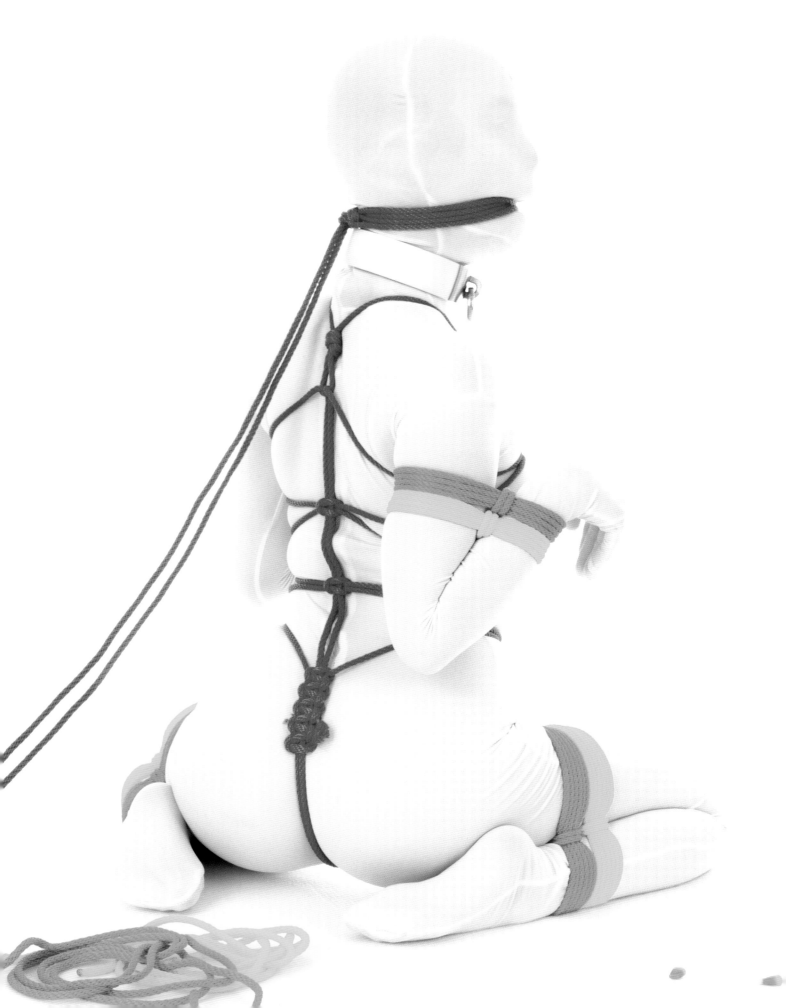

# 11 Building Great Scenes Using Multiple Ties

Going through this book, you learned several versions of single columns, double columns, chest harnesses, and hip harnesses. You now have command of many techniques that can be combined in literally thousands of ways to make amazing scenes.

In this chapter we will show you a few examples of what you can do using just the ties in this book! Use these as roadmaps for cool scenes or for inspiration to create new and wonderful things! Here are a few samples of what you find in the next few pages!

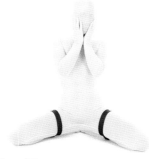

**Frog Tie**

**Kneeling Strappado**

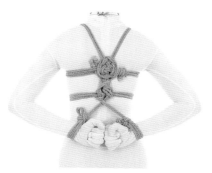

**Adjustable Box Tie**

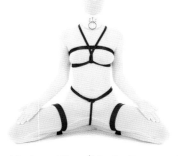

**Various Ties (Nadu Position)**

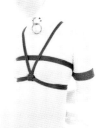

**Box Tie**

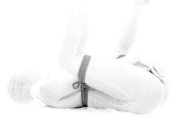

**Malasana Tie**

# A Survey of Foundation Ties

You could tie these two examples on any surface that has two anchor points separated by enough space; on a bed, on a couch, or between two pillars in a basement, for example.

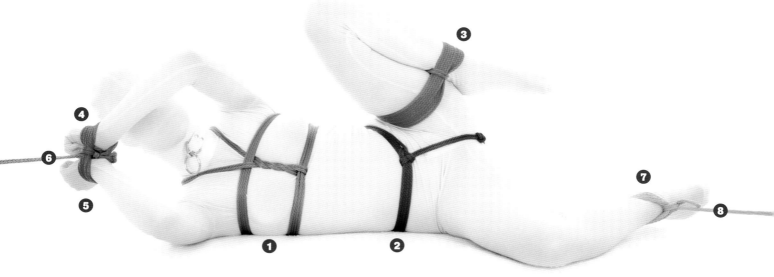

## Example 1

**1** Start with a **Bikini Harness**.

**2** Add a **Crotch Rope** with optional **Happy Knot**.

**3** Add a **Double Column**. This one happens to be a **Lark's Head Double Column**.

**4** Add a **Double Column**. This one happens to be a **Wrap & Cinch Double Column**.

**5** Convert (4) to load-bearing version of a **Double Column**.

**6** Run that tail from (5) to an anchor point and tie it off with two **Half Hitches**.

**7** Add a **Sommerville Bowline**.

**8** Run the tail from (7) to an anchor point and tie it off with two **Half Hitches**.

### Tie *and* Order
The number lists throughout this chapter indicate what the tie is and the order in which they were tied for that given scene.

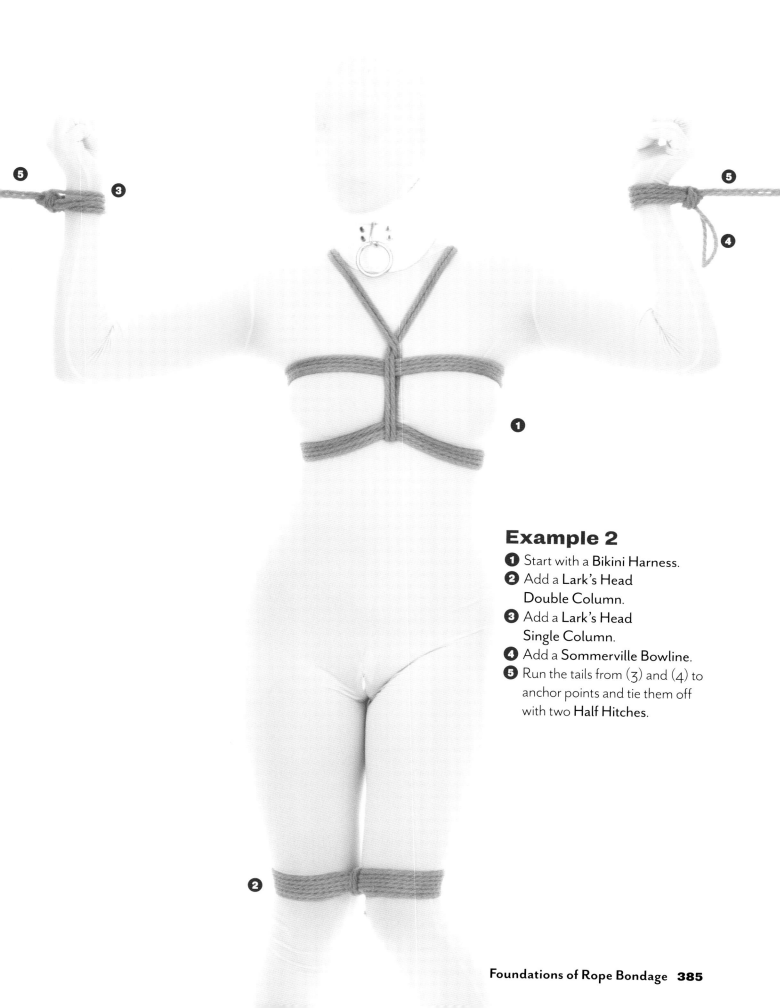

## Example 2

**1** Start with a **Bikini Harness**.

**2** Add a **Lark's Head Double Column**.

**3** Add a **Lark's Head Single Column**.

**4** Add a **Sommerville Bowline**.

**5** Run the tails from (3) and (4) to anchor points and tie them off with two **Half Hitches**.

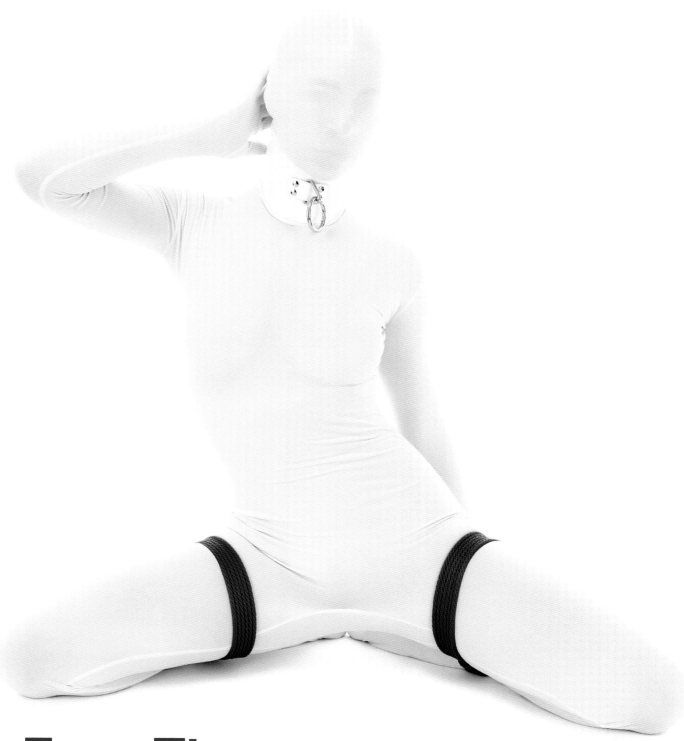

# Frog Tie

A **Frog Tie** is simply a **Lark's Head Double Column** or
**Wrap & Cinch Double Column** on each leg, tying ankle to thigh.

This can be done tying wrist to upper arm as well. If you do both at the
same time, you have converted your partner into a quadruped. For an
example of this, see p. 396.

# Classic Hog Tie

This is another classic position, but it has issues, so use caution:

- No matter how you tie the wrist cuffs, they will slide down to the hand and rest on the wrist joint. If too much tension is added, this can cause injury. This is why many people like to tie to a chest harness instead of the wrists, see **Adjustable Hog Tie** (p. 409).
- This position can make breathing difficult for some people. This is called positional asphyxia. As always, play within your partner's limits and keep communication open.

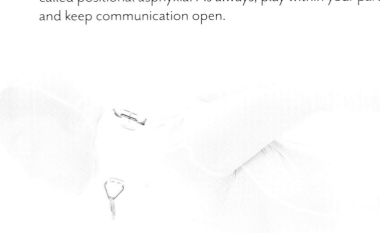
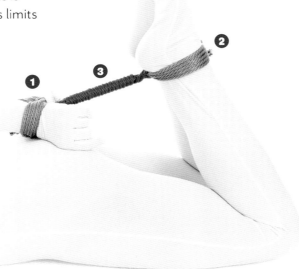

❶ Start with a **Lark's Head Double Column** around the wrists, behind the back.

❷ Add a **Lark's Head Double Column** around the ankles.

❸ Add a new rope to connect (1) to (2). Be sure to connect to the cuffs in a way that they do not tighten on the wrists or ankles when under tension. Here is one way to do that:

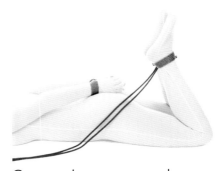
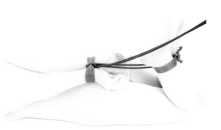
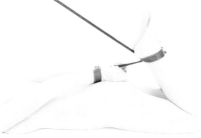

Connect the new rope to the closer side of the ankle cuffs, running one strand on each side of the cinch. This approach allows you to add tension without tightening the ankle cuffs.

Run the tail down to the wrist cuffs. Run it though one cuff and back through the other, load-bearing style (p. 248).

Tighten. Take care when doing so that you do not tighten so much that it puts too much strain on your partner's arms and wrists, or that it bends them so far back that they have trouble breathing. Wrap the tail around to use it up. Lock off.

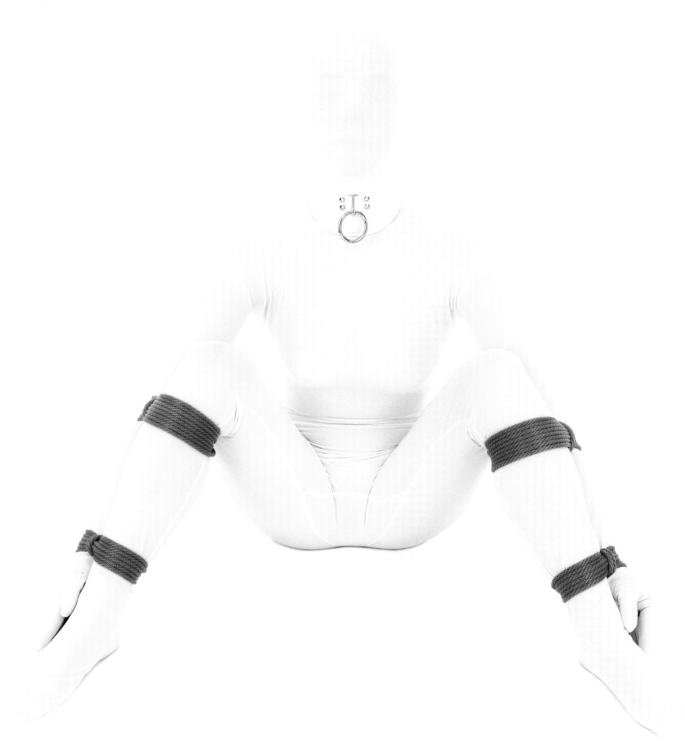

# Crab Tie

This is simply a series of **Double Columns** attaching the wrist to ankle on both sides, then attaching the knee to elbow. In this example, I chose **Lark's Head Double Columns** for their clean appearance.

It is important to note that this position can be stressful for some people. As always, keep good communication and adjust or untie them if needed.

# Malasana Tie

The **Malasana** (ma-LAH-sa-na) **Tie** opens your bottom's legs by binding the knees up near the shoulders. It is named after a yoga pose with a similar position. The tie features a cuff around each leg, just above the knee, and a band across the back to connect the two cuffs.

This tie can be done as shown below on people with good hip flexibility. If you have trouble with the back band sliding down (as can be the case with less hip flexibility), you can anchor it in place with ropes from another layer of bondage, if present. For example, you could put a chest harness on your partner first and then run the back band ropes from this tie through the ropes of the chest harness to keep them from sliding down.

## Risks and Safety

- **Back:** This tie should not be done on a person with any sort of back trouble or pain.
- **Positional Asphyxiation:** Keep in mind that this tie puts a person into a position that can be challenging for some. When folded like this, it can be difficult for some people to breathe. This is one reason it can be good to have the rapid release feature.
- **Communication:** If your partner will not be able to speak during the scene, give them some other means to signal distress.

❶ Start with a **Slipped Somerville Bowline** to allow for quick release.
❷ Run the tail across the back to the other leg.
❸ Add a **Hojo Cuff** to the other leg.
❹ Run the tail back and forth between the two cuffs until it is used up, then tie it off.

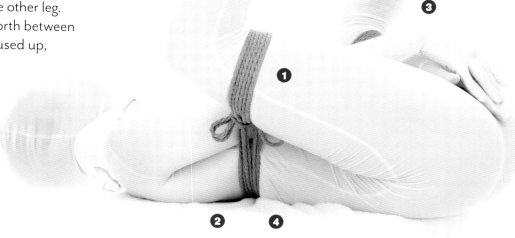

# How To Tie This

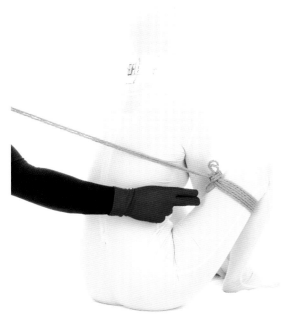

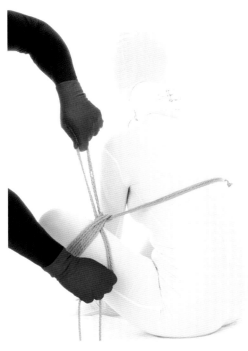

**1.** Start with a **Somerville Bowline** around one of your partner's legs. Consider three wraps instead of two to distribute the force across a wider area. Position the knot so that it points to your partner's back and then...

**2.** ...run the tail straight across their back. Tie a **Hojo Cuff** around this leg. Use the same number of wraps you used for Step 1.

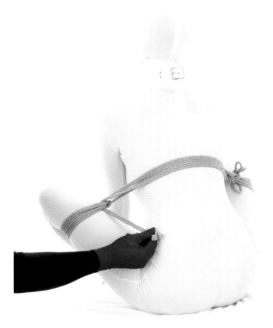

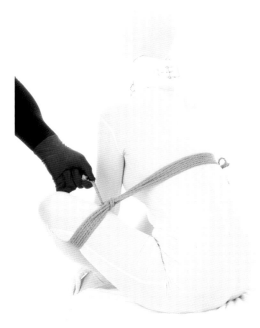

**3.** Run the tail back and forth between the cuffs until you are almost out of rope.

**4.** Wrap the tail around the band.

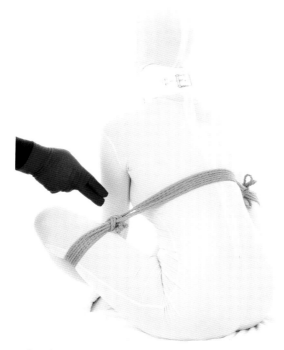

**5.** Lock off.

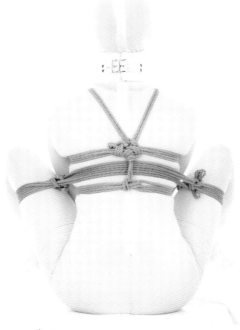

**6.** (Optional) If adding a chest harness, tie it first and then run the **Malasana** band under the stem to keep it from moving.

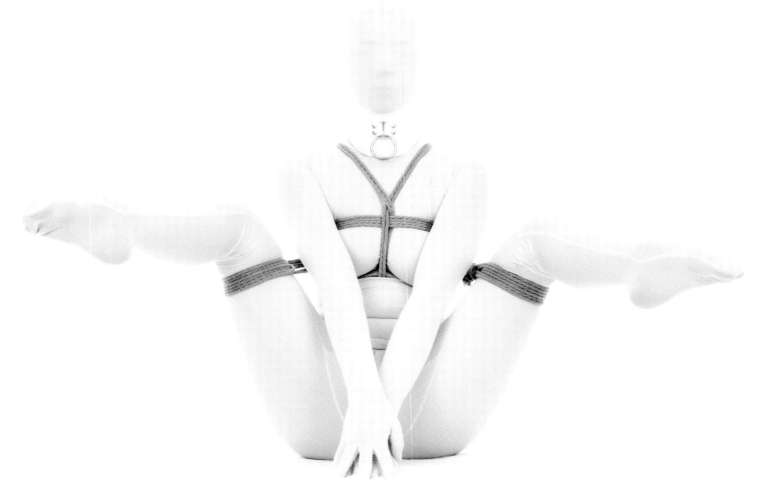

# Kneeling Strappado

"Strappado" or "corda" means to tie a person's wrists behind their back, then connect the tied wrists to an overhead hard point, pulling them up.

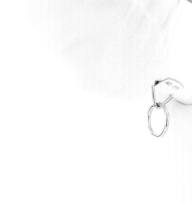

❶ (Optional) Start with a **Crotch Rope**.
❷ Add a **Frog Tie**.
❸ Add a **Lark's Head Double Column**.
❹ Add a new rope to convert (3) into a **Load-bearing Double Column**, then run it up to an overhead point. In this example, the tail is brought back to the wrists and then tied off by wrapping the tail around the up line and then tucking the ends through the lines periodically.

## Alternatives

• The tail can be brought down to the waist band and tied off there instead, adding a small predicament element, that is, if they pull down with their arms, it will pull the **Crotch Rope** into them more tightly.
• You can add a chest harness before you begin and anchor (4) to the chest band.

# The Bound Nadu

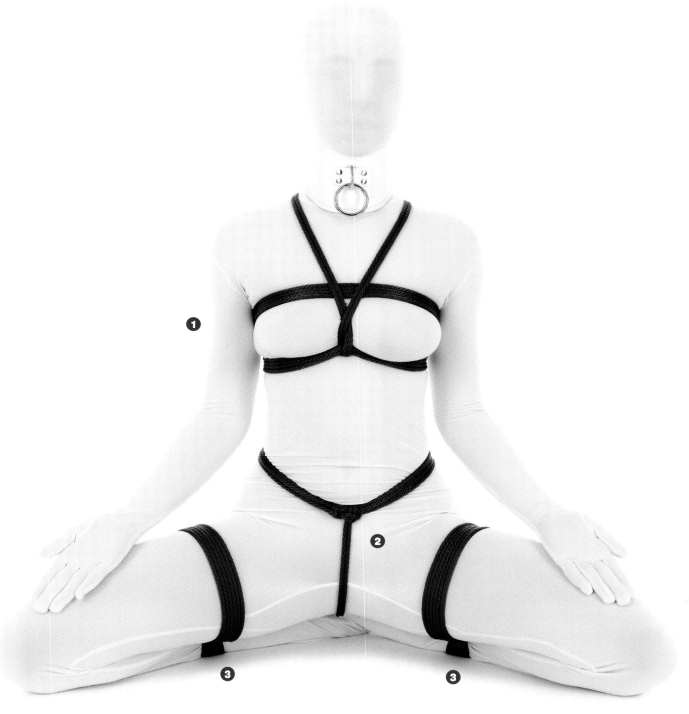

This is Nadu, a classic slave/sub position made popular by John Norman's *Gor* novels.

**1** Start with a **Bikini Harness**.
**2** Add a **Crotch Rope**.
**3** Add a **Frog Tie**.

# Standing Strappado

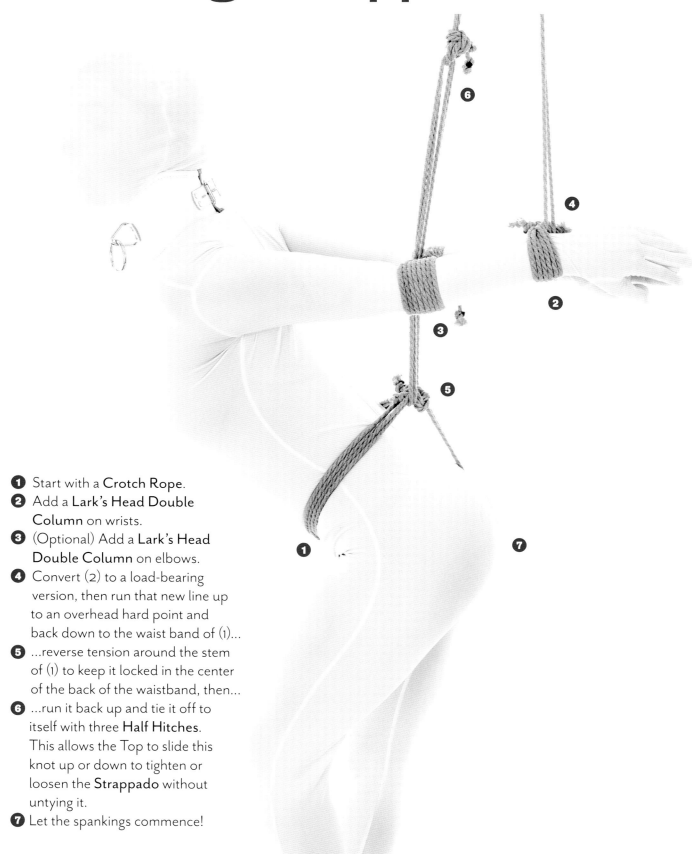

1. Start with a **Crotch Rope**.
2. Add a **Lark's Head Double Column** on wrists.
3. (Optional) Add a **Lark's Head Double Column** on elbows.
4. Convert (2) to a load-bearing version, then run that new line up to an overhead hard point and back down to the waist band of (1)...
5. ...reverse tension around the stem of (1) to keep it locked in the center of the back of the waistband, then...
6. ...run it back up and tie it off to itself with three **Half Hitches**. This allows the Top to slide this knot up or down to tighten or loosen the **Strappado** without untying it.
7. Let the spankings commence!

# Holiday Inspiration

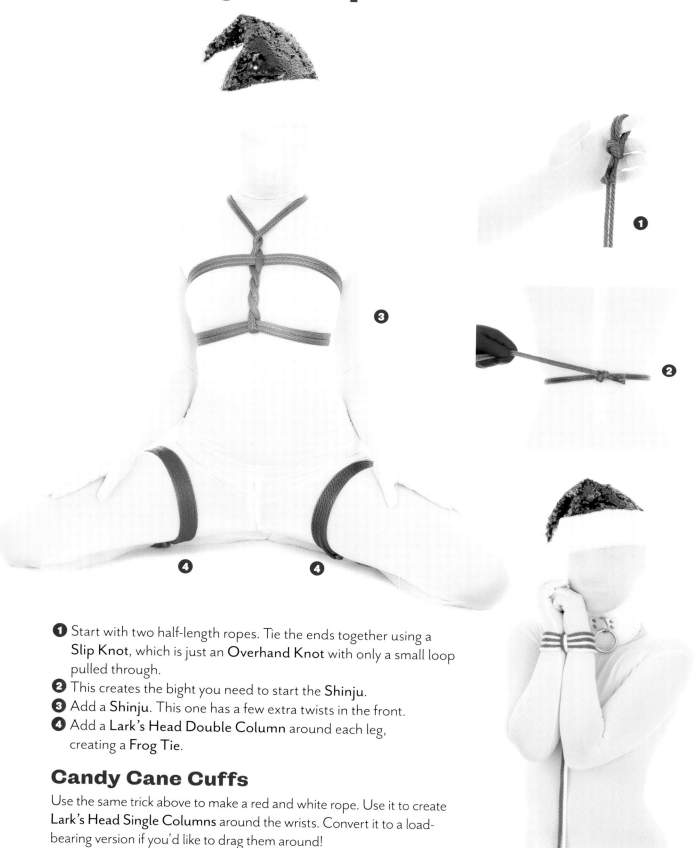

1. Start with two half-length ropes. Tie the ends together using a **Slip Knot**, which is just an **Overhand Knot** with only a small loop pulled through.
2. This creates the bight you need to start the **Shinju**.
3. Add a **Shinju**. This one has a few extra twists in the front.
4. Add a **Lark's Head Double Column** around each leg, creating a **Frog Tie**.

## Candy Cane Cuffs

Use the same trick above to make a red and white rope. Use it to create **Lark's Head Single Columns** around the wrists. Convert it to a load-bearing version if you'd like to drag them around!

# Autumn Quadruped

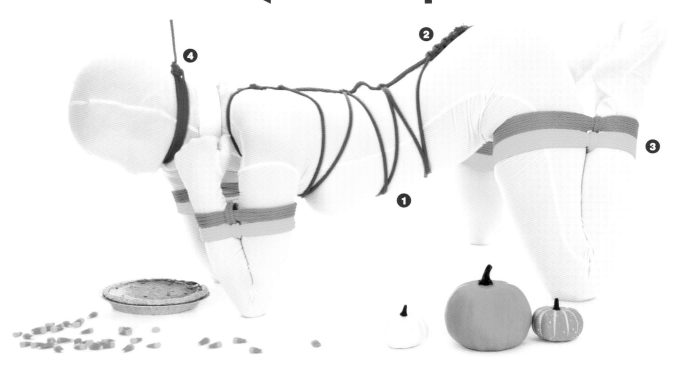

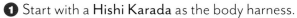

1. Start with a **Hishi Karada** as the body harness.
2. (Optional) Use **Cored Square Knots** for rear connection points and to use up rope.
3. Add a festival of **Lark's Head Double Columns** on the legs and arms, using different color ropes just for the fun of it!
4. (Optional) Add a **Lark's Head Single Column** as a gag and lead.

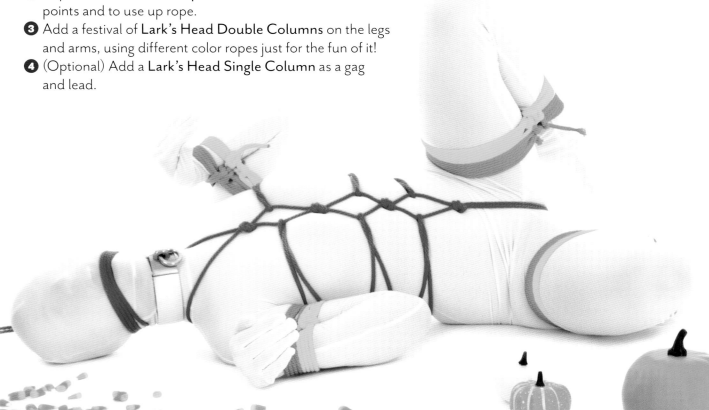

# One Type of Box Tie

You now know everything you need to make a simple **Box Tie**!

This example was done with a short rope on the wrists:

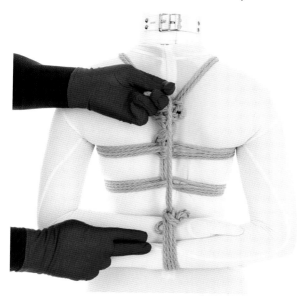

**1.** Start with a **Shinju** on the chest, then add a **Slipped Somerville Bowline** around both wrists. The single cuff should be around both wrists.

The above was shown using a **Slipped Somerville Bowline** with two wraps around the wrists. This is so you can more easily compare it to the core technique. In practice, I always like to do three wraps around my partner's wrists when doing a **Box Tie** because it distributes the force across a greater area, making it more comfortable for longer-term wear.

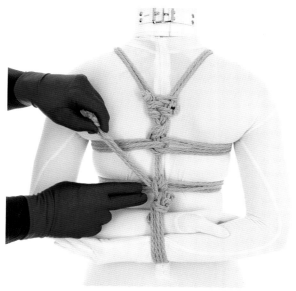

**2.** Run the tail up and connect it to one of the horizontal bands of the chest harness.

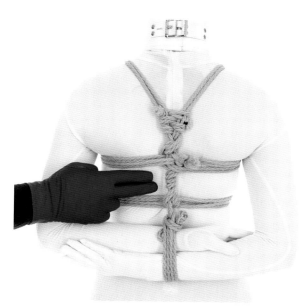

**3.** Lock it off and use up the remaining rope.

# Good Box Tie Position — Protect Your Wrists!

**Important!** Note the hand and wrist position shown in these pictures. The insides of the wrists are facing each other.

## Don't do This!

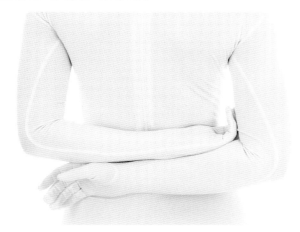 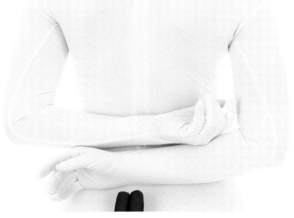

Don't let your partner place their arms in just any position...

...this exposes the sensitive part of the wrist to pressure on both arms against the rope.

## Do This!

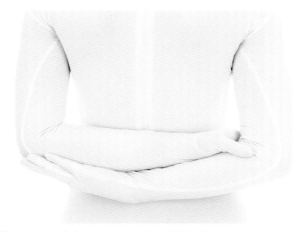 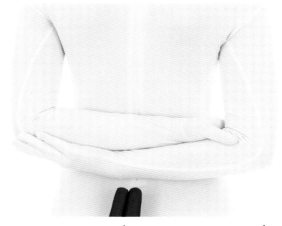

The wrist of the top arm should be facing downward and the wrist of the lower arm should be facing upward.

This position protects the sensitive inner part of the wrist from pressure from the rope.

**Also important:** Sometimes just having arms behind the back can put pressure on nerves or blood vessels and cause issues. Direct your partner to tell you if they feel anything strange. If they do so, adjust their position. If the issue does not go away in 15 seconds, untie them.

If a person cannot get into this position, consider using a **Single Column** around each wrist independently so the tie can be adjusted to meet their needs. See p. 405 for an example.

If the person would like to be able to get into this position, there are shoulder flexibility exercises that can be helpful.

# A Box and Elbow Tie

You can also add one more layer to turn this into a very hot and very secure **Box Tie**!

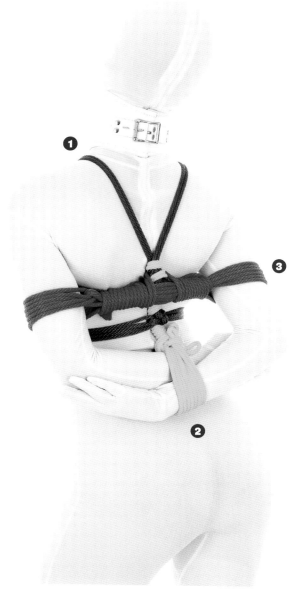

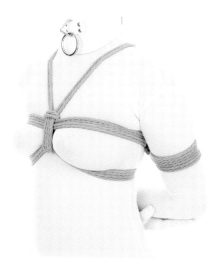

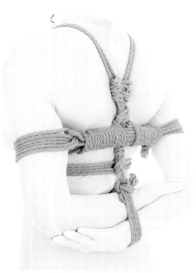

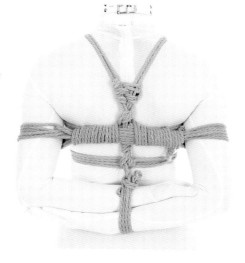

❶ Start with a **Shinju**.

❷ Add a **Slipped Somerville Bowline** around wrists. Tie the tail to the bands of the **Shinju**.

❸ Add an **Extended Lark's Head Double Column** around the elbows. Wrap the tail around the upper chest band of the **Shinju** in addition to the lines normally wrapped. This keeps it from migrating down your partner's arms as they move around.

**Important!** Remember the nerve safety information you learned in the **Extended Lark's Head Double Column** tutorial. See *Important Safety Information* (p. 403) for a reminder.

# How To Tie This

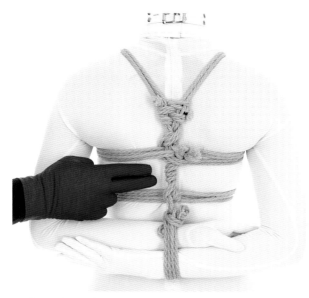

**1.** Complete the **Box Tie** above.

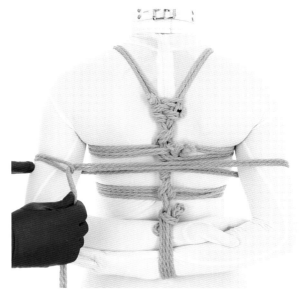

**2.** Begin tying the **Extended Lark's Head Double Column**. Place it just a bit below the upper chest band of the **Shinju**.

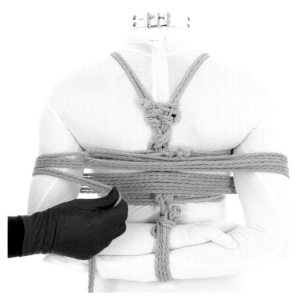

**3.** Finish the elbow wraps. See page 403 for important safety information.

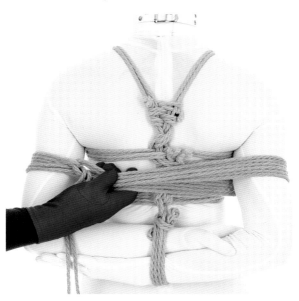

**4.** Complete the first wrap or two just around the lines of the **Extended Lark's Head Double Column**.

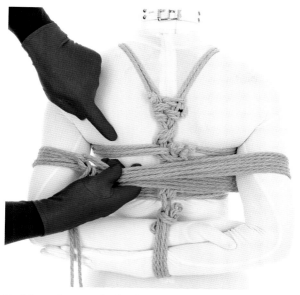

**5.** After that, include the lines from the **Shinju** as well.

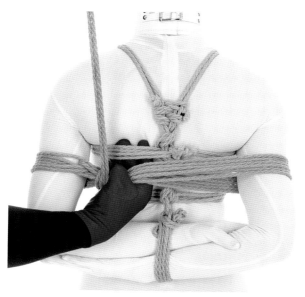

**6.** Starting with the second or third wrap, place your fingers behind the chest band of the **Shinju**...

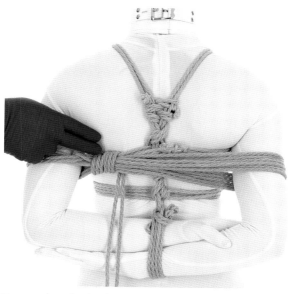

**7.** ...and include those lines in the wrap as well.

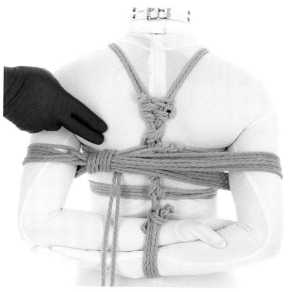

**8.** Continue wrapping around all those lines.

*continues...*

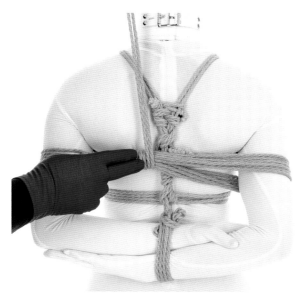

**9.** When you get to the stem...

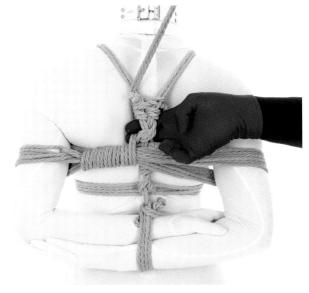

**10.** ...run the tail around it.

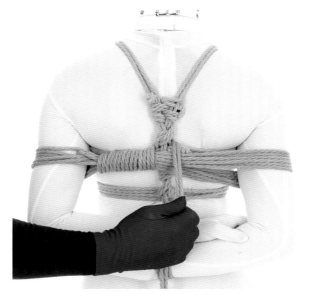

**11.** Like this.

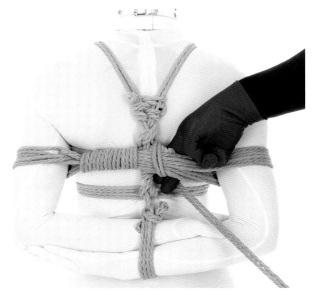

**12.** Then keep wrapping around the other side. It doesn't matter that the direction of the wrapping changes.

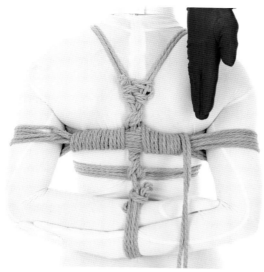

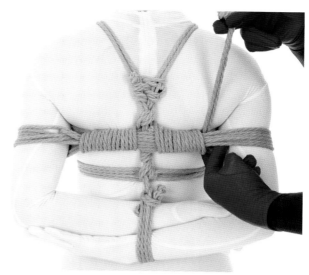

**13.** When you get to the point that the lines from the **Extended Lark's Head Double Column** begin to pull away from the lines of the **Shinju**...

**14.** ...switch to wrapping around the lines of the **Extended Lark's Head Double Column**, the way you started on the other side.

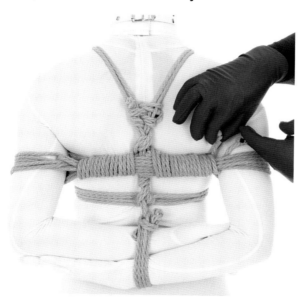

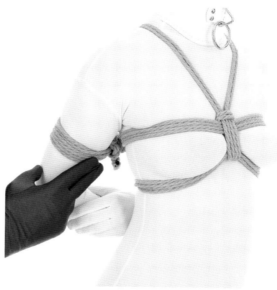

**15.** When you get to the end, split the tails and tie off just as you normally do for an **Extended Lark's Head Double Column**. Then use up the remaining rope however you wish.

**16.** Now that the lines are separated, you can lock off with a **Square Knot**.

## Important Safety Information!

Don't make this too tight or pull the elbows closer together than is comfortable for your partner.

Remember that there are nerves running through the outside of the upper arm between the deltoid and the elbow. Too much pressure in the wrong place can compress those nerves (p. 60, 70).

If your partner reports any strange sensations — e.g. numbness, tingling, etc. — move this band up or down an inch or so immediately.

If the sensation doesn't stop in 15 seconds, untie this element.

## A Box and Elbow Tie

**Or, Color Coded:**

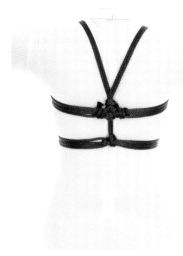

Shinju.

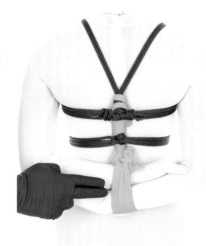

Slipped Somerville Bowline.

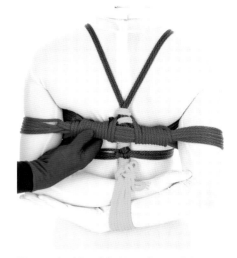

Extended Lark's Head Double Column.

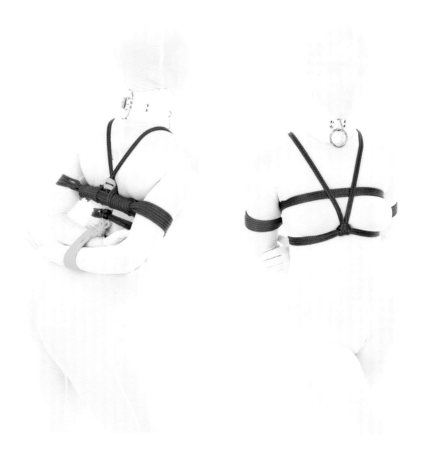

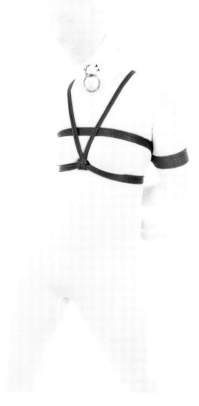

# An Adjustable Box Tie

You can modify this **Box Tie** to tie people that are not able to put their arms into a **Box Tie Position** (p. 398). This simple change allows you to adjust the tie to whatever position they are able to comfortably adopt!

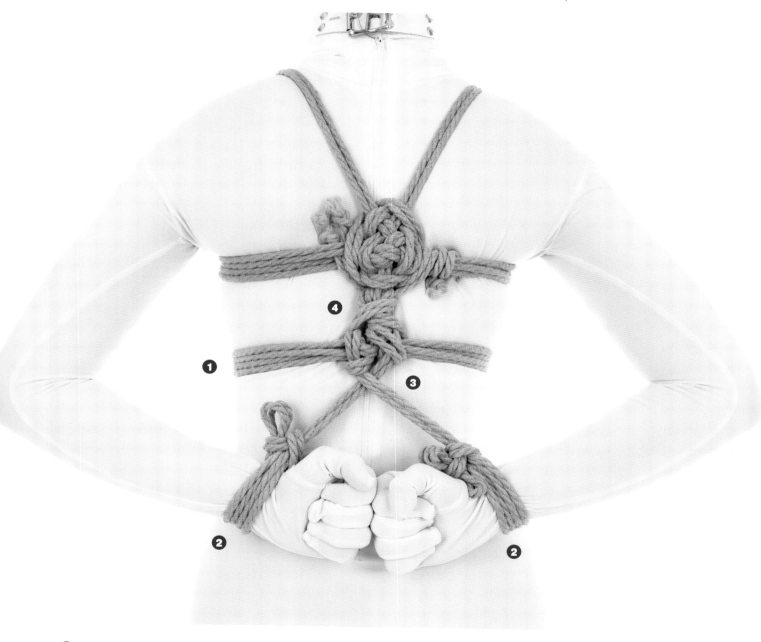

❶ Start with a **Shinju** on the chest.
❷ Add a **Slipped Somerville Bowline** around each wrist.
❸ Run the tails from (2) up to the opposite side of the **Shinju**, then under the band or stem. Adjust the position as appropriate for your partner's level of comfort and capability.
❹ Lock the tail off however you wish.

## An Adjustable/Accessible Box Tie

### How to Tie This

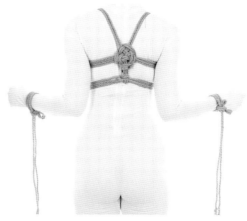

**1.** Add a **Slipped Somerville Bowline** to each wrist.

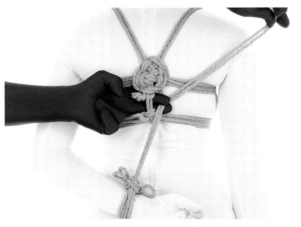

**2.** Work with one wrist at a time. Bring the tail up over the lower chest band on the other side. Reach under the stem with your other hand and hook the tail.

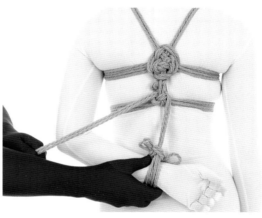

**3.** Pull the tail through. Then position your partner's wrist where you want it to be, pulling the tail at the same time.

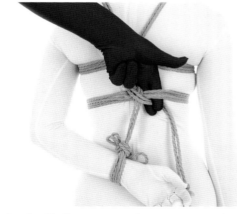

**4.** Lock off. One way to do so is to run the tail over itself to the other side again, then up under the band.

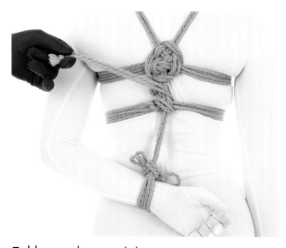

**5.** Use up the remaining rope.

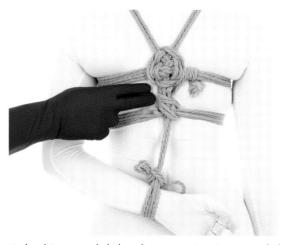

**6.** In this case, I did so by wrapping it around the stem, then...

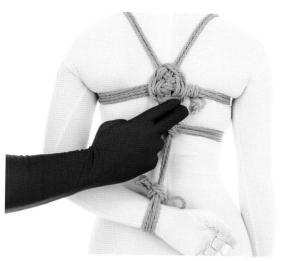

**7.** ...up to the upper chest band, where I wrapped it a few times.

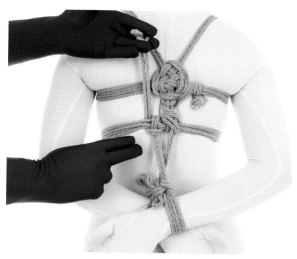

**8.** Repeat on the other side.

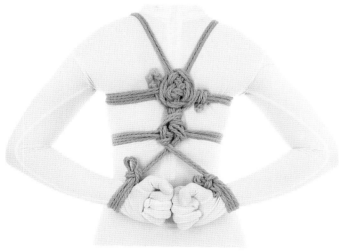

**9.** Done!

# Waitress

Waitress is a classic BDSM position command.
Here we help enforce it with rope.

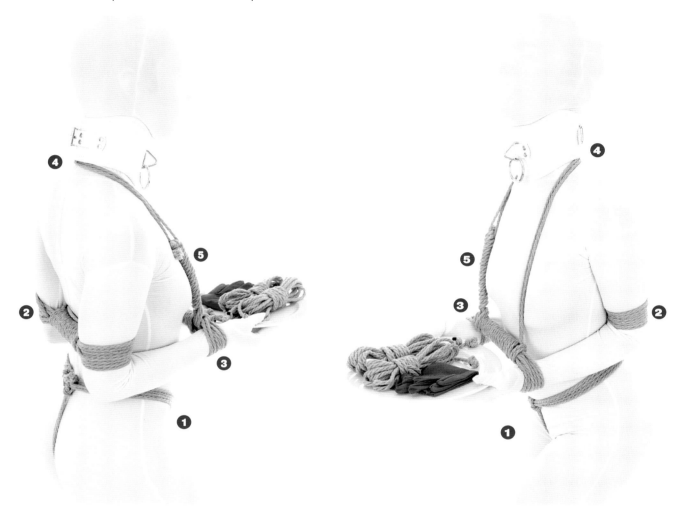

❶ Start with a **Crotch Rope**.
❷ Add an **Extended Lark's Head Double Column** around the elbows.*
❸ Add an **Extended Lark's Head Double Column** around the wrists.
❹ Run the tail from (3) around the back of the neck and down through the cuff of the other wrist.
❺ Lock off the tie. One way is to wrap the remainder of tail around itself and tuck the ends between the strands or add a **Half Hitch** to tie off.

* **Important!** Don't make this too tight or pull the elbows closer together than is comfortable for your partner. Remember the nerve safety information you learned in the **Extended Lark's Head Double Column** tutorial. Too much pressure can compress those nerves. If your partner reports any strange sensations — e.g. numbness, etc. — move this band up or down an inch immediately. If the sensation doesn't stop in 15 seconds, untie this element.

# An Accessible Hog Tie

A **Hog Tie** can be a lot of fun, but it is also a very challenging position. A strict **Hog Tie** is when the person is bent backward to the point of stress. *Be careful with Hog Ties*. For some people, such a position can make it difficult to breathe and can lead to positional asphyxiation.

Always remember the rule:
**Never leave a person alone when they are in bondage.**
   This version of the **Hog Tie** can be easily adjusted to make it more or less strict, as needed.

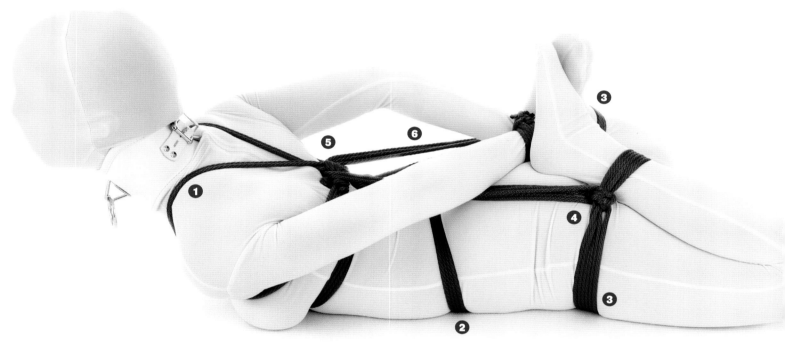

❶ Start with a **Shinju** on the chest.
❷ (Optional) Add an **Crotch Rope**.
❸ Add a **Frog Tie**. This is just a **Lark's Head Double Column** on each leg, tying the ankle to the thigh on each side.
❹ Add a new rope around the cinch of the left **Frog Tie**, converting it to a **Load-bearing Double Column**.
❺ Run the tail you added in (4) up to the upper chest band, then back down and around the cinch lines of the right **Frog Tie**. Pull that rope to force your partner into a back bend (be careful and move slowly).
❻ Use up the rest of the rope by going back and forth from ankle to chest band to ankle until it runs out. Tie off.

# Lambda

**1** Start with **Lark's Head Double Columns** tying wrists to thighs.

**2** Add a **Somerville Bowline** on each ankle.

**3** Add a **Lark's Head Single Column** tied around the head and through the mouth as a cleave gag.

**4** Run the tails from (2) and (3) to points on the side and overhead, and tie them off using two **Half Hitches** for each connection.

You could do this same position on a bed if the frame has appropriate anchor points!

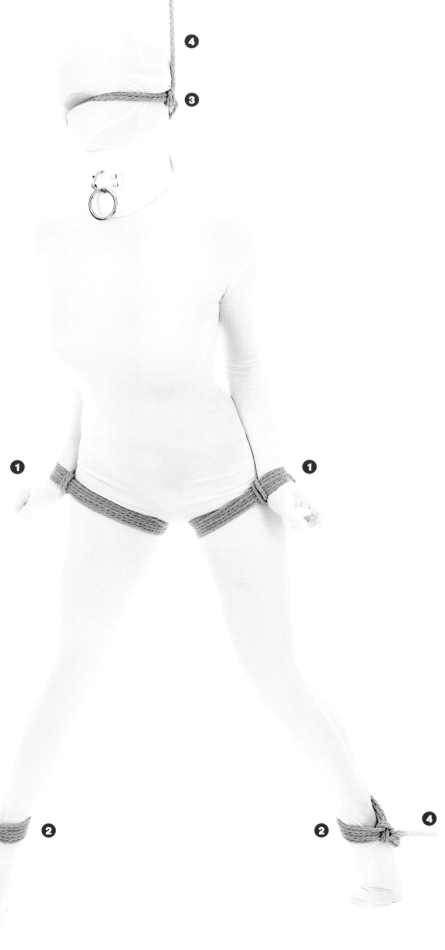

# Tying to a Chair or Wheelchair

## There are many ways to tie someone to a chair!

Despite what you have seen in countless movies and TV shows, it is kind of difficult to make a chair tie secure. Often, they show someone with just wrists tied to the arms of a chair, or maybe wrists and ankles, or — if they are really advanced — wrists, ankles, and a band around the chest. If a determined person was trying to work themselves free, none of these would hold for more than a few minutes.

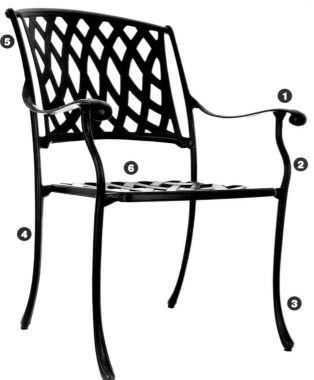

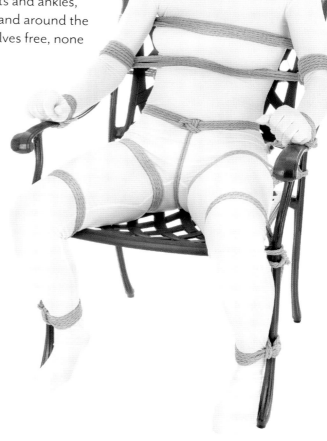

Here are a few options for each part of the body, so you can mix and match them to fit your vision!

Find anchor points on the chair. Make more if you need them.

If you want your partner to be able to fight and thrash, you need a sturdy chair. There are many anchor points on one!

**1** Armrest for wrists.
**2** Armrest support for the knees.
**3** Front chair legs for ankles.
**4** Rear chair legs for ankles and/or wrists.
**5** Back for chest.
**6** Seat or back for waist or hips.
**7** Cross brace as a middle anchor for hips or ankles but this chair doesn't have a cross brace, so...

...if you need an anchor point located in the middle, just create one yourself!

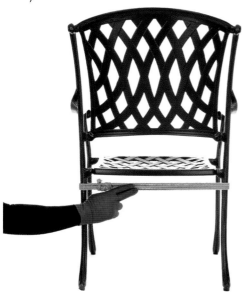

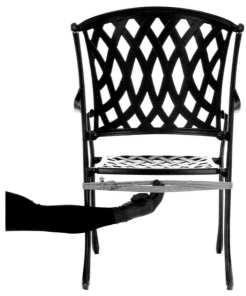

**1.** Tie a **Lark's Head Single Column** (p. 181) tightly around the legs or back of the chair.

**2.** Connect to the part of the band opposite where the tension will be coming from. We want that tension to tighten the band.

Wheelchairs also offer many great anchor points!

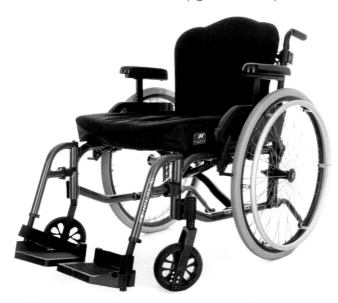

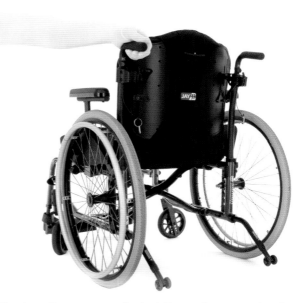

The braces and supports are great anchor points.

The handles are great for holding a chest rope in place.

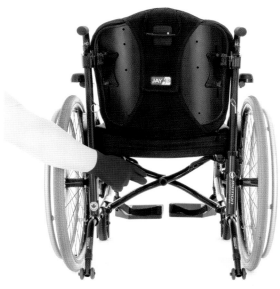

The lower cross brace is good for connecting a waist band.

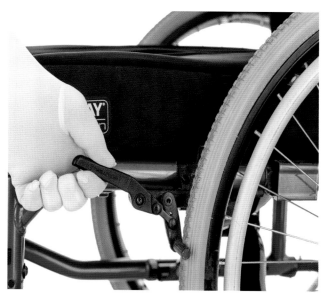

Be sure to lock the wheels!

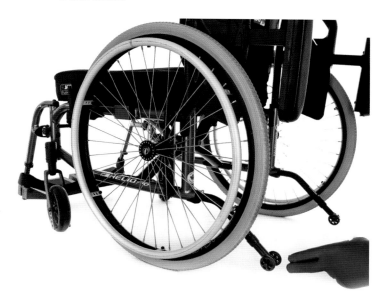

Look for rear kick stands so the chair can't flip over backward.

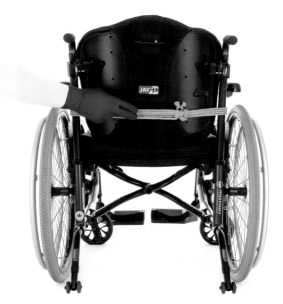

Just as with any other chair, if you need another central point, add one!

To tie a person to a chair securely, you need to make sure they can't wriggle into other positions. This means making sure their core is locked down. When I do chair ties, I like to start with the waist/hips, *then* move to the chest, and then deal with the arms and legs.

# Waist/Hips

A tie around the waist or hips helps keep them from sliding forward in the chair or thrashing back and forth too much to try to knock the chair over or to get better access to knots.

### Use a Belt (Belt Knot on Back)

...and tie it to the back of the chair or to a point you create.

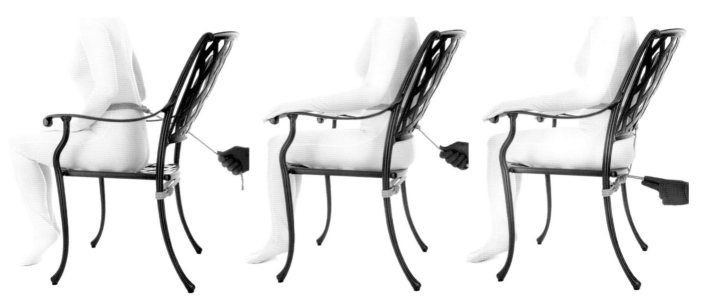

**1.** Tie a belt with the knot on the back.

**2.** Run the tail behind the chair.

**3.** Tie off to some central point. You can tie off to a slat on the back of the chair itself, or to a point you create, if needed.

## Use a Belt (Belt Knot on Front)

...then run the tail between the legs to be even more restrictive.

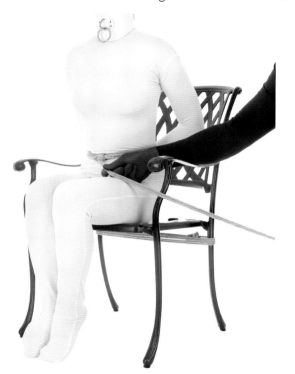

**1.** Tie a belt with the knot on the front.

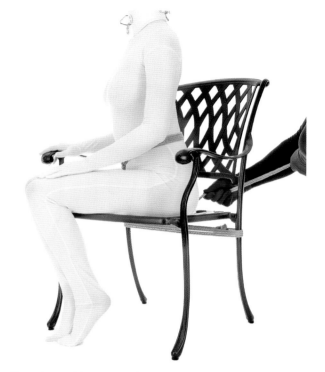

**2.** Run the tail between their legs.

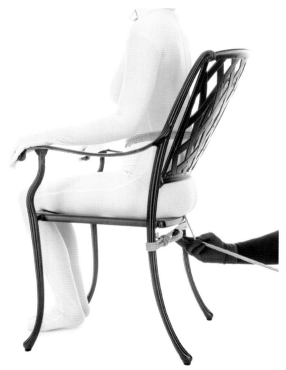

**3.** Run it to the back and tie off.

## Waist/Hips

### Use a Crotch Rope or Other Hip Harness

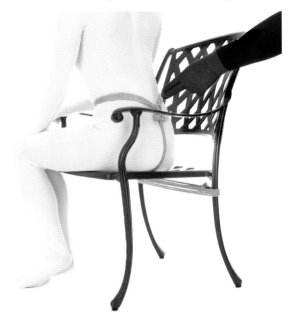 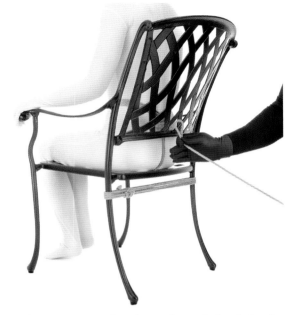

**1.** If you already have some form of waist or hip harness in place...

**2.** ...attach a new rope, then have them sit firmly back and tie them to the back of the chair.

### Tie Them Back by the Legs Instead of the Waist

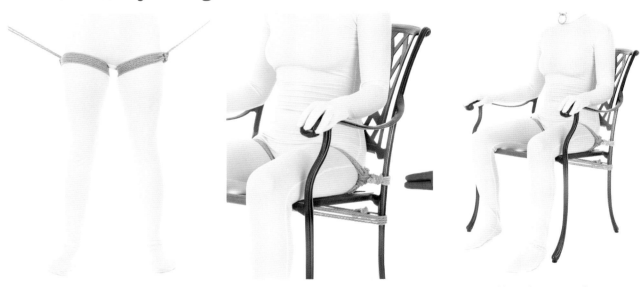

**1.** Start with a *loose* **Single Column** on each leg.

**2.** Run the tail across the hips to the back and...

**3.** ...tie off to chair uprights.

Safety Note: This approach may put pressure on the crease where the leg meets the torso. There are nerves in that area that can be sensitive to being compressed if the ropes are too tight or if your partner puts sustained pressure on them while struggling. Tell your partner to report any strange sensations (numbness, burning, etc.) in their legs or tops of their feet. If that happens, loosen these ropes.

# Chest

Controlling the chest is helpful for two reasons: One, to keep your partner from leaning forward to try to untie their wrists using their teeth. Two, to prevent them from thrashing around too much and possibly moving or knocking over the chair, as this could result in injury.

## Wrap a New Rope Around a Band and Elements on the Chair

The classic way to achieve this is to have them sit firmly back in the chair and tie them directly to the chair back in whatever way you wish. Here is one way. This method is only effective if you also have their hips or waist tied as described before. Otherwise, they can just sink down to work their way out.

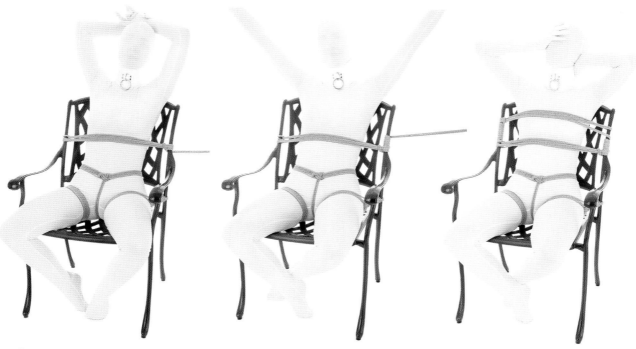

**1.** Put a **Lark's Head** around one side of the chair, then run the rope back and forth, then tie off.

**2.** If you have rope left, bring it to another location by wrapping it around one side a few times.

**3.** Then add another band and tie off.

## Chest

### Use the Tail From a Chest Harness or Band Around the Chest

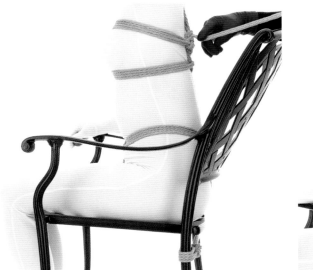

**1.** Complete a chest harness or just a band around the chest, but don't use up the tail in the harness itself.

**2.** Use it to connect to the chair and tie off.

Knots on the spine can be uncomfortable if the chair has a hard back. Consider adding a pillow if needed, to cushion the back.

Alternatively, you can not use a chest harness at all and instead have them sit fully back in the chair and tie their chest directly to the chair back.

### Wrap a New Rope Around a Band and Elements on the Chair

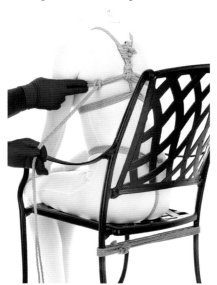 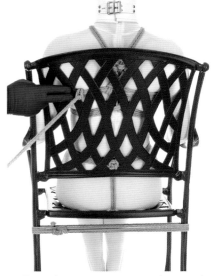 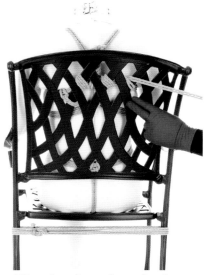

**1.** Put a **Lark's Head** around a band.

**2.** Run the new rope over/around any available place on the back of the chaair, attaching the band of the chest harness to the chair in multiple places.

**3.** This chair has a fancy back, so I wrapped the rope into that pattern. Tie off using a **Half Hitch** or by separating the tails and using a **Square Knot**.

## Wrap a New Rope Between Two Bands or Two Points on the Same Band

This can be helpful if the chair's back is solid.

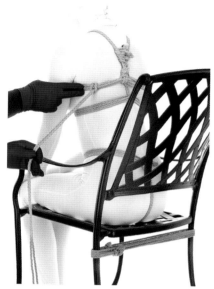

**1.** Put a **Lark's Head** around the band.

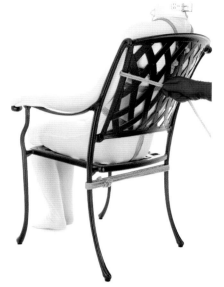

**2.** Run the new rope over or around any convenient point on the back of the chair.

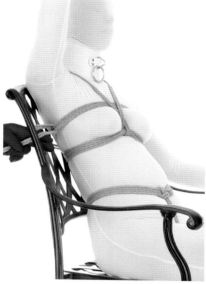

**3.** Run under the other band (or a different point on the same band).

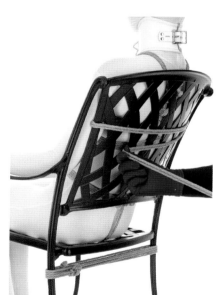

**4.** Bring the rope back to the side.

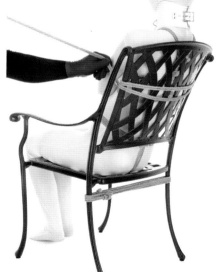

**5.** Bring it back under the band where you started. If you have more rope, you can repeat until the rope is consumed, or...

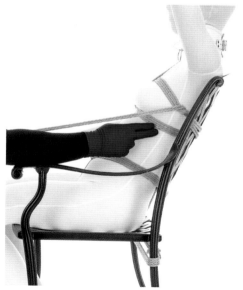

**6.** ...you can move the tail to a different band and repeat there.

# Legs and Ankles

### Legs Together

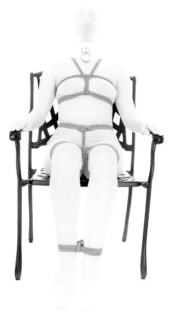
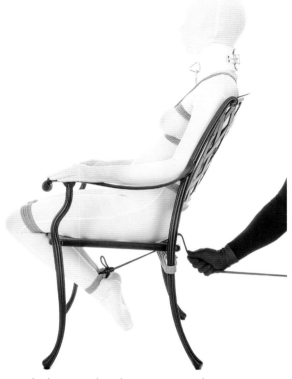

**1.** Use **Double Columns** on the ankles and (optionally) knees. You can leave the legs otherwise free if you want your partner to be able to kick and struggle, or...

**2.** ...attach them to the chair at a cross brace underneath the seat, or a point in the back (which you can create if needed).

### Legs Apart, Ankles Tied to the Front Legs of the Chair

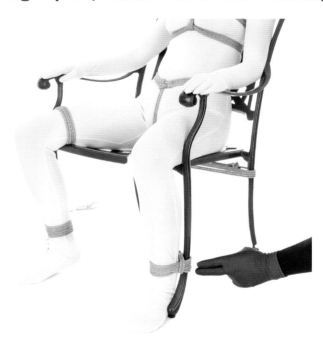
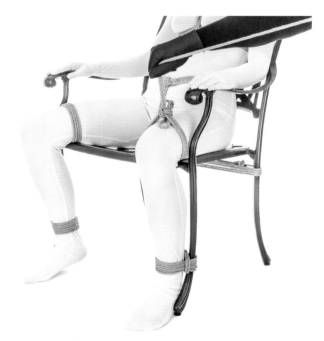

**1.** Tie the ankles to the front chair legs using a **Single** or **Double Column**. underneath the chair.

**2.** (Optional) Add **Single Column** around knees and attach either...

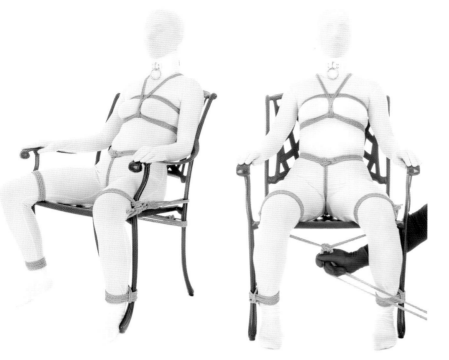
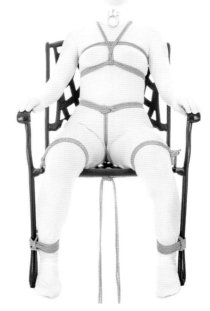

**3.** ...to the armrest supports, or...

**4.** ...to each other underneath the seat.

**5.** With this arrangement, when they pull one leg, it pulls on the other.

### Legs Apart, Ankles Tied to the Back of the Chair, Keeping the Feet Off the Ground

This can keep your partner from trying to kick the chair over. It also provides some... access.

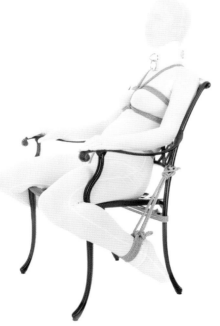
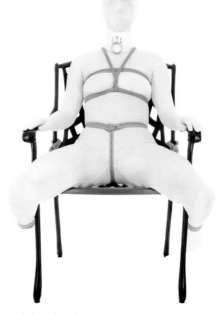

**1.** Tie the ankles using a **Single Column**. Run the tails up to the backrest of the chair. If you have more rope, you can run the tail back and forth from there through the cuff.

**2.** Tie off when you run out of rope.

# Arms and Wrists

### Wrists to Armrests

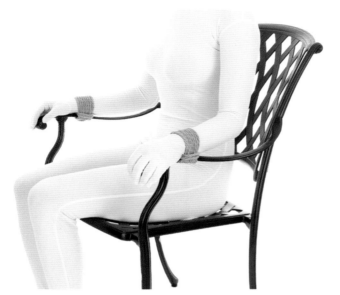

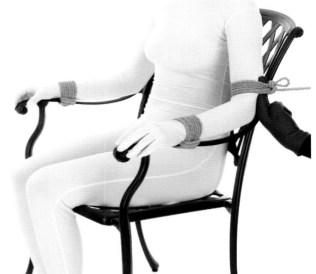

**1.** Tie **Double Columns** on wrists, tying them to the arms of the chair.

**2.** Consider also adding loose **Single Columns** around the upper arms and...

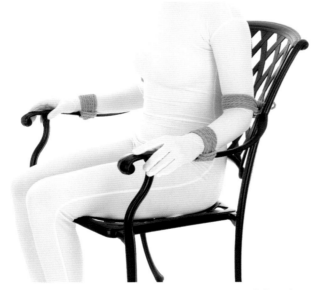

**3.** ...tying them together behind the back of the chair.

## Wrists to Back Legs

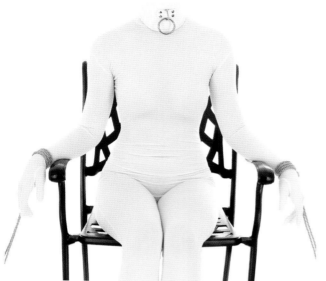

**1.** Tie a **Single Column** around each wrist.

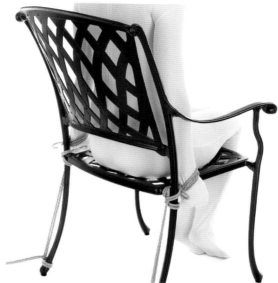

**2.** Run the tail to the back leg of the chair and anchor in place.

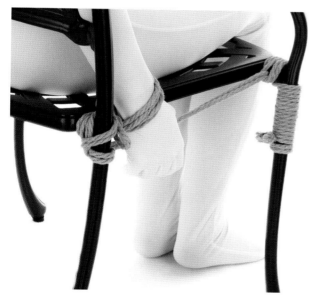

**3.** Then find another location out of reach to tie off the end; perhaps the front leg of the chair just to taunt them.

## Adjustable Box Tie

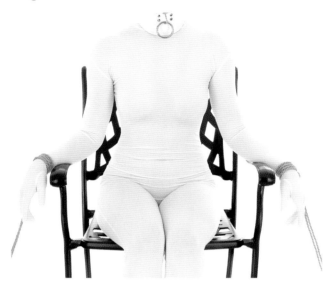

**1. Single Column** around each wrist.

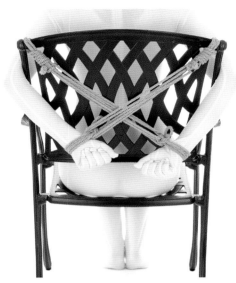

**2.** Tie off on the opposite sides. This provides a great deal of ability to adjust the position and level of tension.

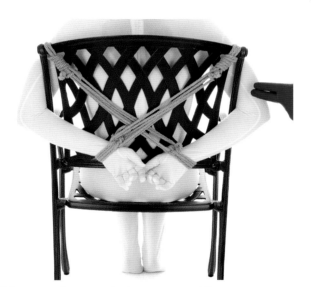

**3.** Take special care with this position. The arm can press into the chair, with the risk of a compression injury.

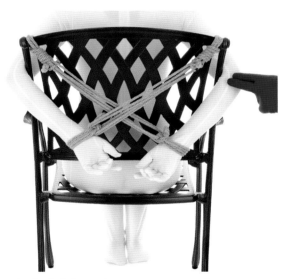

**4.** It can be helpful to adjust your partner's position, so the edges press on different locations. In this case, it was more comfortable for my partner to lean forward. If I had been doing this as part of a scene, I might have supplied a cushion to assist.

Tell your partner to inform you immediately if they feel anything strange in their thumb or fingers. If this occurs, change their position to something else.

## Bunny Tie

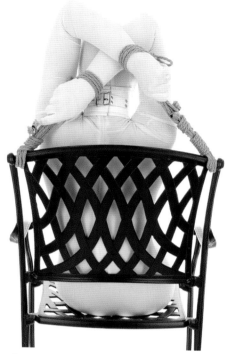

**1.** With a **Single Column** on each wrist, bring the wrists to the back of your partner's head. Tie the tails somewhere below that, on the opposite sides of the chair. To be secure, this needs to be combined with chest and hip anchors.

---

## Straightjacket Position

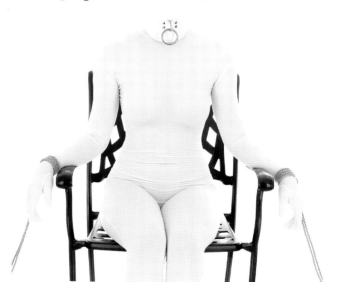

**1.** Tie a **Single Column** around each wrist.

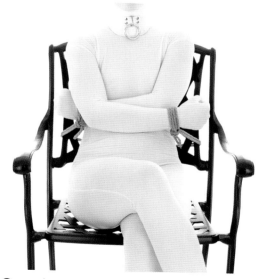

**2.** Cross the arms across the front of the body.

*continues...*

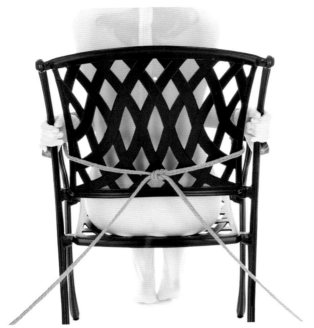

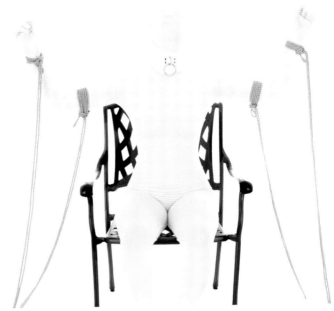

**3.** Tie off the ends somewhere in the back, out of reach.

**4.** Consider adding a **Single Column** to the upper arms as well.

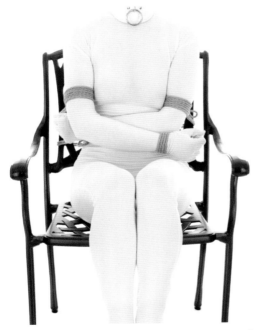

**5.** When combined with a hip harness connected to the back of a chair, this can be quite secure.

## Sarcophagus/Egyptian Position

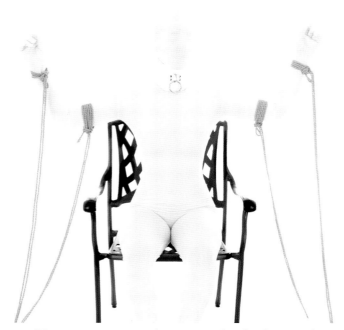

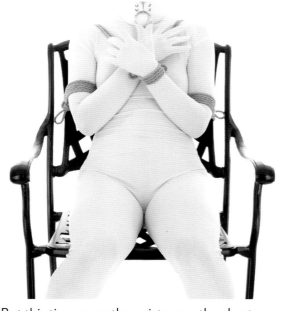

**1.** The starting point is the same as for the **Straitjacket**.

**2.** But this time cross the wrists over the chest, running the tails over the shoulders and tying them off in the back.

Make sure the cuffs on the upper arms are not pulling the arms back too far. You don't need this to be especially tight.

Optional: Add a band around the entire torso and chair when done to make this even more of a hug.

Add a hip harness to increase security.

# Keep Learning!

This book includes enough ties for you to plan *thousands* of different scenes. For many, this is enough; it teaches them the specific things they want to know.

If that is the case for you, you can always keep getting better by doing the following things:

- Practicing these techniques to build muscle memory, so you don't need to refer to the book to tie them and can do them more smoothly and with greater speed and confidence.
- Finding a partner to practice on/with.
- Finding a mentor.
- Increasing your medical knowledge and thus your ability to apply your skills to a greater variety of possible partners.

## How to Build Confidence and Competence

Confidence comes with competence. Competence comes with practice. When you practice, you build experience and muscle memory. You make mistakes and learn from them. You refine your technique. You earn that confidence through the innate and demonstrated knowledge.

## How to Progress Faster

### Find Someone to Practice on!

You can practice the techniques in this book on pool noodles or couch cushions or mannequins, and that can be great to help you memorize the rote steps, but until you practice them on a *person* and get live feedback on how what you are doing *feels*, you will only be learning half of what there is to know.

### Find a Local Mentor or Rope Group!

If you have not already done so, we strongly recommend you find a local mentor to work with (p. 11). Start by finding your local BDSM community and a local rope group, if there is one. There you can ask people to watch what you are doing and provide feedback. If you connect well with someone, perhaps they will be willing to work with you regularly. But even if that does not happen, different people in the group can help with different things and you will continue to build your skills.

## Take the Opportunities When They are Offered, and be Grateful!

We live in the real world. Things happen. Plans change. Practice sessions or scenes sometimes get canceled or have to change. This is just part of life. Don't let it frustrate you. When you have the opportunity to do rope, enjoy that time; be grateful for it. Especially if it was because someone else was joining you. That is a gift! A gift from and for both of you. Be grateful to them for that gift.

## Take the Next Step!

You have all the tools you need. The next step is up to you!

If you want to learn more, check out TheDuchy.com for a wide variety of other fun tutorials:

- Courses on a variety of topics: TheDuchy.com/courses/
- Tutorials on individual ties: TheDuchy.com/tutorials/
- Tutorials showing examples and how to layer ties: TheDuchy.com/layered-ties/
- Tutorials on how to create floggers made from rope: TheDuchy.com/flogger-forge/

# Other Helpful Resources

A Kinky Education List:
TheDuchy.com/education-list/

Scene Negotiation Forms (pg. 432)
TheDuchy.com/negotiation-forms/

A BDSM Experience and Curiosity Checklist (pg. 435)
TheDuchy.com/bdsm-checklist/

Kink and Non-monogamy Aware Professionals (KAP):
kapprofessionals.org

*Psychology Today* maintains a list of counselors that are kink allied:
psychologytoday.com/us/therapists/sex-positive-kink-allied

National Coalition for Sexual Freedom:
ncsfreedom.org

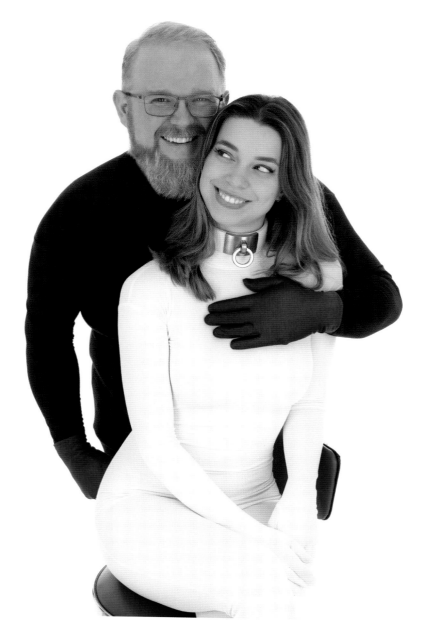

## Meet the Authors

Hi! My name is Lazarus Redmayne; bondage enthusiast and creator of TheDuchy.com. I started TheDuchy in 2000 to teach people the fun and erotic art of rope bondage. Cuffs, rope, and other kinky things have fascinated me since before I knew what sex was. By teaching the basics of rope bondage both online and in person for several decades, I have honed a unique teaching style that people find easy to understand. Joining me is Kajira Blue, who co-authored portions of this book and is the person in most of the pictures.

Hello! My name is Kajira Blue. I am relatively new to the rope scene, having begun exploring it roughly one year before writing this book. My introduction to the world of bondage came as a side effect of my fascination with human sexuality and psychology. Lazarus and I hope that by combining our very different perspectives and skill levels, we have made a book that is accessible and helpful to you.

# Appendices

## Negotiation Form

This form is the *beginning* of negotiations. You still need to *talk*!

There are no right or wrong answers. If you answer honestly, you are more likely to have a good time. You may not get everything on your list, but honesty *plus* conversation with your partner should help you find common ground.

- Remember the phrase, "What do you mean by _____?"
- My definition of "heavy impact" may be very different than yours!
- Don't up-negotiate during a scene. If you didn't talk about it before, don't do it.
- You can revoke consent at any time before or during an activity. You *cannot* revoke consent *after* the fact.

Name: ...........................................................................................

Playing with: ..............................................................................

### Today, I want to be a...
☐ Top  ☐ Bottom  ☐ Switch

### Today I want...
Check things you know you want. Put a line though the entire line for things you know you *don't* want (hard/soft limits for this scene).
Lines left blank are items to be discussed and agreed before the scene.

The forms presented in this appendix are available to download for free at:
THEDUCHY.COM/negotiation-forms/
THEDUCHY.COM/bdsm-checklist/

| **Bondage** | **Sensation Play** | **Impact Play** | **Role Play** | **Touching, Intimacy, Sex** |
|---|---|---|---|---|
| ☐ Blindfolds | ☐ Biting | ☐ Spanking | ☐ Boss/Employee | ☐ Cuddling |
| ☐ Collar/Lead | ☐ Edge Play | ☐ Punching | ☐ Burglar/Victim | ☐ Dirty Talk |
| ☐ Leather Cuffs | ☐ Electricity | ☐ Paddles | ☐ Doctor/Patient | ☐ Groping |
| ☐ Metal Cuffs | ☐ Hair Pulling | ☐ Canes | ☐ Human Furniture | ☐ Kissing |
| ☐ Gags | ☐ Knives | ☐ Floggers | ☐ Kidnapper/ Captive | ☐ Open Mouth Kissing |
| ☐ Rope | ☐ Licking | ☐ Whips | ☐ Law Enforcer/ Convict | ☐ Exhibitionism |
| ☐ Box Tie/TK | ☐ Mind Fucks | ☐ Intro | ☐ Little | ☐ Hands On Genitals |
| ☐ Floor Bondage | ☐ Nipples | ☐ Light | ☐ Consensually non-consensual | ☐ Orgasms |
| ☐ Suspension | ☐ Playing with Hair | ☐ Heavy | ☐ Owner/Pet | ☐ Giving Oral Sex |
| ☐ Cross | ☐ Pressure Points | ☐ Stingy | ☐ Royalty/Servant | ☐ Receiving Oral Sex |
| ☐ Bench | ☐ Scratching | ☐ Thuddy | ☐ Teacher/Student | ☐ Condoms/ Dent Dams |
| ☐ Table | ☐ Sensory Deprivation | ☐ Other | ☐ Wealthy/ Commoner | ☐ Fluid Exchange |
| ☐ Cages | ☐ Sharp | | ☐ Other | |
| ☐ Hoods | ☐ Tickling | | | |
| ☐ Decorative | ☐ Other | | | |
| ☐ Restrictive | | | | |
| ☐ Mental | | | | |
| ☐ Other | | | | |

## Marks
☐ None
☐ For Today
☐ For the Week
☐ Longer (discuss)

## Safewords
☐ Plain Language
☐ Red/Yellow/
  Green
☐ The word
  "Safeword"
☐ Other (discuss)

## Penetration
☐ Fingers
☐ Penis
☐ Toys
☐ Oral
☐ Vaginal
☐ Anal

## I want to feel...
☐ Beautiful
☐ Catharsis
☐ Controlled
☐ Degraded
☐ Dominant
☐ Energetic
☐ Erotic
☐ Helpless
☐ Masochistic
☐ Overwhelmed
☐ Peaceful
☐ Platonic
☐ Playful
☐ Sadistic
☐ Serious
☐ Submissive

## Aftercare
☐ ~ ____ - ____ mins
☐ Water
☐ Electrolytes
☐ Salt
☐ Sugar
☐ Snack
☐ Let me be
☐ Blanket
☐ Cuddling
☐ Comfort Item
☐ Conversation
☐ Service
☐ Snuggly Clothes
☐ Socialize
☐ Check in Tomorrow

## I do not want to be touched here:

## You should know about my:

Partners:...............................................

Triggers: ...............................................

Medical Conditions & Meds:....................

Injuries: .................................................

STI status: ..............................................

Allergies: ................................................

Safe Call: ...............................................

Other Considerations: .............................

## Disclosure of Any Relevant Medical Conditions
- Do you have any medical conditions? Particularly any that may cause fainting or seizures?
- Do you have impaired circulation, musculoskeletal injuries or conditions, sprains, breaks, flexibility limitations, etc.?
- Have you had any surgeries or have sensitive or weakened areas, hernias, metal plates or pins, any implants or devices (including breast implants), piercings or joint replacements?
- Do you have any contraceptive implants? If so, where are they located?
- Do you have any concerns related to pregnancy or menstruation that might pertain to this scene that you would like to share?
- Do you have any allergies (grass, lanolin, natural fiber rope, medication, etc.)?
- Have you had problems with nerve damage or previously sustained a rope-related injury?

### Very Important
The Top/rigger and the bottom are equally responsible for having a complete, thorough, and honest pre-rope negotiation to reduce the risk of accidental breaches of trust or consent, or accidental injury. Both parties must ask questions of the other and provide accurate and complete information on everything relevant.

## Negotiation Form

### Intake of Medication, Alcohol or Drugs

- Are you taking any medication that may affect play, such as blood thinners (may increase marking/bruising), painkillers (may mask 'bad' pain) or beta-blockers (may cause fainting)?
- Have you taken all prescribed medication that could affect this scene?
- Are you in an impaired state now ('under the influence')?
- What is your current consumption of alcohol or drugs? Anything that may impair your ability to deal with the play in any way?

### Personal Boundaries and Physical Limits

- Do you have any emotional or verbal triggers I need to know about?
- Do you currently have any issues with certain positions, flexibility issues or anything else that restricts where the rope can freely go?
- Do you currently have any tender spots?
- Which areas are okay for me to touch?
- Which areas are NOT okay for me to touch?
- Where, if anywhere, would you like to touch me?
- Rope play can leave various marks ranging from simple pressure lines to bruises, welts, and petechial hemorrhaging. Are you okay with marks? If so, which areas are okay and which are not?

### Style of Play

- What is your experience level with rope?
- What type of scene would you like?
  - ☐ Basic/Instructional (Just want to be tied up)
  - ☐ Sensual (Slow and gentle tying)
  - ☐ Rough (Fight and forceful tying)
  - ☐ Sadistic (Tight and forceful ties with extra pain inflicted via ropes and other implements)
  - ☐ Suspension (Entire body weight supported by rope; requires special negotiation in addition to this sheet)

### Safe Words, Consent, and In-Play Communication Methods

☐ Standard language       ☐ Red, Yellow, Green
☐ The word "Safeword"    ☐ Other (discuss): ..........................

### Clothing

- What level of dress or undress are you comfortable with?

I have read, understand and I agree to take 100% responsibility for my part in this scene:

Signature: ...................................................................

Date: ...................................................................

---

### Additional Considerations

Potential dangers of a rope scene include bruising, abrasions, nerve damage, loss of circulation, allergic reactions and more. Alert your Top immediately if you feel *anything* 'weird', for instance if something starts to tingle or go numb. This could be a sign of circulation or a nerve issue.

Untying takes some time, please keep this in mind if things start to get uncomfortable. If you think you may need to be untied soon, please alert your partner immediately, so they can start to untie you BEFORE the rope becomes unbearable. DO NOT BE AFRAID TO SPEAK UP if something doesn't feel right physically or mentally.

# BDSM Checklist

Name: ............................................ Date: ...............................................

**Rate your Pleasure of that Activity**

**1** = Disliked | **2** = Gave no pleasure | **3** = Was OK | **4** = Liked it | **5** = Extremely enjoyed | **6** = Essential

**Would you Like to Do it (again)?**

**Never** = A hard limit | **No Desire** = A soft limit | **Forced** = If you were forced to you (might) like it
**Maybe** = If under the right conditions | **Yes** = Absolutely
**Fetish Need** = this really turns you on and you can't live without it

| Activity | Tried | | Rate Activity 1-6 | Would You Like to Try or do Again? | | | | | | | | |
|---|---|---|---|---|---|---|---|---|---|---|---|---|
| | Yes | No | | Never | No Desire | Maybe | Yes | Fetish Need | Forced | Give | Receive | Either/Both |
| **Bondage** | | | | | | | | | | | | |
| Arm and leg sleeves ("armbinders") | | | | | | | | | | | | |
| Breast bondage | | | | | | | | | | | | |
| Blindfolds | | | | | | | | | | | | |
| Bondage – Light | | | | | | | | | | | | |
| Bondage – Heavy | | | | | | | | | | | | |
| Bondage – All day/multi day | | | | | | | | | | | | |
| Cages/cells/closets (being locked inside of) | | | | | | | | | | | | |
| Chains (bound with) | | | | | | | | | | | | |
| Chastity device/belts | | | | | | | | | | | | |
| Collars – Worn in private | | | | | | | | | | | | |
| Collars – Worn in public | | | | | | | | | | | | |
| Cuffs – Leather | | | | | | | | | | | | |
| Cuffs – Metal | | | | | | | | | | | | |
| Cuffs – Handcuff style | | | | | | | | | | | | |
| Ear plugs (sound deprivation) | | | | | | | | | | | | |
| Gags – Ball | | | | | | | | | | | | |
| Gags – Bit | | | | | | | | | | | | |
| Gags – Cloth | | | | | | | | | | | | |
| Gags – Inflatable | | | | | | | | | | | | |
| Gags – Phallic | | | | | | | | | | | | |
| Gags – Ring | | | | | | | | | | | | |
| Gags – Tape | | | | | | | | | | | | |
| Harnessing – Leather | | | | | | | | | | | | |
| Harnessing – Rope | | | | | | | | | | | | |
| Hoods (full head) | | | | | | | | | | | | |
| Immobilisation | | | | | | | | | | | | |

**Rate: 1** = Disliked | **2** = Gave no pleasure | **3** = Was OK | **4** = Liked it | **5** = Extremely enjoyed | **6** = Essential

# BDSM Checklist

| Activity | Tried | | Rate Activity 1-6 | Would You Like to Try or do Again? | | | | | | | | |
|---|---|---|---|---|---|---|---|---|---|---|---|---|
| | Yes | No | | Never | No Desire | Maybe | Yes | Fetish Need | Forced | Give | Receive | Either/Both |
| **Bondage** *continued* | | | | | | | | | | | | |
| Leash | | | | | | | | | | | | |
| Leather restraints | | | | | | | | | | | | |
| Manacles & Irons | | | | | | | | | | | | |
| Mummification | | | | | | | | | | | | |
| Muzzles | | | | | | | | | | | | |
| Rope bondage – Simple | | | | | | | | | | | | |
| Rope bondage – Intricate (Shibari) | | | | | | | | | | | | |
| Spreader bars | | | | | | | | | | | | |
| Stocks (head & hands) | | | | | | | | | | | | |
| Straightjackets | | | | | | | | | | | | |
| Suspension – Upright | | | | | | | | | | | | |
| Suspension – Horizontal | | | | | | | | | | | | |
| Suspension – Inverted | | | | | | | | | | | | |
| Sleep sacks | | | | | | | | | | | | |
| **Bodily Fluids & Functions** | | | | | | | | | | | | |
| Chamber pot use | | | | | | | | | | | | |
| Creampie | | | | | | | | | | | | |
| Cum – In anus | | | | | | | | | | | | |
| Cum – In mouth | | | | | | | | | | | | |
| Cum – In vagina | | | | | | | | | | | | |
| Cum – On body | | | | | | | | | | | | |
| Cutting – Blood play | | | | | | | | | | | | |
| Golden showers (being urinated on) | | | | | | | | | | | | |
| Human toilet | | | | | | | | | | | | |
| Injections (saline) | | | | | | | | | | | | |
| Milking (being made to produce breast milk) | | | | | | | | | | | | |
| Pearl necklace (cum on chest/throat) | | | | | | | | | | | | |
| Pearl shower (cum on face) | | | | | | | | | | | | |
| Rimming (oral/anal play) | | | | | | | | | | | | |
| Scat (brown showers) | | | | | | | | | | | | |
| Swallowing semen | | | | | | | | | | | | |
| Swallowing urine | | | | | | | | | | | | |

**Rate: 1** = Disliked | **2** = Gave no pleasure | **3** = Was OK | **4** = Liked it | **5** = Extremely enjoyed | **6** = Essential

| Activity | Tried | | | Would You Like to Try or do Again? | | | | | | | | |
| --- | --- | --- | --- | --- | --- | --- | --- | --- | --- | --- | --- |
| | Yes | No | Rate Activity 1-6 | Never | No Desire | Maybe | Yes | Fetish Need | Forced | Give | Receive | Either/Both |

**Fetishes**

| | | | | | | | | | | | | |
| --- | --- | --- | --- | --- | --- | --- | --- | --- | --- | --- | --- | --- |
| Boot worship | | | | | | | | | | | | |
| Cock/penis worship | | | | | | | | | | | | |
| Corsets | | | | | | | | | | | | |
| Cross dressing | | | | | | | | | | | | |
| Diapers | | | | | | | | | | | | |
| Foot worship | | | | | | | | | | | | |
| Gas masks | | | | | | | | | | | | |
| High heels (wearing) | | | | | | | | | | | | |
| High heel worship | | | | | | | | | | | | |
| Leather (wearing) | | | | | | | | | | | | |
| Lingerie (wearing) | | | | | | | | | | | | |
| Pussy worship | | | | | | | | | | | | |
| Rubber/latex clothing (wearing) | | | | | | | | | | | | |
| Slutty clothing | | | | | | | | | | | | |
| Spandex clothing | | | | | | | | | | | | |

**Humiliation**

| | | | | | | | | | | | | |
| --- | --- | --- | --- | --- | --- | --- | --- | --- | --- | --- | --- | --- |
| Forced dressing | | | | | | | | | | | | |
| Forced feminization | | | | | | | | | | | | |
| Forced homosexuality | | | | | | | | | | | | |
| Forced masturbation | | | | | | | | | | | | |
| Forced nudity | | | | | | | | | | | | |
| Forced servitude | | | | | | | | | | | | |
| Humiliation in private | | | | | | | | | | | | |
| Humiliation in public | | | | | | | | | | | | |
| Lecturing for misbehaviors | | | | | | | | | | | | |
| Shaving head hair | | | | | | | | | | | | |
| Shaving or depilation of body hair | | | | | | | | | | | | |
| Standing in corner (punishment) | | | | | | | | | | | | |
| Verbal humiliation | | | | | | | | | | | | |

**Impact & Rough Play**

| | | | | | | | | | | | | |
| --- | --- | --- | --- | --- | --- | --- | --- | --- | --- | --- | --- | --- |
| Breast whipping | | | | | | | | | | | | |
| Caning – English | | | | | | | | | | | | |
| Caning – Sensation | | | | | | | | | | | | |
| Face slapping | | | | | | | | | | | | |
| Punching | | | | | | | | | | | | |
| Pussy punching | | | | | | | | | | | | |
| Pussy kicking | | | | | | | | | | | | |

**Rate: 1** = Disliked | **2** = Gave no pleasure | **3** = Was OK | **4** = Liked it | **5** = Extremely enjoyed | **6** = Essential

# BDSM Checklist

| Activity | Tried | | | Would You Like to Try or do Again? | | | | | | | | |
|---|---|---|---|---|---|---|---|---|---|---|---|---|
| | Yes | No | Rate Activity 1-6 | Never | No Desire | Maybe | Yes | Fetish Need | Forced | Give | Receive | Either/Both |

### Impact & Rough Play *continued*

| Activity | Yes | No | Rate | Never | No Desire | Maybe | Yes | Fetish Need | Forced | Give | Receive | Either/Both |
|---|---|---|---|---|---|---|---|---|---|---|---|---|
| Pussy spanking (smacking) | | | | | | | | | | | | |
| Pussy whipping | | | | | | | | | | | | |
| Riding crops | | | | | | | | | | | | |
| Spanking – Hairbrush | | | | | | | | | | | | |
| Spanking – Hand | | | | | | | | | | | | |
| Spanking – Leather slappers | | | | | | | | | | | | |
| Spanking – Wooden paddles | | | | | | | | | | | | |
| Spanking – (OTK) Over The Knee | | | | | | | | | | | | |
| Whipping – Belt | | | | | | | | | | | | |
| Whipping – Cat o' nine tails | | | | | | | | | | | | |
| Whipping – Flogger | | | | | | | | | | | | |
| Whipping – Single tail | | | | | | | | | | | | |
| Wrestling | | | | | | | | | | | | |

### Non-monogamy

| Activity | Yes | No | Rate | Never | No Desire | Maybe | Yes | Fetish Need | Forced | Give | Receive | Either/Both |
|---|---|---|---|---|---|---|---|---|---|---|---|---|
| Fantasy gang rape | | | | | | | | | | | | |
| Group play – Multiple men "gang bang" | | | | | | | | | | | | |
| Group play – Multiple partners | | | | | | | | | | | | |
| Group play – Orgy | | | | | | | | | | | | |
| Shared (given to another only temp) | | | | | | | | | | | | |
| Swapping (with one other couple) | | | | | | | | | | | | |
| Swinging (multiple couples) | | | | | | | | | | | | |

### Marking

| Activity | Yes | No | Rate | Never | No Desire | Maybe | Yes | Fetish Need | Forced | Give | Receive | Either/Both |
|---|---|---|---|---|---|---|---|---|---|---|---|---|
| Branding | | | | | | | | | | | | |
| Scarification (cutting, making scars) | | | | | | | | | | | | |
| Tattooing (inking) | | | | | | | | | | | | |

### Role Play

| Activity | Yes | No | Rate | Never | No Desire | Maybe | Yes | Fetish Need | Forced | Give | Receive | Either/Both |
|---|---|---|---|---|---|---|---|---|---|---|---|---|
| Abandonment (fantasy) | | | | | | | | | | | | |
| Age play (not pedophilia) | | | | | | | | | | | | |
| Animal roleplay (not bestiality) | | | | | | | | | | | | |
| Auctioned for charity | | | | | | | | | | | | |
| Fear play | | | | | | | | | | | | |
| Human puppy-dog play | | | | | | | | | | | | |
| Infantilism (baby play) | | | | | | | | | | | | |
| Initiation rites | | | | | | | | | | | | |

**Rate: 1** = Disliked | **2** = Gave no pleasure | **3** = Was OK | **4** = Liked it | **5** = Extremely enjoyed | **6** = Essential

| Activity | Tried | | Rate Activity 1-6 | Would You Like to Try or do Again? | | | | | | | | |
|---|---|---|---|---|---|---|---|---|---|---|---|---|
| | Yes | No | | Never | No Desire | Maybe | Yes | Fetish Need | Forced | Give | Receive | Either/Both |
| **Role Play** *continued* | | | | | | | | | | | | |
| Interrogations | | | | | | | | | | | | |
| Kidnapping | | | | | | | | | | | | |
| Medical scenes | | | | | | | | | | | | |
| Name change | | | | | | | | | | | | |
| Pony play | | | | | | | | | | | | |
| Psych ward play | | | | | | | | | | | | |
| Prison scenes | | | | | | | | | | | | |
| Prostitution fantasy | | | | | | | | | | | | |
| Religious scenes | | | | | | | | | | | | |
| Schoolroom scenes | | | | | | | | | | | | |
| Switching roles (Top/bottom) | | | | | | | | | | | | |
| Total Power Exchange (TPE) | | | | | | | | | | | | |
| Other roleplaying | | | | | | | | | | | | |
| **Sensation Play (non-impact)** | | | | | | | | | | | | |
| Abrasion (scraping, sanding) | | | | | | | | | | | | |
| Asphyxiation | | | | | | | | | | | | |
| Ball (testicle) stretching | | | | | | | | | | | | |
| Biting (being bitten) | | | | | | | | | | | | |
| Beating hard | | | | | | | | | | | | |
| Beating soft | | | | | | | | | | | | |
| Breath control (Choking) | | | | | | | | | | | | |
| Breath control (Mild restriction) | | | | | | | | | | | | |
| Clamps – Labia/clit area | | | | | | | | | | | | |
| Clothespins | | | | | | | | | | | | |
| Dilation | | | | | | | | | | | | |
| Electricity – Internal (egg or probe) | | | | | | | | | | | | |
| Electricity – TENS unit | | | | | | | | | | | | |
| Electricity – Violet Wand | | | | | | | | | | | | |
| Enemas – For cleansing | | | | | | | | | | | | |
| Enemas – Retention/training | | | | | | | | | | | | |
| Finger claws | | | | | | | | | | | | |
| Fire cupping | | | | | | | | | | | | |
| Fire play | | | | | | | | | | | | |
| Hair pulling | | | | | | | | | | | | |
| Hot wax – Dripping on body/genitals | | | | | | | | | | | | |
| Hot waxing – Hair removal | | | | | | | | | | | | |

**Rate: 1** = Disliked | **2** = Gave no pleasure | **3** = Was OK | **4** = Liked it | **5** = Extremely enjoyed | **6** = Essential

# BDSM Checklist

| Activity | Tried | | | Would You Like to Try or do Again? | | | | | | | | |
|---|---|---|---|---|---|---|---|---|---|---|---|---|
| | Yes | No | Rate Activity 1-6 | Never | No Desire | Maybe | Yes | Fetish Need | Forced | Give | Receive | Either/Both |
| **Sensation Play (non-impact)** *continued* | | | | | | | | | | | | |
| Ice cubes | | | | | | | | | | | | |
| Kicking | | | | | | | | | | | | |
| Knife play (blood drawn) | | | | | | | | | | | | |
| Knife play (no blood)(sensation) | | | | | | | | | | | | |
| Needle play | | | | | | | | | | | | |
| Nipple clamps | | | | | | | | | | | | |
| Nipple piercing | | | | | | | | | | | | |
| Nipple play – Pulls, tugs, twists | | | | | | | | | | | | |
| Pain – Mild | | | | | | | | | | | | |
| Pain – Severe | | | | | | | | | | | | |
| Piercing (permanant) | | | | | | | | | | | | |
| Piercing (temporary) | | | | | | | | | | | | |
| Punishment scene | | | | | | | | | | | | |
| Riding the horse (crotch torture) | | | | | | | | | | | | |
| Scratching | | | | | | | | | | | | |
| Sensory deprivation | | | | | | | | | | | | |
| Sleep deprivation | | | | | | | | | | | | |
| Strapping (full body beating) | | | | | | | | | | | | |
| Suction cups | | | | | | | | | | | | |
| Teasing | | | | | | | | | | | | |
| Tickling | | | | | | | | | | | | |
| Vampire gloves | | | | | | | | | | | | |
| Water torture (waterboarding) | | | | | | | | | | | | |
| Wartenburg pinwheel | | | | | | | | | | | | |
| Zippers – Clothespins | | | | | | | | | | | | |
| Zippers – Clamps | | | | | | | | | | | | |
| Zippers – Needles | | | | | | | | | | | | |
| **Service & Restricted/Controlled Behavior** | | | | | | | | | | | | |
| Auctioned for charity | | | | | | | | | | | | |
| Bathroom use control (permission) | | | | | | | | | | | | |
| Begging | | | | | | | | | | | | |
| Chauffeuring (driving) | | | | | | | | | | | | |
| Chores (domestic service/ housework) | | | | | | | | | | | | |
| Having clothing chosen | | | | | | | | | | | | |
| Having food chosen | | | | | | | | | | | | |
| Contract slave | | | | | | | | | | | | |
| Daily diary | | | | | | | | | | | | |

**Rate: 1** = Disliked | **2** = Gave no pleasure | **3** = Was OK | **4** = Liked it | **5** = Extremely enjoyed | **6** = Essential

| Activity | Tried | | | Would You Like to Try or do Again? | | | | | | | | |
|---|---|---|---|---|---|---|---|---|---|---|---|---|
| | Yes | No | Rate Activity 1-6 | Never | No Desire | Maybe | Yes | Fetish Need | Forced | Give | Receive | Either/Both |
| **Service & Restricted/Controlled Behavior** *continued* | | | | | | | | | | | | |
| Exercise – Forced/required | | | | | | | | | | | | |
| Erotic dancing | | | | | | | | | | | | |
| Eye contact restrictions | | | | | | | | | | | | |
| Following orders | | | | | | | | | | | | |
| Gor Slave Training (positions) | | | | | | | | | | | | |
| Harems (serving with other subs) | | | | | | | | | | | | |
| Hypnotism | | | | | | | | | | | | |
| Kneeling | | | | | | | | | | | | |
| Manicures | | | | | | | | | | | | |
| Mantra and meditation | | | | | | | | | | | | |
| Massage | | | | | | | | | | | | |
| Pedicures & foot massages | | | | | | | | | | | | |
| Personality modification | | | | | | | | | | | | |
| Phone sex | | | | | | | | | | | | |
| Rituals | | | | | | | | | | | | |
| Serving as a maid | | | | | | | | | | | | |
| Serving as furniture | | | | | | | | | | | | |
| Serving as art | | | | | | | | | | | | |
| Serving other Doms (supervised only) | | | | | | | | | | | | |
| Speech restrictions (when, what, to whom) | | | | | | | | | | | | |
| Uniform (wearing) | | | | | | | | | | | | |
| Wearing symbolic jewelry | | | | | | | | | | | | |
| Weight control | | | | | | | | | | | | |
| **Sexual Activity & Penetration** | | | | | | | | | | | | |
| Anal beads | | | | | | | | | | | | |
| Anal play | | | | | | | | | | | | |
| Anal plugs – Small | | | | | | | | | | | | |
| Anal plugs – Medium | | | | | | | | | | | | |
| Anal plugs – Large | | | | | | | | | | | | |
| Anal plugs – Public, under clothes | | | | | | | | | | | | |
| Anal sex | | | | | | | | | | | | |
| Breast fucking | | | | | | | | | | | | |
| Catheterization | | | | | | | | | | | | |
| Cunnilingus (giving oral to a woman) | | | | | | | | | | | | |
| Cunnilingus (receiving oral) | | | | | | | | | | | | |

**Rate: 1** = Disliked | **2** = Gave no pleasure | **3** = Was OK | **4** = Liked it | **5** = Extremely enjoyed | **6** = Essential

# BDSM Checklist

| Activity | Tried | | | Would You Like to Try or do Again? | | | | | | | |
|---|---|---|---|---|---|---|---|---|---|---|---|
| | Yes | No | Rate Activity 1-6 | Never | No Desire | Maybe | Yes | Fetish Need | Forced | Give | Receive | Either/Both |

**Sexual Activity & Penetration** *continued*

| Activity | | | | | | | | | | | |
|---|---|---|---|---|---|---|---|---|---|---|---|
| Dildos – Anal | | | | | | | | | | | |
| Dildos – Oral | | | | | | | | | | | |
| Dildos – Vaginal | | | | | | | | | | | |
| Double penetration | | | | | | | | | | | |
| Fantasy rape play | | | | | | | | | | | |
| Fellatio (oral sex on a penis) | | | | | | | | | | | |
| Fisting – Anal | | | | | | | | | | | |
| Fisting – Vaginal | | | | | | | | | | | |
| Genital sex | | | | | | | | | | | |
| Masturbation | | | | | | | | | | | |
| Orgasm control | | | | | | | | | | | |
| Orgasm denial | | | | | | | | | | | |
| Sexual deprivation | | | | | | | | | | | |
| Sounding | | | | | | | | | | | |
| Speculums | | | | | | | | | | | |
| Strap-on-dildos (sucking on) | | | | | | | | | | | |
| Strap-on-dildos (being penetrated by) | | | | | | | | | | | |
| Strap-on-dildos (wearing) | | | | | | | | | | | |
| Triple penetration | | | | | | | | | | | |
| Vibrator - Anal | | | | | | | | | | | |
| Vibrator - External genital | | | | | | | | | | | |
| Vibrator - Internal vaginal | | | | | | | | | | | |

**Voyeurism/Exhibitionism**

| Activity | | | | | | | | | | | |
|---|---|---|---|---|---|---|---|---|---|---|---|
| Examinations | | | | | | | | | | | |
| Exhibitionism (friends) | | | | | | | | | | | |
| Exhibitionism (strangers) | | | | | | | | | | | |
| Forced nudity (private) | | | | | | | | | | | |
| Forced nudity (public) | | | | | | | | | | | |
| Modeling for erotic photos | | | | | | | | | | | |
| Outdoor scenes | | | | | | | | | | | |
| Video (watching others) | | | | | | | | | | | |
| Video (recordings of you) | | | | | | | | | | | |
| Voyeurism (watching others) | | | | | | | | | | | |
| Voyeurism (your Dom w/others) | | | | | | | | | | | |

**Rate: 1** = Disliked | **2** = Gave no pleasure | **3** = Was OK | **4** = Liked it | **5** = Extremely enjoyed | **6** = Essential

List any allergies that I should be aware of (latex, grass, food, scents, oils, lotions, wool, feathers, etc.):

......................................................................................................................................................

Any medical problems/issues? If yes, give details:

......................................................................................................................................................

Do you have any known STI's?

......................................................................................................................................................

When were you last tested?

......................................................................................................................................................

Any specific subject not described in this list that should be discussed? Describe:

......................................................................................................................................................
......................................................................................................................................................

Fantasies:

......................................................................................................................................................
......................................................................................................................................................

Comments:

......................................................................................................................................................
......................................................................................................................................................

References:

......................................................................................................................................................

Questions:

......................................................................................................................................................
......................................................................................................................................................

## Acknowledgements:

This list was originally compiled from many sources by **Master Guardian** of SinCity D/s Network in Las Vegas, who gave his very kind permission for us to reuse it. We at TheDuchy.com added a few things, split them into categories to lower context switching and updated the formatting a bit. We now make this version available to the community under the Creative Commons Attribution-ShareAlike 4.0 International license, details below.

## Permissions

We make this available to the community under the Creative Commons Attribution-ShareAlike 4.0 International license. Summary of the license: creativecommons.org/licenses/by-sa/4.0/
Full details: creativecommons.org/licenses/by-sa/4.0/legalcode